CLINICAL GASTROENTEROLOGY

Series Editor
George Y. Wu
University of Connecticut Health Center, Farmington, CT, USA

For further volumes:
http://www.springer.com/series/7672

S. Devi Rampertab • Gerard E. Mullin
Editors

Celiac Disease

Humana Press

Editors
S. Devi Rampertab
Department of Medicine
Rutgers-Robert Wood Johnson Medical School
New Brunswick, NJ, USA

Gerard E. Mullin
Division of Gastroenterology
Johns Hopkins University School of Medicine
Baltimore, MD, USA

ISSN 2197-7399 ISSN 2197-7704 (electronic)
ISBN 978-1-4614-8559-9 ISBN 978-1-4614-8560-5 (eBook)
DOI 10.1007/978-1-4614-8560-5
Springer New York Heidelberg Dordrecht London

Library of Congress Control Number: 2013957056

Printed on acid-free paper

Humana Press is a brand of Springer
Springer is part of Springer Science+Business Media (www.springer.com)

This book is dedicated to my family:
Most notably my parents, Renie and Madhoo Rampertab, for instilling within me a passion for excellence, hard work, dedication, and perseverance toward achieving a goal. Their tremendous love and support have nurtured me over the years and have allowed me to reach higher and higher.
My two brothers, Deo and Victor Rampertab, who have been my role models throughout life. They have been instrumental in my professional development as I sought to emulate them.
My husband, Nake Pooran, for his undying love and encouragement.
My two darling sons, Ajay and Sanjay Pooran, for filling my life with joy and happiness.
"A man's reach should exceed his grasp ..."
–Robert Browning

S. Devi Rampertab, M.D., F.A.C.G.

To the loving memory of my mother and father.
To my family and loved ones for their unwavering support.
To those afflicted with celiac disease and gluten intolerance, the clinicians who care for them, the researchers who are dedicated to pursue a cure, and the foundations and philanthropists who promote awareness and support research.

To my colleagues, administrators, and support staff at Johns Hopkins, the finest institution in the world. To Dr. Tony Kalloo for his continued guidance and inspiration.

Gerard E. Mullin, M.D.

Foreword

Celiac disease is an emerging disease. Studies have shown that the prevalence of celiac disease has increased in the last 50 years. Stored serum, collected 50 years ago from mainly 20-year-old white men in the USA (Warren Air Force Base Cohort), had a seroprevalence of tissue transglutaminase and endomysial IgA antibodies of about 0.2 %. Their current day cohorts of 20-year-old or 70-year-old white men have a seroprevalence approaching 1%, a 4- to 5-fold increase [1]. Similar studies that have compared cohorts over shorter time intervals revealed a similar increase in prevalence in the USA [2] and Finland [3]. Worldwide it is now considered that celiac disease occurs in about 1 % of the population [4, 5].

Celiac disease occurs in genetically predisposed individuals due to the interaction of gluten and other environmental events [6]. The required HLA haplotypes DQ2 or DQ8 actually occur in 30–40 % of the population, yet >90 % of us consume gluten. Thus, two questions arise:

1. Why don't more people have celiac disease?
2. What is responsible for the recent increase in prevalence?

The risk for the development of celiac disease appears to increase as one lives longer. Celiac disease is being increasingly recognized in the elderly [7], and 2.5 % of the elderly in Finland have celiac disease compared to 1 % in children [8, 9]. It is unlikely that genes have changed, and there is evidence that gluten has not either [10]. While we may be consuming more gluten, other environmental factors have been incriminated. They include the protective role of breast-feeding [11, 12], timing of gluten ingestion [13], role of cesarean section [14], effect of season of birth [15], and infections [16]. However, there needs to be more work on determining predisposing factors for the acquisition of celiac disease.

Despite increasing awareness of celiac disease and gluten-related disorders among the general public [17], the latest analysis of the US NHANES dataset revealed that merely 17 % of those with celiac disease were diagnosed and aware that they had celiac disease [18].

There are several reasons why the rate of celiac disease may be so low. While many patients may be asymptomatic [6], others experience a long symptomatic period and see many physicians [19–21]. Physician awareness about the variety of clinical presentations and the use of serological tests appears to be a factor in the under-diagnosis of celiac disease. A primary care study conducted in North America revealed a 40-fold increase in diagnosis after targeted testing of patients with a variety of common symptoms and diagnoses such as IBS, constipation, and fatigue was performed [22]. In addition, a study from Finland attributed a high rate of celiac disease diagnosis to the education of primary care physicians [23].

Currently the gold standard of diagnosis is via endoscopic biopsy of the duodenum; however, even when patients are undergoing endoscopy for diarrhea, weight loss, or anemia (i.e., probable celiac disease), they frequently do not receive a duodenal biopsy [24], or they receive an inadequate number of biopsies [25], or they may not receive duodenal bulbar biopsies, which in our study increased the rate of celiac disease diagnosis by 13 % [26]. Even after biopsy, the pathologist may fail to recognize the diagnostic features [27]. While duodenal biopsy is considered the gold standard in diagnosis of celiac disease, recent guidelines from Europe suggest that a subset of children may not need a biopsy [28]. It is unclear whether or not these guidelines will be accepted in the USA.

While the rate of celiac disease diagnosis lags behind the actual prevalence of the disease, it is ironic that a large proportion of the population (about 0.6 %) has adopted a gluten-free diet without a doctor diagnosis of celiac disease [29]. The reason for this is not clear. Some may have non-celiac gluten sensitivity, a recently described condition in which individuals experience an improvement in symptoms on withdrawal of gluten [30–32]. However, even among these individuals with gluten sensitivity, it is not clear that it is gluten that is the culprit in their diet [31]. We have much to learn about celiac disease and other gluten-related conditions such as non-celiac gluten sensitivity.

New York, NY Peter H.R. Green

References

1. Rubio-Tapia A, Kyle RA, Kaplan EL, Johnson DR, Page W, Erdtmann F, et al. Increased prevalence and mortality in undiagnosed celiac disease. Gastroenterology. 2009;137(1):88–93.
2. Catassi C, Kryszak D, Bhatti B, Sturgeon C, Helzlsouer K, Clipp SL, et al. Natural history of celiac disease autoimmunity in a USA cohort followed since 1974. Ann Med. 2010;42(7):530–8.
3. Lohi S, Mustalahti K, Kaukinen K, Laurila K, Collin P, Rissanen H, et al. Increasing prevalence of coeliac disease over time. Aliment Pharmacol Ther. 2007;26(9):1217–25.
4. Hovell CJ, Collett JA, Vautier G, Cheng AJ, Sutanto E, Mallon DF, et al. High prevalence of coeliac disease in a population-based study from Western Australia: a case for screening? Med J Aust. 2001;175(5):247–50.
5. Mustalahti K, Catassi C, Reunanen A, Fabiani E, Heier M, McMillan S, et al. The prevalence of celiac disease in Europe: results of a centralized, international mass screening project. Ann Med. 2010;42(8):587–95.
6. Green PH, Cellier C. Celiac disease. N Engl J Med. 2007;357(17):1731–43.

7. Mukherjee R, Egbuna I, Brar P, Hernandez L, McMahon DJ, Shane EJ, et al. Celiac disease: similar presentations in the elderly and young adults. Dig Dis Sci. 2010;55(11):3147–53.
8. Vilppula A, Kaukinen K, Luostarinen L, Krekelä I, Patrikainen H, Valve R, et al. Increasing prevalence and high incidence of celiac disease in elderly people: A population-based study. BMC Gastroenterol. 2009;9(1):49.
9. Maki M, Mustalahti K, Kokkonen J, Kulmala P, Haapalahti M, Karttunen T, et al. Prevalence of celiac disease among children in Finland. N Engl J Med. 2003;348(25):2517–24.
10. Kasarda DD. Can an increase in celiac disease be attributed to an increase in the gluten content of wheat as a consequence of wheat breeding? J Agric Food Chem. 2013;61(6):1155–9.
11. Ivarsson A, Hernell O, Stenlund H, Persson LA. Breast-feeding protects against celiac disease. Am J Clin Nutr. 2002;75(5):914–21.
12. D'Amico MA, Holmes J, Stavropoulos SN, Frederick M, Levy J, DeFelice AR, et al. Presentation of pediatric celiac disease in the United States: prominent effect of breastfeeding. Clin Pediatr (Phila). 2005;44(3):249–58.
13. Norris JM, Barriga K, Hoffenberg EJ, Taki I, Miao D, Haas JE, et al. Risk of celiac disease autoimmunity and timing of gluten introduction in the diet of infants at increased risk of disease. JAMA. 2005;293(19):2343–51.
14. Marild K, Stephansson O, Montgomery S, Murray JA, Ludvigsson JF. Pregnancy outcome and risk of celiac disease in offspring: a nationwide case–control study. Gastroenterology. 2012;142(1):39–45 e3.
15. Lebwohl B, Green PH, Murray JA, Ludvigsson JF. Season of birth in a nationwide cohort of coeliac disease patients. Arch Dis Child. 2013;98(1):48–51.
16. Stene LC, Honeyman MC, Hoffenberg EJ, Haas JE, Sokol RJ, Emery L, et al. Rotavirus infection frequency and risk of celiac disease autoimmunity in early childhood: a longitudinal study. Am J Gastroenterol. 2006;101(10):2333–40.
17. Simpson S, Lebwohl B, Lewis S, Tennyson C, Sanders DS, Green P. Awareness of gluten-related disorders: a survey of the general public, chefs and patients. e-SPEN. 2011;b:e1–5.
18. Rubio-Tapia A, Ludvigsson JF, Brantner TL, Murray JA, Everhart JE. The prevalence of celiac disease in the United States. Am J Gastroenterol. 2012 Oct;107(10):1538–44.
19. Dickey W, McConnell JB. How many hospital visits does it take before celiac sprue is diagnosed? J Clin Gastroenterol. 1996;23(1):21–3.
20. Green PHR, Stavropoulos SN, Panagi SG, Goldstein SL, Mcmahon DJ, Absan H, et al. Characteristics of adult celiac disease in the USA: results of a national survey. Am J Gastroenterol. 2001;96(1):126–31.
21. Rampertab SD, Pooran N, Brar P, Singh P, Green PH. Trends in the presentation of celiac disease. Am J Med. 2006;119(4):355 e9-14.
22. Catassi C, Kryszak D, Louis-Jacques O, Duerksen DR, Hill I, Crowe SE, et al. Detection of Celiac disease in primary care: a multicenter case-finding study in North America. Am J Gastroenterol. 2007;102(7):1454–60.
23. Collin P, Huhtala H, Virta L, Kekkonen L, Reunala T. Diagnosis of celiac disease in clinical practice: physician's alertness to the condition essential. J Clin Gastroenterol. 2007;41(2): 152–6.
24. Lebwohl B, Tennyson CA, Holub JL, Lieberman DA, Neugut AI, Green PH. Sex and racial disparities in duodenal biopsy to evaluate for celiac disease. Gastrointest Endosc. 2012.
25. Lebwohl B, Kapel RC, Neugut AI, Green PH, Genta RM. Adherence to biopsy guidelines increases celiac disease diagnosis. Gastrointest Endosc. 2011;74(1):103–9.
26. Gonzalez S, Gupta A, Cheng J, Tennyson C, Lewis SK, Bhagat G, et al. Prospective study of the role of duodenal bulb biopsies in the diagnosis of celiac disease. Gastrointest Endosc. 2010;72(4):758–65.
27. Arguelles-Grande C, Tennyson CA, Lewis SK, Green PH, Bhagat G. Variability in small bowel histopathology reporting between different pathology practice settings: impact on the diagnosis of coeliac disease. J Clin Pathol. 2012 Mar;65(3):242–7.

28. Husby S, Koletzko S, Korponay-Szabo IR, Mearin ML, Phillips A, Shamir R, et al. European Society for Pediatric Gastroenterology, Hepatology, and Nutrition guidelines for the diagnosis of coeliac disease. J Pediatr Gastroenterol Nutr. 2012;54(1):136–60.
29. Ludvigsson JF, Rubio-Tapia A, van Dyke CT, Melton LJ 3rd, Zinsmeister AR, Lahr BD, et al. Increasing incidence of celiac disease in a North American population. Am J Gastroenterol. 2013 May;108(5):818–24.
30. Vazquez-Roque MI, Camilleri M, Smyrk T, Murray JA, Marietta E, O'Neill J, et al. A controlled trial of gluten-free diet in patients with irritable bowel syndrome-diarrhea: effects on bowel frequency and intestinal function. Gastroenterology. 2013;144(5):903–11 e3.
31. Biesiekierski JR, Peters SL, Newnham ED, Rosella O, Muir JG, Gibson PR. No effects of gluten in patients with self-reported non-celiac gluten sensitivity following dietary reduction of low-fermentable, poorly-absorbed, short-chain carbohydrates. Gastroenterology. 2013;145(2):320–8.
32. Ludvigsson JF, Leffler DA, Bai JC, Biagi F, Fasano A, Green PH, et al. The Oslo definitions for coeliac disease and related terms. Gut. 2013 Jan;62(1):43–52.

Acknowledgments

As I complete this gratifying undertaking, it is only fitting that I reflect on the scope of the accomplishment and acknowledge those without whom this task would be near impossible. Throughout the writing, my thoughts have been with those patients suffering with celiac disease, both diagnosed and undiagnosed. I would like to thank Dr. George Wu for granting me the opportunity to create a resource that will hopefully serve as an invaluable tool to practitioners on the front line to better diagnose and treat patients suffering from celiac disease. I would also like to thank Diane Lamsback, our developmental editor, for her untiring patience and her expertise as she skillfully guided us every step of the way through the writing and editorial process. I do owe Dr. Peter Green from the Celiac Disease Center at Columbia University Medical Center a special tribute, since it is he who first sparked my strong interest in celiac disease and further fueled my journey into academic medicine and writing. He was my very first professional mentor and continues to play a prominent role in my development as an academician. I must also thank my mentor and coeditor, Dr. Gerry Mullin, for the multiple collaborative opportunities we have had over the years as well as his tireless work toward this book. Our contributors also deserve a special acknowledgment for sharing their expertise in the furtherance of diagnosis and treatment of patients with celiac disease. They are all leading experts in this very important field, and we are truly indebted to them for their insight and enlightenment. The sharing of information from all sources is one of the hallmarks of medicine as a whole, and so thank you to all of my past instructors and mentors, colleagues, fellows, residents, and students for fostering the spirit of inquiry and the insatiable quest for knowledge.

S. Devi Rampertab, M.D., F.A.C.G.

My sincere thanks to Drs. S. Devi Rampertab and George Wu for choosing me to coedit this first textbook on celiac disease. My deepest appreciation to Ms. Diane Lamsback from Springer publishing for her tireless efforts. I would like to express my gratitude to the many experts whose outstanding contributions made this book possible. There are many individuals I would like to recognize who have guided my career and sparked my interest in celiac disease and gluten intolerance. To my mentors who have guided my career over the years, in particular, Drs. Anthony Kalloo, Andrew Weil, Victoria Maizes, Ben Caballero, and Theodore Bayless. To the nutritionists whose collaborations have fostered career development and friendships over the years: Drs. Laura Matarese, Carol Irenton-Jones, Mark DeLegge, Kelly Tappenden, Jeanette Hassee, Deborah Rubin, Alan Buchmann, Tim Lipman, Ron Koretz, Amy Brown, and Ms. Kathy Swift. A special thank you to those who have supported my clinical practice at Johns Hopkins: my medical office assistant Julie McKenna-Thorpe, Ms. Erin O'Keefe, and Ms. Trudee Wooden; nurse clinicians Julee Dennis and Rose Fusco; administrators Ms. Lisa Bach-Burdsall and Mr. Nathan Smith; administrative director Ms. Tiffany Boldin; Dr. Myron L. Weisfeldt, chairman of medicine at Johns Hopkins; and Dr. Linda A. Lee, clinical director of the Johns Hopkins Division of Gastroenterology and Hepatology.

Gerard E. Mullin, M.D.

Contents

Contributors

Imad Absah Division of Gastroenterology and Hepatology, Department of Pediatrics, Mayo Clinic, Rochester, MN, USA

Federico Biagi Department of Internal Medicine, IRCCS Policlinico San Matteo, University of Pavia, Pavia, Italy

Erica Boettcher Division of Gastroenterology, Department of Medicine, University of California, San Diego, La Jolla, CA, USA

Christophe Cellier Department of Gastroenterology, Hôpital Européen Georges Pompidou, Paris, France

Paul J. Ciclitira Rayne Institute, Gastroenterology Department, St. Thomas' Hospital, London, UK

Gino Roberto Corazza Department of Internal Medicine, IRCCS Policlinico San Matteo, University of Pavia, Pavia, Italy

Sheila E. Crowe Department of Medicine, University of California, San Diego, La Jolla, CA, USA

Esther C. de Haas Department of Genetics, University Medical Center Groningen, University of Groningen, Groningen, The Netherlands

David E. Elliott Division of Gastroenterology/Hepatology, Department of Internal Medicine, University of Iowa Carver College of Medicine and Iowa City VAHC, Iowa City, IA, USA

Alessio Fasano Department of Pediatrics, Massachusetts General Hospital for Children, Massachusetts General Hospital East, Charlestown, Boston, MA, USA

Peter H.R. Green Department of Medicine, Columbia University Medical Center, Celiac Disease Center at Columbia University, New York, NY, USA

Stefano Guandalini Department of Pediatric Gastroenterology, University of Chicago Comer Children's Hospital, Chicago, IL, USA

Margot L. Herman Division of Gastroenterology and Hepatology, Department of Internal Medicine, Mayo Clinic, Rochester, MN, USA

Geoffrey K.T. Holmes Department of Gastroenterology, Royal Derby Hospital, Derby, Derbyshire, UK

Vinod Kumar Department of Genetics, University Medical Center Groningen, University of Groningen, Groningen, The Netherlands

Karen M. Lammers Department of Pediatrics, Massachusetts General Hospital for Children, Massachusetts General Hospital East, Charlestown, Boston, MA, USA

Benjamin Lebwohl Department of Gastroenterology, Columbia University Medical Center, New York, NY, USA

Nina Ruth Lewis Nottingham Digestive Diseases Centre, Queen's Medical Centre, Nottingham University Hospital, Nottingham, Nottinghamshire, UK

José Moisés Laparra Microbial Ecology, Nutrition and Health, Institute of Agrochemistry and Food Technology, National Research Council (IATA-CSIC), Paterna, Valencia, Spain

Jonas F. Ludvigsson Department of Medical Epidemiology and Biostatistics, Karolinska Institutet, Stockholm, Sweden

Örebro University Hospital, Örebro, Sweden

Georgia Malamut Department of Gastroenterology, Hôpital Européen Georges Pompidou, Paris, France

Eric V. Marietta Division of Gastroenterology and Hepatology, Mayo Clinic, Rochester, MN, USA

Joachim Messing Waksman Institute of Microbiology, Rutgers University, Piscataway, NJ, USA

Gerard E. Mullin Division of Gastroenterology, Johns Hopkins University School of Medicine, Baltimore, MD, USA

Joseph A. Murray Division of Gastroenterology and Hepatology, Mayo Clinic, Rochester, MN, USA

Ikram Nasr Gastroenterology Department, St. Thomas' Hospital, London, UK

Marta Olivares Microbial Ecology, Nutrition and Health, Institute of Agrochemistry and Food Technology, National Research Council (IATA-CSIC), Paterna, Valencia, Spain

Amy S. Oxentenko Department of Gastroenterology and Hepatology, Department of Internal Medicine, Mayo Clinic, Rochester, MN, USA

Michelle Maria Pietzak Department of Pediatric Gastroenterology, University of Southern California Keck School of Medicine, Los Angeles, CA, USA

S. Devi Rampertab Department of Medicine, Rutgers-Robert Wood Johnson Medical School, New Brunswick, NJ, USA

Norelle Rizkalla Reilly Division of Pediatric Gastroenterology, Columbia University Medical Center, Celiac Disease Center at Columbia University, New York, NY, USA

Alberto Rubio-Tapia Division of Gastroenterology and Hepatology, Department of Internal Medicine, Mayo Clinic, Rochester, MN, USA

Yolanda Sanz Microbial Ecology, Nutrition and Health, Institute of Agrochemistry and Food Technology, National Research Council (IATA-CSIC), Paterna, Valencia, Spain

Suzanne Simpson Columbia University, Celiac Disease Center, New York, NY, USA

Anna Tavakkoli Department of Internal Medicine, Columbia University Medical Center, New York, NY, USA

Tricia Thompson Gluten Free Watchdog, LLC, Manchester, MA, USA

Brintha Vasagar Department of Pediatrics, Massachusetts General Hospital for Children, Massachusetts General Hospital East, Charlestown, Boston, MA, USA

Cisca Wijmenga Department of Genetics, University Medical Center Groningen, University of Groningen, Groningen, The Netherlands

Sona Young Department of Pediatric Gastroenterology, University of Chicago Comer Children's Hospital, Chicago, IL, USA

Chapter 1
Introduction

Gerard E. Mullin and S. Devi Rampertab

Celiac disease (CD) is an autoimmune disease that is characterized by an aberrant response to dietary gluten in genetically susceptible individuals that results in small intestinal injury and can be associated with diverse systemic consequences. CD usually resolves on a gluten-free diet (GFD); however, ongoing pharmacological and vaccine trials hold promise for the future. Historically, CD was once considered a rare condition seen predominantly in those of northern European ancestry. Today, we now recognize that CD is quite common, yet it remains underdiagnosed by clinicians despite the increased attention it has been receiving in the public sector due in large part to investigations by the various contributors of this book as well as by CD foundations and support groups (see Appendix A).

Epidemiology

Chapter 3 by Ludvigsson et al. describes in detail the epidemiology of CD. The U.S. prevalence of CD in several studies is approximately 1 %, whereas the prevalence in European populations varies from a high of 2.4 % in Finland to a low of 0.3 % in Germany. Interestingly, there are data showing that the incidence and prevalence of CD have increased in the USA, as well as in Europe, over the last 30 years. Murray et al. reported that the incidence rate of CD rose from 0.9 per 100,000 in the 1950s to 9 per 100,000 person-years after 2000 [1, 2].

G.E. Mullin, M.D. (✉)
Division of Gastroenterology, Johns Hopkins University School of Medicine, 600 N Wolfe Street CARN 464 B, Baltimore, MD 21287, USA
e-mail: gmullin1@jhmi.edu

S.D. Rampertab, M.D., F.A.C.G.
Department of Medicine, Rutgers-Robert Wood Johnson Medical School, One Robert Wood Johnson Place MEB 478, New Brunswick, NJ 08903, USA
e-mail: rampersd@rutgers.edu

S.D. Rampertab and G.E. Mullin (eds.), *Celiac Disease*, Clinical Gastroenterology, DOI 10.1007/978-1-4614-8560-5_1,

Rubio-Tapia et al. compared age- and calendar-matched cohorts of individuals using historical data and banked sera from the Warren Air Force Base as baseline. They concluded that during 45 years of follow-up, the prevalence of undiagnosed CD in the USA is likely to have increased fourfold [3]. Thus, the rise in the prevalence of CD is not likely to merely result from a greater access to serological testing and public awareness. As discussed in Chaps. 3 and 13, additional risk factors in the early postnatal period that may play a role in development of CD include birth by cesarean section, lack of breast-feeding, early introduction of gluten, and possibly high numbers of rotavirus infections.

Pathobiology

The discussion of pathophysiology of CD spans four chapters in this book. Chapter 4 by Elliott focuses on the role of gluten as an antigen and describes in elaborate detail the mechanisms involved in antigen presentation and the importance of HLA-DQ2/DQ8 as well as tissue transglutaminase in allowing for the intense inflammatory reaction to occur which ultimately leads to the villous atrophy that characterizes celiac disease.

Dietary gluten storage proteins from wheat, rye, and barley contain protein sequences that elicit a diverse array of immunological response. Oats do not typically elicit an immunological response unless there is sufficient cross-contamination from milling and handling of gluten-rich grains (i.e., wheat). Alpha-2 gliadin (α2-gliadin) contains a 33 amino acid sequence that is resistant to digestion by human gut and pancreatic enzymes and is a classic CD antigen.

In order to mount an immunological response to gluten proteins, a number of events need to take place. The antigen must breach the protective barrier of the small intestine to be presented to the B and T cells of the mucosal immune system by major histocompatibility complex molecules (MHCs) present on antigen-presenting cells (APCs) such as dendritic cells. Gluten proteins appear to traverse the cells and leak between cells due to defective regulation of tight junction proteins such as zonulin-1, providing a target for therapy [4]. A number of agents can initiate a breach in barrier function (i.e., infections, nonsteroidal medications, bacterial overgrowth); thus, defective permeability may be an antecedent to disease development as proposed by Fasano. The resultant processing of indigestible gluten antigens by the mucosal immune system leads to active small intestine inflammation whose inflammatory cytokines can further loosen the tight junctions and promote further entry of more gluten peptides to perpetuate the vicious cycle as shown by Elliott in Chap. 4, Fig. 4.2.

The enzyme tissue transglutaminase (TTG) removes the amide group from glutamine of gluten peptides such α2-gliadin, leaving it in a highly negatively charged state, which increases its affinity and binding to MHC HLA-DQ2.5 or DQ8. The aforementioned antibodies against TTG and deamidated gliadin become an important screening tool for CD.

The APC containing the altered gluten peptide on its surface then engages receptors on T and B cells to mount a vigorous immune response, including a Th1/Th17 dominant proinflammatory response (interferon gamma, interleukin-17). Interleukin-15 (IL-15), made by mucosal APCs activated by gluten and injured epithelial cells expanding the intraepithelial cell (IEL) population, induces the expression of natural killer cell receptors and promotes their cytolytic capabilities, which destroys epithelial cells and results in villous atrophy. These cytokines are additional targets of therapy; for example, IL-15 blockade would be an attractive target due to its central role in driving the damaging immune response in CD [5]. Such novel therapies are further discussed in Chap. 14 by Nasr et al. and outlined in Table 14.1.

CD, like many autoimmune disorders, is the result of a complex interaction of environmental, genetic, and immunological factors to produce disease. Chapter 5 by de Haas et al. hones in on the association between CD and HLA-DQ2/DQ8 haplotypes. It underscores the fact that while virtually all those with CD have one of these haplotypes, neither haplotype is sufficient to develop the disease as evidenced by the fact that although 40 % of Caucasians possess one of these haplotypes, only 3 % of them will go on to develop CD.

The human leukocyte antigen (HLA)-DQ genotype, specifically HLA-DQ2 and HLA-DQ8, is the strongest genetic risk factor. Genome-wide association studies (GWAS) have identified 57 associated non-HLA variants, located in 39 regions with mainly immunological functions. Together with HLA, these variants explain approximately 54 % of the disease's heritability.

The most relevant application of HLA testing is for potential screening of high-risk groups since a negative HLA-DQ2.5 and HLA-DQ8 would essentially rule out CD with over a 95 % certainty. The positive predictive value of HLA-DQ 2.5/DQ8 testing limits its utility in confirming the diagnosis of CD. A higher prevalence of CD observed in siblings of children with CD (10 %) and in first (4.5 %)- and second (2.6 %)-degree relatives when compared to the general population (0.9 %) and a stronger concordance in monozygotic (83 %) vs. dizygotic (16 %) twin pairs all speak of a strong heritability for CD, which has been reported to be 57–87 % [6].

"Using Animal Models of Celiac Disease to Understand the Role of MHC II," Chap. 6 by Marietta et al. reviews the spontaneous and induced non-transgenic animal models along with transgenic models that have been utilized to study the role of HLA and non-HLA factors in the pathogenesis of CD and their potential role in testing novel therapies.

Chapter 7 by Laparra et al. provides a comprehensive review concerning the potential role of the microbiota in the pathogenesis of CD. Moreover, it makes a compelling argument that the gut microbial environment early in life as determined by antibiotic intake, mode of delivery, type of milk feeding, and early gastrointestinal infections is crucial in determining future disease development. Interestingly, the microbiota of infants at high risk of developing CD showed reduced numbers of *Bifidobacterium* spp., a type of bacteria whose growth is enhanced by breastfeeding. Formula-fed infants at high genetic risk of developing CD also showed increased numbers of the *Bacteroides fragilis* group.

CD pathogenesis appears to be associated with intestinal dysbiosis, as there are abundant data that show pathogenic skewing of the gut microbiome in CD patients when compared to controls. Given the potential role of dysbiosis in the pathogenesis of CD and the ability of probiotics to downregulate proinflammatory responses and regulate autoimmunity, basic investigations have been conducted in animal models to potentially provide the basis for future human clinical trials. Certain lactobacilli, when added to sour dough for fermentation, hydrolyze the gluten peptide and render them less immunotoxic. A combination bacterial probiotic supplement, VSL#3, has shown ability to decrease the toxicity of wheat flour by completely hydrolyzing the α2-gliadin-derived epitopes 62–75 and 33-mer in vitro [7]. The probiotic yeast *Saccharomyces boulardii* has been shown to hydrolyze the 28-kDa gliadin fraction and improve enteropathy in gluten-sensitive mice [8]. Oral administration of probiotic bacteria *Lactobacillus casei* induced a complete recovery of villus blunting and improved gut-associated lymphoid tissue GALT homeostasis in a mouse model of gliadin-induced enteropathy [9].

Presentation, Screening, and Diagnosis

The clinical presentation of CD is highly variable, including typical (gastrointestinal symptoms), atypical (extra-intestinal symptoms), latent (no intestinal damage despite ingesting gluten, but later develops villous change; retrospective diagnosis), and silent (asymptomatic, discovered via screening) forms. The typical and atypical presenting symptoms of CD are extensively described in Chap. 8 by Reilly and Green.

The growth in public awareness of gluten-related illness has led to an explosion in the gluten-free food industry. Packaged Facts has reported that gluten-free packaged foods are a $4.2 billion industry with a projection of $6.6 billion in 2017 (http://www.foxnews.com/health/2012/10/23/gluten-free-foods-industry-worth-42-billion/). A Gluten Free Diet (GFD) is challenging and expensive and should be recommended based upon the best available evidence, thus defining that gluten intolerance is critical. Lammers et al. in Chap. 2 and Tavakkoli and Lebwohl in Chap. 9 provide a firm foundation for diagnosing the spectrum of gluten-related illness. Collectively, these authors report that the reactions to gluten represent a heterogeneous set of conditions, including CD, non-celiac gluten sensitivity, and wheat allergy, which combined affect about 10 % of the general population. As outlined by Tavakkoli and Lebwohl, the diagnosis of CD is currently made through a combination of serological, genetic, and endoscopic testing.

Lammers et al. have proposed that the diagnosis of CD can be confirmed by a "four out of five rule" to account for the variability in celiac disease presentation [10]. Under this rule, patients must meet at least four of the following five criteria to be diagnosed with CD: typical symptoms seen in CD, positive serological markers such as serum anti-transglutaminase (TTG) antibodies or antigliadin antibodies, small intestine biopsy showing absent or blunted villi (Marsh II–III a–c) and increased numbers of CD3+ intraepithelial cells, positive genetic screening for HLA-DQ2 or -DQ8, or improvement of symptoms with a GFD.

The chapter by Tavakkoli and Lebwohl also outlines the high-risk groups that should be considered for screening, including first-degree relatives (10 % prevalence), unexplained anemia, osteoporosis, type 1 diabetes mellitus (DM), Hashimoto's thryoiditis, autoimmune liver disease, irritable bowel syndrome, Down and Turner syndromes, IgA deficiency, and pancreatic insufficiency (Chap. 9, Table 9.2).

The recently published American College of Gastroenterology Celiac Disease Guidelines recommended screening for CD in patients with typical symptoms, signs, and/or laboratory evidence of CD and patients with a first-degree family member having confirmed CD. Screening is also recommend for asymptomatic relatives with a first-degree family member with confirmed CD, those with unexplained serum aminotransferase elevation, and those with type 1 DM with typical symptoms and or laboratory evidence suggesting CD [11].

Populations in which CD occurs more frequently than the general population for whom a GFD may be beneficial may include symptomatic malabsorption, diarrhea with weight loss, chronic diarrhea, chronic iron deficiency anemia, metabolic bone disease, unexplained weight loss, postprandial bloating and gaseousness, abnormal liver enzymes, dermatitis herpetiformis, incidental discovery of villous atrophy endoscopically or histologically, peripheral neuropathy, oral aphthous ulcers, growth failure, discolored teeth or developmentally synchronous enamel loss, irritable bowel syndrome, and Down and Turner syndromes.

Tavakkoli and Lebwohl summarized the diagnostic approach to CD. The serological evaluation is the first step in making the diagnosis of CD and the IgA anti-tissue transglutaminase antibody (anti-TTG) is the initial test of choice. IgG anti-TTG is also available for commercial use; however, the sensitivity and specificity of this test are widely variable and are reserved for use in patients with IgA deficiency. IgA anti-EMA antibody testing is not currently recommended as the first-line therapy due to the high cost, variability, and subsequent development of IgA anti-TTG. IgA anti-TTG performs better and is less costly than the IgA-deamidated gliadin peptide (DGP) IgA-DGP. Genetic testing provides an almost 100 % negative predictive value for the diagnosis of CD. However, the routine addition of genetic testing to the standard serological evaluation described above does not increase diagnostic performance; thus, genetic testing was not recommended by Tavakkoli and Lebwohl in the initial evaluation of CD. Duodenal biopsies (two from the bulb at 9 and 12 O'clock positions, four biopsies post-bulbar) remain the gold standard for diagnosing CD in particular, since 10 % of CD patients may be seronegative and up to a third of CD patients with histologically active disease have a normal-appearing mucosa on endoscopic examination during endoscopy [12, 13]. The Marsh–Oberhuber histological criteria for diagnosing CD are presented in Chap. 9, Table 9.3, by Tavakkoli and Lebwohl.

Non-celiac Gluten Sensitivity

Non-celiac gluten sensitivity (NCGS) is a reaction to gluten that is not mediated by an allergic or an immune-mediated response. Non-celiac gluten-sensitive patients usually present with the same variety of symptoms as CD. Lammers and Fasano reported that the prevalence of NCGS is estimated to be between 3 and 6 %. There are six criteria of NCGS, all of which are required for making the diagnosis:

- Celiac disease, IgE-mediated wheat allergy, and other clinically overlapping diseases (type 1 DM, inflammatory bowel diseases, *Helicobacter pylori* infection) have been ruled out
- Negative skin prick test for wheat
- Negative autoantibody serology (EMA-IgA and TTG-IgA)
- Small intestine biopsy demonstrates normal mucosa (Marsh 0) or increased intraepithelial lymphocytes (Marsh I)
- Symptoms are triggered by gluten exposure
- Improvement of symptoms within a few days of a GFD

The pathogenesis of CD and NCGS are distinct based upon lack of serological, tissue, and immunopathology as well as preserved intestinal barrier function in NCGS [14].

Special Considerations in Children

The prevalence of CD in children and adults is similar, approximately 1 % in the USA. Guandalini and Young in Chap. 13 remark that the pathobiology of CD is also quite similar in both populations; however, there are some notable exceptions. T cells from children are reactive to multiple epitopes of gluten and glutenin while in adults a single region of deaminated alpha-gliadin serves as the dominant epitope to cause an immunologic response. Interestingly, both deamidation-dependent and deamidation-independent responses to alpha-gliadin are seen in the pediatric CD population. Compared to children, adults and adolescents are more likely to have a longer duration of symptoms prior to the diagnosis of celiac disease and be diagnosed based upon asymptomatic or targeted screening. In contrast, children and teens with CD often present with the aforementioned gastrointestinal symptoms, extra-intestinal presentations (most commonly growth maturation issues such as delayed puberty, idiopathic short stature, dental enamel defects, failure to thrive, iron deficiency anemia, neurologic issues, behavioral symptoms), or asymptomatic disease diagnosed by targeted screening of the aforementioned high-risk groups. In fact, problems such as dental enamel hypoplasia, aphthous ulcers, and delayed teeth eruption are common in children with CD, while anemia is more frequently seen at presentation in adults compared to children. Down syndrome appears to have a high risk of CD, since up to 16 % of these patients are affected [15]. An overall decrease in the prevalence of diarrheal presentations over the past two decades, accompanied by an increase in atypical manifestations of the disease, has been well described in both adults and children.

The North American Society for Pediatric Gastroenterology, Hepatology, and Nutrition (NASPGHAN) recommends that testing be done in children with gastrointestinal symptoms, non-gastrointestinal symptoms (including dermatitis herpetiformis, short stature, and delayed puberty), and asymptomatic patients who reside in a high-risk population such as type 1 DM, autoimmune thyroiditis, Down syndrome, Turner syndrome, Williams syndrome, and first-degree relatives of CD patients. Testing of these asymptomatic patients is recommended to begin around 3 years of age as long as the child has been on a gluten-containing diet for at least 1 year prior to testing. The initial screening test of choice is the IgA antibody to TTG. Anti-TTG and anti-EMA antibodies are often negative in children with CD who are younger than 2 years of age, and the histological changes can be more commonly due to other causes such as cow's milk-sensitive enteropathy, post-enteric syndrome, *Giardia* infection, autoimmune enteropathy, and common variable immune deficiency [16].

According to European Society for Pediatric Gastroenterology, Hepatology, and Nutrition (ESPGHAN), children with symptoms suggestive of CD, an IgA anti-TTG antibody level greater than ten times the upper limit of normal, and a positive HLA haplotype do not need a duodenal biopsy to diagnose CD.

Therapy and Monitoring

In CD, the primary nutrition intervention is the education and implementation of a strict GFD, currently the only treatment for CD. The GFD requires complete elimination of the gluten protein found in wheat, barley, and rye. All foods containing these grains as ingredients or through contamination must be removed from the diet. A referral to a dietitian with expertise in CD is essential. Chapter 10 outlines the tools for evaluating the nutritional status of CD patients, describes when to refer to an experienced registered dietitian, and emphasizes the importance of educating patients about the foods to avoid as well as alternatives to improve compliance with a GFD. GFD impacts quality of life, morbidity, and mortality. Nutritional deficiencies can occur in patients with CD due to malabsorption of nutrients from loss of small intestine absorptive capacity, pancreatic insufficiency, lack of fortification of gluten-free food products, and restrictive dietary practices. In Chap. 11, Pietzak reviews the nutritional manifestations and therapy of CD. Since anemia is a common presentation and manifestation of CD, consideration of iron deficiency in the setting of microcytic anemia and vitamin B_{12} or folate deficiency in the presence of macrocytosis is warranted. Fat-soluble vitamin deficiencies (A, D, E, and K) can occur in CD from decreased absorptive surface area, from pancreatic insufficiency, and even from associated liver disease from lack of bile flow. Monitoring of fat-soluble vitamins should be done at least annually, except for vitamin D—seasonally, given the risk of osteoporosis in CD and widespread prevalence of vitamin D deficiency in the USA and in CD patients. Micronutrient screening for zinc, copper, and selenium should be performed at least annually and sooner, if deficiency is suspected. Finally, patients on a GFD tend to have a paucity of dietary fiber. The recommended dietary reference intake (DRI) for fiber in the US diet is 25 g daily.

A number of novel and experimental therapeutic trials for the treatment of CD are ongoing and reviewed in Chap. 14 by Nasr et al. The areas of research include the development of gluten products with low immunogenicity, oral enzymes to detoxify ingested gluten, probiotics, tight junction regulatory peptides, tissue transglutaminase enzyme blockage, regulatory cytokines, proinflammatory cytokine blockade, HLA-DQ groove blockade, anti-adhesion molecule therapy, intestinotrophic mitogens, and gluten peptide vaccination.

CD is a lifelong chronic disease requiring long-term follow-up; thus, monitoring is a critical aspect of treating the CD patient. Monitoring of CD is addressed in Chap. 10 by Simpson and Thompson and in Chap. 12 by Herman et al. Rapid resolution of the clinical symptoms is usually noted within a few weeks after starting the GFD.

In Chap. 12, Herman et al. review the currently published recommendations for longitudinal follow-up of patients with celiac disease in Table 12.1 and Fig. 12.1. The authors suggest a first follow-up visit in 3–6 months, then annually from date of diagnosis including serology, and in some cases even every 2 years if otherwise doing well on a GFD. Unfortunately, the use of anti-TTG or related (anti-EMA, anti-DPG) antibodies should not be the sole tool for the monitoring of compliance to a GFD. Patients with normalized serology may continue to have ongoing intestinal inflammation and gluten contamination in their diets, and a patient who continues to consume gluten may have falsely normal serology. Mucosal recovery generally requires several years of strict gluten avoidance in adults, and is often patchy or incomplete; thus, mucosal biopsy after the first year of a GFD as well as when patients fail to improve or have recurrent symptoms despite a GFD is advocated. At diagnosis, it is recommended that patients be assessed for anemia, malnutrition, vitamin or mineral deficiencies, liver test abnormalities, and thyroid dysfunction. Other recommendations for the patient with CD include immunization for encapsulated organisms, screening for bone mineral density, and prompt attention to those with alarm symptoms such as lymphoma-type symptoms (i.e., fevers), refractory symptoms, or persisting serological titers on a GFD to evaluate potential complications.

Morbidity and Mortality

Lewis and Holmes discuss the morbidity and mortality associated with CD in Chap. 15. The disease associations with CD are numerous and diverse across all systems, and their recognition as being potentially treatable with a GFD may prevent, improve, and even reverse complications. It is incumbent on those who care for patients with CD to be aware of these associations so that patients receive optimum management.

Type 1 DM is the most common autoimmune disease association, occurring in 3.5–5 % of celiacs and usually precedes the development of CD. Thyroiditis causing hypothyroidism is ten times more common in CD than in the general population. In adults, gluten withdrawal in adults may normalize thyroid tests in those with subclinical hypothyroidism. A spectrum of liver pathology has been associated with CD, including isolated transaminitis, sclerosing cholangitis, and autoimmune hepatitis (AIH) and its complications (i.e., cirrhosis). GFD improves transaminitis and hepatic histology (i.e., inflammation, steatosis) in AIH. Other autoimmune diseases associated with CD include psoriasis, Addison's disease, systemic lupus erythematosus, Sjögren's syndrome, hypoparathyroidism, hypopituitarism, dermatomyositis, scleroderma, alopecia areata, ulcerative colitis, Crohn's disease, microscopic colitis, and myasthenia gravis. Patients with CD are at an increased risk of disease development and mortality from cardiovascular disease. Like in the general population, vascular disease is the most important single cause of mortality in diagnosed CD, accounting for 39 % of all deaths [17].

Chapter 16 by Malamut and Cellier reviews the complication of refractory celiac disease (RCD). Diagnosis of RCD relies on persistent malabsorption and villous atrophy after 1 year of strict GFD ascertained by a dietitian. Most cases of nonresponsive CD are related to continuing ingestion of gluten either deliberately or inadvertently, and this should be checked by a skilled dietitian. Serological tests and repeat small bowel biopsies will help in the assessment. Primary RCD is a failure to induce a response to a GFD after the initial diagnosis of CD, while secondary RCD represents a return of symptoms after a period of quiescence. Once surreptitious gluten ingestion is ruled out, conditions causing RCD associated with CD should be considered such as intestinal lymphoma, pancreatic insufficiency, small intestine bacterial overgrowth, microscopic colitis, irritable bowel syndrome, inflammatory bowel disease, lactose intolerance, and thyroid dysfunction. The diagnosis of RCD is made after exclusion of other small bowel diseases with villous atrophy such as autoimmune enteropathy and common variable immunodeficiency.

RCD has been subdivided into two subgroups according to the normal-type 1 RCD or abnormal phenotype of intraepithelial lymphocytes (IEL)-type 1I RCD. Type 1 RCD has a phenotypically normal T-cell population on duodenal histology and carries a good prognosis, responds to corticosteroids and azathioprine, and the 5-year survival is over 90 %. In type 2 RCD there is an aberrant intraepithelial T-cell population that carries intracytoplasmic but not surface CD3, usually lacks CD8, and has clonal rearrangements of the T-cell receptor-γ gene. Type 2 RCD resembles a low-grade lymphoma. The prognosis for type 2 RCD is poor, with no satisfactory treatments.

Malignancies have been related to CD for over five decades with enteropathy-associated T-cell lymphoma type 1 (EATL-1) and small bowel adenocarcinoma being the most prominent cancers. CD is associated not only with EATL but also with a wide variety of other lymphomas. Paradoxically, CD patients have a decreased risk of developing breast cancer. Increased risks of oropharyngeal cancer, esophageal cancer, colon, liver, pancreas [18], and papillary cancer of the thyroid have been demonstrated, but in contrast to lymphomas, where there is evidence that a GFD will reduce the risk for these malignancies, there is no evidence at present that a GFD will reduce their occurrence [19].

There is a modest increased risk of metabolic bone disease and fracture in patients with CD. The risk of developing a number of neurological and psychiatric disorders is increased in patients with CD. Depression and anxiety, epilepsy, and migraine disorders are increased in CD, and improvement is seen in many following a GFD. Other neurological conditions including spinocerebellar and cerebellar disorders, peripheral neuropathy, myelopathy, brainstem encephalitis and chronic progressive leukoencephalopathy, ADHD, dementia, and cognitive decline are also increased in CD. There is no formal link between CD and either schizophrenia, autism, or multiple sclerosis. It has to be concluded that a neurological or psychiatric disorder specific for CD has not been identified; however, there is growing evidence for gluten ataxia that improves on a GFD.

Reduced fertility and increased adverse pregnancy-related outcomes are seen more commonly in women with CD. Hyposplenism leading to an increased risk of mortality from sepsis and pneumonia from encapsulated organisms is seen in patients with CD. Thus, vaccination against pneumococcus is recommended for all CD patients with hyposplenism. The main dermatological association with CD is dermatitis herpetiformis (DH). Most individuals with DH have CD, but DH is rarely found in patients with CD.

Other gastrointestinal conditions that can be associated with CD include the irritable bowel syndrome (IBS), although the two conditions can have overlapping symptomatology. A meta-analysis of five case–control studies employing biopsy diagnosis of CD found a fourfold increase among patients with IBS meeting the Rome II criteria [20]. This association between IBS and dietary gluten is more extensively reviewed in Chap. 2 by Lammers and Fasano and in Chap. 8 by Reilly and Green. Interestingly, the prevalence of eosinophilic esophagitis, pancreatitis, enamel defects, glossitis, angular stomatitis, and recurrent aphthous ulcers appears to be increased in CD.

As discussed in Chap. 15 by Lewis and Holmes, Rubio-Tapia et al. reported that the mortality of untreated CD is increased fourfold but was not confirmed in European studies [3]. In contrast, a recent meta-analysis suggests that there is a strong link between diagnosed CD to increased all-cause mortality [21]. The degree of compliance with a GFD correlates with mortality as do the severity of the clinical presentation and the length of time from onset of symptoms to the diagnosis of CD.

There is abundant literature to show that there is no increase in mortality with strict adherence to the GFD; however, Lebwohl et al. report that CD patients with persistent villus atrophy did not have an increased all-cause mortality [22].

Misconceptions and Myths: Separating Fact from Fiction

Boettcher and Crowe dispel many misconceptions and myths about CD in Chap. 17. Misconceptions that were refuted include CD is rare, only symptomatic individuals should be tested for CD, only Caucasians are susceptible to CD, women are more often affected by CD, you cannot have CD if you are overweight, CD is not a serious condition, CD signs and symptoms are easy to recognize, CD is easy to diagnose, everyone knows how to biopsy for CD and CD is easy to treat, a positive response to a GFD is suggestive of CD, and getting information about a GFD is straightforward. Myths of management were dispelled: you cannot use gluten-containing beauty products and cosmetics having CD; the consumption of oats can trigger CD; a separate set of utensils, dishes, and other kitchen goods is necessary; gluten-free cleaning products are recommended; and pets should eat gluten-free.

In summary, celiac disease is a very common condition, affecting 1 % of the population worldwide. Our knowledge of this disease has grown tremendously in the last three decades due to the hard work and dedication of researchers, educators, and clinicians, including all the contributors to our book. This production represents a compilation of the most up-to-date information presented by prominent experts in the field from around the world. We trust that this book will be an excellent resource to you in recognizing the myriad presentations of this disease, understanding the pathophysiology of the disease, and educating and treating your patients effectively to prevent long-term complications and allow them to have better quality of life.

References

1. Catassi C, Kryszak D, Bhatti B, Sturgeon C, Helzlsouer K, Clipp SL, et al. Natural history of celiac disease autoimmunity in a USA cohort followed since 1974. Ann Med. 2010;42(7):530–8.
2. Murray JA, Van Dyke C, Plevak MF, Dierkhising RA, Zinsmeister AR, Melton 3rd LJ. Trends in the identification and clinical features of celiac disease in a North American community, 1950–2001. Clin Gastroenterol Hepatol. 2003;1(1):19–27.
3. Rubio-Tapia A, Kyle RA, Kaplan EL, Johnson DR, Page W, Erdtmann F, et al. Increased prevalence and mortality in undiagnosed celiac disease. Gastroenterology. 2009;137(1): 88–93.
4. Fasano A. Zonulin, regulation of tight junctions, and autoimmune diseases. Ann N Y Acad Sci. 2012;1258:25–33.
5. Sollid LM, Khosla C. Novel therapies for coeliac disease. J Intern Med. 2011;269(6):604–13.
6. Nisticò L, Fagnani C, Coto I, Percopo S, Cotichini R, Limongelli MG, et al. Concordance, disease progression, and heritability of coeliac disease in Italian twins. Gut. 2006;55:803–8.
7. De Angelis M, Rizzello CG, Fasano A, Clemente MG, De Simone C, Silano M, et al. VSL#3 probiotic preparation has the capacity to hydrolyze gliadin polypeptides responsible for celiac sprue. Bioenergetics. 2006;1762(1):80–93.
8. Papista C, Gerakopoulos V, Kourelis A, Sounidaki M, Kontana A, Berthelot L, et al. Gluten induces coeliac-like disease in sensitised mice involving IgA, CD71 and transglutaminase 2 interactions that are prevented by probiotics. Lab Invest. 2012;92(4):625–35.

9. D'Arienzo R, Stefanile R, Maurano F, Mazzarella G, Ricca E, Troncone R, et al. Immunomodulatory effects of *Lactobacillus casei* administration in a mouse model of gliadin-sensitive enteropathy. Scand J Immunol. 2011;74(4):335–41.
10. Catassi C, Fasano A. Celiac disease diagnosis: simple rules are better than complicated algorithms. Am J Med. 2010;123(8):691–3.
11. Rubio-Tapia A, Hill I, Kelly CP, Calderwood AH, Murray JA. ACG clinical guidelines: diagnosis and management of celiac disease. Am J Gastroenterol. 2013;108:656–76.
12. Leffler DA, Schuppan D. Update on serologic testing in celiac disease. Am J Gastroenterol. 2010;105(12):2520–4. PubMed PMID: 21131921.
13. Kurien M, Evans KE, Hopper AD, Hale MF, Cross SS, Sanders DS. Duodenal bulb biopsies for diagnosing adult celiac disease: is there an optimal biopsy site? Gastrointest Endosc. 2012;75(6):1190–6. PubMed PMID: 22624810.
14. Sapone A, Lammers KM, Casolaro V, Cammarota M, Giuliano MT, De Rosa M, et al. Divergence of gut permeability and mucosal immune gene expression in two gluten-associated conditions: celiac disease and gluten sensitivity. BMC Med. 2011;9:23.
15. Carlsson A, Axelsson I, Borulf S, Bredberg A, Forslund M, Lindberg B, et al. Prevalence of IgA-antigliadin antibodies and IgA-antiendomysium antibodies related to celiac disease in children with Down syndrome. Pediatrics. 1998;101(2):272–5. PubMed PMID: 9445503.
16. Hill ID, Dirks MH, Liptak GS, Colletti RB, Fasano A, Guandalini S, et al. Guideline for the diagnosis and treatment of celiac disease in children: recommendations of the North American Society for Pediatric Gastroenterology, Hepatology and Nutrition. J Pediatr Gastroenterol Nutr. 2005;40(1):1–19. PubMed PMID: 15625418.
17. Peters U, Askling J, Gridley G, Ekbom A, Linet M. Causes of death in patients with celiac disease in a population-based Swedish cohort. Arch Intern Med. 2003;163(13):1566–72.
18. Landgren AM, Landgren O, Gridley G, Dores GM, Linet MS, Morton LM. Autoimmune disease and subsequent risk of developing alimentary tract cancers among 4.5 million US male veterans. Cancer. 2011;117(6):1163–71.
19. Holmes GK, Prior P, Lane MR, Pope D, Allan RN. Malignancy in coeliac disease–effect of a gluten free diet. Gut. 1989;30(3):333–8.
20. Ford AC, Chey WD, Talley NJ, Malhotra A, Spiegel BM, Moayyedi P. Yield of diagnostic tests for celiac disease in individuals with symptoms suggestive of irritable bowel syndrome: systematic review and meta-analysis. Arch Intern Med. 2009;169(7):651–8.
21. Tio M, Cox MR, Eslick GD. Meta-analysis: coeliac disease and the risk of all-cause mortality, any malignancy and lymphoid malignancy. Aliment Pharmacol Ther. 2012;35(5):540–51.
22. Lebwohl B, Granath F, Ekbom A, Montgomery SM, Murray JA, Rubio-Tapia A, et al. Mucosal healing and mortality in coeliac disease. Aliment Pharmacol Ther. 2013;37(3):332–9. doi:10.1111/apt.12164.

Chapter 2
Definition of Celiac Disease and Gluten Sensitivity

Karen M. Lammers, Brintha Vasagar, and Alessio Fasano

Introduction

As an important component of wheat, rye, and barley, gluten can be found in a large variety of foods consumed throughout the world. However, the introduction of gluten-containing grains in the human diet about 10,000 years ago created the conditions for human disease related to gluten exposure. These reactions to gluten represent a heterogeneous set of conditions, including celiac disease (CD), non-celiac gluten sensitivity, and wheat allergy, which combined affect about 10 % of the general population [1].

The immune-reactive component of gluten is gliadin, a complex glycoprotein rich in proline and glutamine. Because of this structure, intestinal enzymes cannot entirely degrade the protein. We do know that undigested or partly digested gliadin can affect a wide range of human cells. The effects of gliadin on the myelocytic leukemia cell line, K562, and various intestinal cell lines are, respectively, its agglutinating activity [2], its capacity to induce rearrangement of the epithelial actin cytoskeleton by redistribution of F-actin [3], and its cytotoxic activities including inhibition of cell growth, induction of apoptosis, and alteration of redox equilibrium [4, 5].

There are three variants of gliadin, the alpha-, gamma-, and omega-variant, with the alpha-gliadin variant being the most prevalent. A 13-mer and a 33-mer alpha-gliadin motif have been reported to exert a cytotoxic effect on intestinal epithelial cells [6] and to be capable of activating gut-derived T-cell lines from CD patients [7],

K.M. Lammers, Ph.D. • B. Vasagar, M.D., M.P.H.
Department of Pediatrics, Massachusetts General Hospital for Children, Massachusetts General Hospital East, Charlestown, Boston, MA, USA

A. Fasano, M.D. (✉)
Department of Pediatrics, Massachusetts General Hospital for Children, Massachusetts General Hospital East, Building 114, 16th Street, Mail Stop 114-3503, Charlestown, Boston, MA 02129-4404, USA
e-mail: AFasano@partners.org

S.D. Rampertab and G.E. Mullin (eds.), *Celiac Disease*, Clinical Gastroenterology, DOI 10.1007/978-1-4614-8560-5_2, © Springer Science+Business Media New York 2014 respectively. Furthermore, two 20-mer intestinal permeating and an immunomodulatory 17-mer alpha-gliadin peptide have recently been identified [8, 9].

CD, non-celiac gluten sensitivity, and wheat allergy represent distinct pathophysiological reactions to gluten ingestion, with differing clinical presentations, serological markers, and long-term treatments. Though current research strives to clarify the boundaries between these entities, their differences can be difficult to distinguish. This chapter provides an overview of the ever-evolving definitions of gluten-related disorders.

Celiac Disease

CD, an autoimmune-mediated enteropathy triggered by gluten ingestion in genetically predisposed individuals, is one of the most common chronic digestive disorders, showing an overall prevalence worldwide of 1 % with large variations between countries [10]. The disease prevalence is even higher amongst first-degree relatives of CD patients (8–15 %) [11, 12] and other at-risk groups, such as patients with other genetic diseases like type 1 diabetes mellitus, Hashimoto's thyroiditis, Down syndrome, or IgA deficiency [13–17]. Importantly and contrary to previous assumption, CD is not confined to Europe; rather it is present worldwide [18] and it is increasing over time [19].

The genetic predisposition to CD is strong but complex (see Chap. 5 on HLA genetics). Human leukocyte antigen (HLA) haplotypes DQ2 and DQ8 are found in at least 95 % of patients with CD [20]. While the presence of these alleles provides a strong negative predictive value, their positive predictive value is low. Indeed, although 30 % of the general population carries the HLA-DQ2 allele [20], the prevalence of CD is currently 1 % [10]. As much as 65 % of the genetic component of CD may be caused by a complex, still undefined, mosaic of over 40 non-HLA genes, each adding a small contribution to the risk of CD development [20, 21].

Clinical Presentation

The clinical presentation of CD is highly variable, including typical (gastrointestinal symptoms), atypical (extra-intestinal symptoms), latent (no intestinal damage despite ingesting gluten, but later develops villous change; retrospective diagnosis), and silent (asymptomatic, discovered via screening) forms [22, 23]. The presenting symptoms may vary from diarrhea, constipation, vomiting, malnutrition, or failure to thrive to chronic fatigue, joint pain, anemia, osteoporosis, or migraines. Many times, the onset of symptoms occurs during the first 24 months of life, usually some months after the introduction of gluten-containing cereals in the infant's diet. A recent study highlights the importance of timing with regard to gluten introduction into the diet in genetically susceptible infants. Those infants to whom gluten was introduced in the diet at 6 months developed CD more frequently than those infants to whom gluten introduction was delayed until 12 months of age [24]. However, it is important to note that initial signs and symptoms of CD can occur at any age, including adults and the elderly [19, 25]. Unlike the relatively rapid reaction seen in wheat allergy, the signs and symptoms of CD usually do not manifest until weeks to years after exposure.

Diagnosis by a "four out of five rule" has been proposed to account for the variability in CD presentation [26]. Under this rule, patients must meet at least four of the following five criteria to be diagnosed with CD:

- Typical symptoms seen in CD
- Positive serological markers such as serum anti-transglutaminase (TTG) antibodies or antigliadin antibodies
- Small intestine biopsy showing absent or blunted villi (Marsh II–III a–c), and increased numbers of CD3+ intraepithelial cells
- Positive genetic screening for HLA-DQ2 or -DQ8
- Improvement of symptoms with a gluten-free diet

Treatment for CD is the lifelong implementation of a gluten-free diet, in which all gluten-containing foods are eliminated from the diet. Compliance with a strict gluten-free diet reverses small intestinal changes in the vast majority of patients and reduces the risk of complications from CD (osteoporosis, lymphoma, infertility). However, this change in diet can be difficult to implement and maintain, not only because gluten-rich products are an important part of the Western diet, but also because of "hidden" gluten in processed foods [27, 28]. Adding to the challenge, designated gluten-free foods are often more expensive than their gluten-containing counterparts. Moreover, eating gluten-free can be exclusionary, as it makes it difficult to eat at restaurants for fear of cross-contamination. Given the negative impact of the gluten-free diet on the quality of life of affected individuals, there is currently a strong interest on possible alternative strategies of treatment or prevention [29, 30].

Non-celiac Gluten Sensitivity

Non-celiac gluten sensitivity is the least clearly defined of the gluten-related disorders as it has only become widely recognized in recent years [1, 31–33]. When the reaction to gluten is not mediated by an allergic or autoimmune response, gluten sensitivity may be considered [1, 34, 35]. The lack of clear diagnostic criteria may have led to non-celiac gluten sensitivity being undiagnosed and underdiagnosed by physicians for many years. The prevalence of non-celiac gluten sensitivity is estimated to be between 3 and 6 % [1, 36]. The genetic component of gluten sensitivity is not yet completely understood. Only 50 % of non-celiac gluten sensitivity patients express the HLA-DQ2 or HLA-DQ8 haplotype, indicating that these genes are not necessary or sufficient to develop gluten sensitivity [1].

Clinical Presentation

Non-celiac gluten-sensitive patients usually present with the same variety of symptoms (diarrhea, stomach pain, etc.) and prevalence of extra-intestinal symptoms (headache, "foggy brain," fatigue, rash, joint pain, depression, anxiety, etc.) as seen in CD [1]. Due to the absence of distinct pathology on biopsy, and lack of identifiable serological markers (e.g., negative CD serology but with possible presence of anti-gliadin antibodies [1, 37]), gluten sensitivity is currently a diagnosis of exclusion. As such, non-celiac gluten-sensitive patients must meet the following criteria for diagnosis:

- CD, IgE-mediated wheat allergy, and other clinically overlapping diseases (type 1 diabetes mellitus, inflammatory bowel diseases, *Helicobacter pylori* infection) have been excluded
- Negative skin prick test for wheat
- Negative autoantibody serology (EMA-IgA and TTG-IgA)
- Small intestine biopsy demonstrates normal mucosa (Marsh 0) or increased intraepithelial lymphocytes (Marsh I)
- Symptoms are triggered by gluten exposure
- Improvement of symptoms within a few days of a gluten-free diet

Gluten and the Irritable Bowel Syndrome Connection

Whether the prevalence of the irritable bowel syndrome (IBS) is higher in CD has been a point of controversy. A meta-analysis of five case–control studies found a fourfold increase of CD among patients with IBS meeting the Rome II criteria compared with controls (OR 4.34 [95 % CI 1.78–10.6]) [38]. However, a subsequent study found a similar prevalence of CD in non-constipated IBS patients when compared to controls [39].

Gluten-free diets are recommended with increasing frequency for IBS symptoms in the absence of CD. Patients who do not have CD, but possess a consistent genotype of HLA-DQ2/8, have also reported benefit from a gluten-free diet. There are several reports linking gluten ingestion with worsening of IBS symptoms and gluten restriction with improvement of IBS [32, 40]. A subgroup of patients with IBS, that is, patients with diarrhea-predominant irritable bowel syndrome (IBS-D), can benefit from a gluten-free diet. Vazquez-Roque et al. report on a randomized, controlled trial designed to explore whether a gluten-free diet benefits patients with IBS-D [41]. Subjects on a gluten-free diet exhibited lower stool frequency than those on a gluten-containing diet ($P=0.04$; 95 % confidence interval [CI], –0.652 to –0.015). In addition, the impact on stool frequency of a gluten-free diet was greater for patients who were HLA-DQ2/8 positive. Gluten ingestion was shown to increase the small intestinal permeability in these patients, and especially those patients who carry the HLA-DQ2/DQ8 haplotype. The implementation of a gluten-free diet in this subgroup of patients restored the intestinal barrier function. Interestingly,

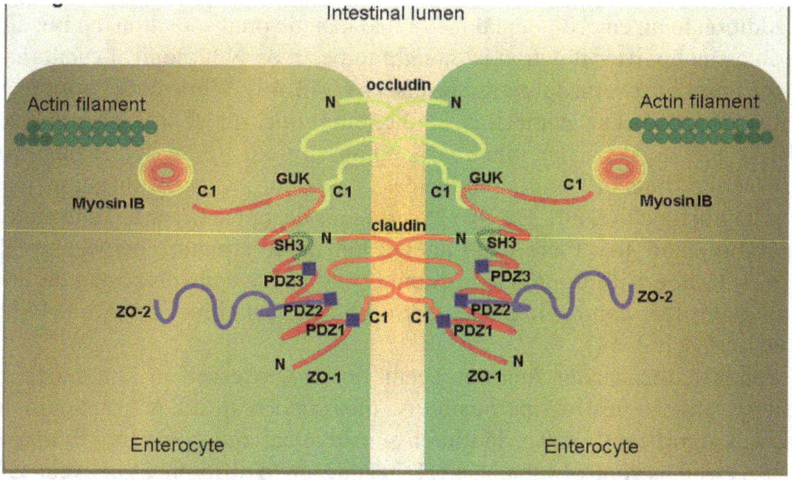

Fig. 2.1 Schematic drawing of the tight junction (TJ) complex. Intestinal epithelial permeability is regulated by the intercellular tight junction protein complex that consists of many components including zonula occludin (ZO)-1, occludin, claudins, and junctional adhesion molecules. These TJ proteins maintain cell–cell adhesion in epithelial monolayers. The overall balance of TJ protein expression is thought to define the regulation of the paracellular path by the TJ complex

decreased expression of tight junction proteins zonula occludens (ZO)-1, claudin-1, and occludin correlated with the increased permeability [41]. Overall there appears to be a connection of gluten ingestion to worsening gastrointestinal symptomatology and improvement upon withdrawal at least in IBS-D.

Pathogenesis

Barrier Function in Celiac Disease and Gluten Sensitivity

Intestinal epithelial permeability is regulated by intercellular tight junction protein complex that consists of many components such as ZO-1, occludin, claudins, and junctional adhesion molecules [42, 43]. These tight junction proteins maintain cell–cell adhesion in epithelial monolayers [44, 45] and the overall balance of tight junction (TJ) protein expression is thought to define the regulation of the paracellular path by the TJ complex (Fig. 2.1).

Zonulin, now identified and characterized as pre-haptoglobin-2 [46], is the human analogue of Zonula occludin toxin derived from *Vibrio cholera* [47]. It is released by the small intestinal mucosa after challenge with gliadin or bacteria [48] and modulates the paracellular intestinal permeability by a PAR2-dependent transactivation of epithelial growth factor receptor and subsequent phosphorylation of TJ proteins [46].

In addition to an environmental factor and genetic predisposition, an impairment of the intestinal barrier function is thought to be an early biological event that precedes the onset of several autoimmune diseases [42, 49]. While under normal physiological circumstances the intestinal epithelium is impermeable to macromolecules, in CD the epithelial barrier function is compromised. In the active phase of the disease, serum titers of zonulin are increased and, consequently, intestinal permeability is augmented [42, 50]. Ex vivo experiments designed to measure the intestinal permeability show that there is an altered junctional structure between epithelial cells [51]. In line with these data, genomic studies have also reported an involvement of genes that control intestinal permeability, including *PARD3*, *MAGI2*, and *MYO9B*, in CD [52–54].

In contrast, the barrier function seems to be conserved in non-celiac gluten sensitivity. Small intestinal permeability, measured with a LA/MA double sugar probe, was significantly lower in gluten-sensitive patients compared to that in CD patients as well as control subjects [31]. In addition to differences between CD and non-celiac gluten sensitivity with regard to intestinal permeability, there are also differences in mucosal TJ protein gene transcripts between the two conditions. The mucosa of subjects affected by gluten sensitivity expresses significantly higher levels of transcripts for claudin-4, a protein involved in TJ-dependent enhancement of the barrier function, relative to that of CD or in healthy individuals [31]. These findings suggest that the distinct clinical and serological features between celiac and gluten-sensitive patients are associated with marked differences in intestinal barrier function and with apparent differences in the expression of *CLDN4* gene expression.

Immune Response of Celiac Disease and Non-celiac Gluten Sensitivity

When the integrity of the intestinal tight junction complex is compromised, an immune response to environmental antigens develops and in genetically predisposed individuals may result in the pathogenesis of CD. CD is considered a classical Th1-mediated disorder because of the increased mucosal gene expression of interferon (IFN)-γ, but not IL-4, in the active phase of the disease [55, 56]. The adaptive immune response in celiac disease is triggered by tissue transglutaminase (TTG)-deamidated gluten peptides that bind with high affinity to HLA-DQ2 or -DQ8 [57]. This involves the mucosal recruitment and activation of Th1 cell clones and production of the Th1 cytokine, IFN-γ (Fig. 2.2).

Another characteristic of CD is the increased numbers of CD3+ intraepithelial lymphocytes. Following the identification of the Th17 T-cell subset [58], and the growing appreciation that these cells are centrally involved in the pathogenesis of autoimmune disorders, recent reports have confirmed the enhanced expression of Th17-active cytokines, IL-1β and IL-23, and the Th17-associated cytokine, IL-17A, in active CD [59–61]. The villous atrophy observed in active CD might be, at least in part, a result of NKG2D (natural killer group 2, member D)-mediated epithelial cell death by intraepithelial cytotoxic T lymphocytes [62]. Reports on regulatory

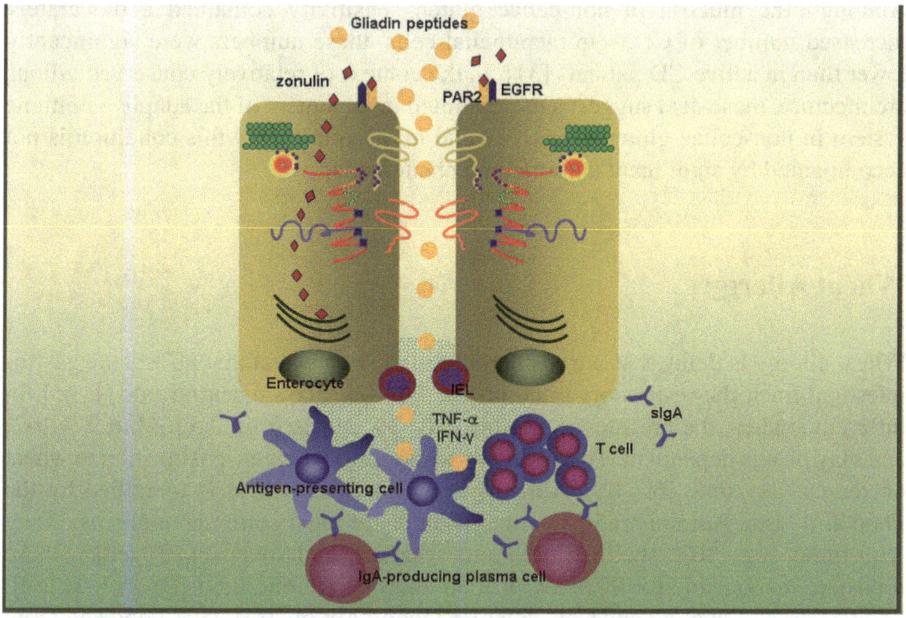

Fig. 2.2 The immune response in the autoimmune enteropathy, celiac disease (CD). In response to undigested gliadin peptides, enterocytes release zonulin that via a PAR2-mediated transactivation of EGFR induces phosphorylation of a major tight junction protein, zonula occludens (ZO)-1. This results in disassembly of the tight junction complex and, hence, increase in intestinal permeability. This allows the gliadin peptides to enter the lamina propria and an immune response is mounted against the gliadin peptides. In response to the accumulation of gliadin peptides in the lamina propria, enterocytes produce IL-15 that recruits intraepithelial lymphocytes (IEL). Histology of active CD shows an increased number of IEL. Tissue transglutaminase (tTG) deamidates the gliadin peptides. The peptides then bind with high affinity to the HLA-DQ2/DQ8 receptor on antigen-presenting cells and are presented to T helper (Th) cells. CD is a Th1-mediated autoimmune disease. The activated Th1 cells secrete inflammatory mediators that attract and activate other immune cells. One key cytokine in this Th1-mediated inflammation is interferon-gamma. The Th1 cells activate natural killer cells to attack enterocytes. B cells mature in IgA antibody producing plasma cells. Hallmark of established CD is the presence of IgA autoantibodies, the anti-TTG, and anti-endomysial (EMA) antibodies in the serum

T cells do suggest that these cells are present in sufficient number in the intestinal tissue, but exert an impaired suppressor function [63, 64].

The pathogenesis of non-celiac gluten sensitivity is not yet understood, but the results we have obtained so far suggest that there is a predominant involvement of the innate immune response rather than the adaptive immune response. Thus far we have observed that in contrast to CD, in non-celiac gluten sensitivity the mucosal expression of IFN-γ, IL-17A, IL-6, and IL-21, cytokines that have an established role in the pathophysiology of Th1 and Th17 responses, is not increased [31, 61]. In addition, we observed a significant reduction in the expression of FoxP3 (fork-head box P3), a T-regulatory cell marker, relative to controls and CD patients.

Although the mucosa in non-celiac gluten sensitivity contained a moderately increased number of CD3+ intraepithelial cells, these numbers were significantly lower than in active CD patients [31]. In the context of relatively conserved villous architecture, these data suggest a more limited involvement of the adaptive immune system in non-celiac gluten sensitivity and may explain why this condition is not accompanied by significant autoimmune phenomena.

Wheat Allergy

Wheat allergy is defined as a true allergic response to wheat that affects the gastrointestinal tract, the respiratory tract, or the skin. IgE plays a central role [1, 65]. In different studies, the prevalence of wheat allergy ranges from 0.5 [66] to 9 % [67] and may be age dependent. There is controversy as to whether sensitization to wheat decreases over time [67, 68]. Amongst food allergies, wheat is identified by the Food and Drug Administration as one of the eight most common allergens, along with milk, eggs, fish, shellfish, tree nuts, peanuts, and soybeans. Together, these foods are responsible for 90 % of all food allergies (Public Law 108-282, Title II, Food Allergen Labeling and Consumer Protection Act of 2004. U.S. Food and Drug Administration, Revised 2004[1]). Positive correlation of food allergy in parents and their children suggests that there is a genetic predisposition for food allergies [69].

Clinical Presentations

Wheat allergy patients typically describe skin, respiratory, or gastrointestinal symptoms, which occur within minutes to hours after wheat ingestion. Symptoms are varied and may include stomach pain, bloating, vomiting, diarrhea, hives, atopic dermatitis, urticaria, rhinitis, and in severe cases, anaphylaxis or death. If wheat allergy is suspected, diagnosis is usually made by elevated IgE serum assay or a positive skin prick test for wheat. However, since the positive predictive value of these tests is only 75 %, in some cases, a food challenge may be necessary for diagnosis [1]. Treatment includes dietary avoidance of wheat and all wheat by-products. Since some studies suggest that wheat allergy may be outgrown, a periodic food challenge regardless of IgE levels to determine if wheat can be tolerated has been suggested [65]. Other studies suggest that less allergenic strains of wheat that are better tolerated by wheat allergy patients may exist [30, 70].

[1] Publication is available at: http://www.fda.gov/food/labelingnutrition/FoodAllergensLabeling/GuidanceComplianceRegulatoryInformation/ucm106187.htm.

Pathogenesis

Most of the studies have been performed on Bakers' asthma, but similarities with the other food allergy conditions, atopic dermatitis, urticaria, and anaphylaxis exist [1]. Wheat allergy is an IgE-mediated allergic reaction and IgE-specific antibodies to alpha-, beta-, gamma-, and omega-gliadins are detected. The adaptive immune reaction to gluten in this condition is mediated by T lymphocyte-driven activation in the gastrointestinal mucosa and repeated sequences in the gluten peptides, for example, Ser-Gln-Gln-Gln-(Gln-)Pro-Pro-Phe, which may induce cross-linking of IgE antibodies and trigger the release of chemical mediators from mast cells in the blood of patients with wheat allergy [71].

Conclusion

Contrary to our previous belief that clinical reaction to gluten was limited to CD, we now appreciate that gluten can instigate different reactions, including wheat allergy and non-celiac gluten sensitivity. While clinically these three conditions overlap and, therefore, make the differential diagnosis much more difficult, the mechanism underlying these conditions is very different. The lack of specific biomarkers and the poor definition of non-celiac gluten sensitivity have created great confusion among healthcare professionals. Progress made during the last few years will hopefully ease this confusion, particularly when a validated biomarker for the diagnosis will become available.

References

1. Sapone A, Bai JC, Ciacci C, Dolinsek J, Green PH, Hadjivassiliou M, et al. Spectrum of gluten-related disorders: consensus on new nomenclature and classification. BMC Med. 2012;10:13.
2. Auricchio S, De Ritis G, De Vincenzi M, Mancini E, Minetti M, Sapora O, et al. Agglutinating activity of gliadin-derived peptides from bread wheat: implications for coeliac disease pathogenesis. Biochem Biophys Res Commun. 1984;121(2):428–33.
3. Clemente MG, De Virgiliis S, Kang JS, Macatagney R, Musu MP, Di Pierro MR, et al. Early effects of gliadin on enterocyte intracellular signalling involved in intestinal barrier function. Gut. 2003;52(2):218–23.
4. Dolfini E, Elli L, Dasdia T, Bufardeci B, Colleoni MP, Costa B, et al. In vitro cytotoxic effect of bread wheat gliadin on the LoVo human adenocarcinoma cell line. Toxicol In Vitro. 2002;16(4):331–7.
5. Dolfini E, Elli L, Roncoroni L, Costa B, Colleoni MP, Lorusso V, et al. Damaging effects of gliadin on three-dimensional cell culture model. World J Gastroenterol. 2005;11(38):5973–7.
6. Maiuri L, Troncone R, Mayer M, Coletta S, Picarelli A, De Vincenzi M, et al. In vitro activities of A-gliadin-related synthetic peptides: damaging effect on the atrophic coeliac mucosa and

activation of mucosal immune response in the treated coeliac mucosa. Scand J Gastroenterol. 1996;31(3):247–53.

7. Shan L, Molberg O, Parrot I, Hausch F, Filiz F, Gray GM, et al. Structural basis for gluten intolerance in celiac sprue. Science. 2002;297(5590):2275–9.
8. Lammers KM, Khandelwal S, Chaudhry F, Kryszak D, Puppa EL, Casolaro V, et al. Identification of a novel immunomodulatory gliadin peptide that causes interleukin-8 release in a chemokine receptor CXCR3-dependent manner only in patients with coeliac disease. Immunology. 2011;132(3):432–40.
9. Lammers KM, Lu R, Brownley J, Lu B, Gerard C, Thomas K, et al. Gliadin induces an increase in intestinal permeability and zonulin release by binding to the chemokine receptor CXCR3. Gastroenterology. 2008;135(1):194–204. e193.
10. Lionetti E, Catassi C. New clues in celiac disease epidemiology, pathogenesis, clinical manifestations, and treatment. Int Rev Immunol. 2011;30(4):219–31.
11. Dogan Y, Yildirmaz S, Ozercan IH. Prevalence of celiac disease among first-degree relatives of patients with celiac disease. J Pediatr Gastroenterol Nutr. 2012;55(2):205–8.
12. Fasano A, Berti I, Gerarduzzi T, Not T, Colletti RB, Drago S, et al. Prevalence of celiac disease in at-risk and not-at-risk groups in the United States: a large multicenter study. Arch Intern Med. 2003;163(3):286–92.
13. Kneepkens CM, von Blomberg BM. Clinical practice: coeliac disease. Eur J Pediatr. 2012;171(7):1011–21.
14. Metso S, Hyytia-Ilmonen H, Kaukinen K, Huhtala H, Jaatinen P, Salmi J, et al. Gluten-free diet and autoimmune thyroiditis in patients with celiac disease. A prospective controlled study. Scand J Gastroenterol. 2012;47(1):43–8.
15. Volta U, Tovoli F, Caio G. Clinical and immunological features of celiac disease in patients with type 1 diabetes mellitus. Expert Rev Gastroenterol Hepatol. 2011;5(4):479–87.
16. Wang N, Shen N, Vyse TJ, Anand V, Gunnarson I, Sturfelt G, et al. Selective IgA deficiency in autoimmune diseases. Mol Med. 2011;17(11–12):1383–96.
17. Wouters J, Weijerman ME, van Furth AM, Schreurs MW, Crusius JB, von Blomberg BM, et al. Prospective human leukocyte antigen, endomysium immunoglobulin A antibodies, and transglutaminase antibodies testing for celiac disease in children with Down syndrome. J Pediatr. 2009;154(2):239–42.
18. Catassi C, Anderson RP, Hill ID, Koletzko S, Lionetti E, Mouane N, et al. World perspective on celiac disease. J Pediatr Gastroenterol Nutr. 2012;55(5):494–9.
19. Catassi C, Kryszak D, Bhatti B, Sturgeon C, Helzlsouer K, Clipp SL, et al. Natural history of celiac disease autoimmunity in a USA cohort followed since 1974. Ann Med. 2010;42(7):530–8.
20. Ahn R, Ding YC, Murray J, Fasano A, Green PH, Neuhausen SL, et al. Association analysis of the extended MHC region in celiac disease implicates multiple independent susceptibility loci. PLoS One. 2012;7(5):e36926.
21. Trynka G, Hunt KA, Bockett NA, Romanos J, Mistry V, Szperl A, et al. Dense genotyping identifies and localizes multiple common and rare variant association signals in celiac disease. Nat Genet. 2011;43(12):1193–201.
22. Fasano A, Catassi C. Clinical practice. Celiac disease. N Engl J Med. 2012;367(25):2419–26.
23. Ludvigsson JF, Leffler DA, Bai JC, Biagi F, Fasano A, Green PH, et al. The Oslo definitions for coeliac disease and related terms. Gut. 2013;62(1):43–52.
24. Sellitto M, Bai G, Serena G, Fricke WF, Sturgeon C, Gajer P, et al. Proof of concept of microbiome-metabolome analysis and delayed gluten exposure on celiac disease autoimmunity in genetically at-risk infants. PLoS One. 2012;7(3):e33387.
25. Kaukinen K, Collin P, Maki M. Latent coeliac disease or coeliac disease beyond villous atrophy? Gut. 2007;56(10):1339–40.
26. Catassi C, Fasano A. Celiac disease diagnosis: simple rules are better than complicated algorithms. Am J Med. 2010;123(8):691–3.

27. Hollon JR, Cureton PA, Martin ML, Puppa EL, Fasano A. Trace gluten contamination may play a role in mucosal and clinical recovery in a subgroup of diet-adherent non-responsive celiac disease patients. BMC Gastroenterol. 2013;13(1):40.
28. Catassi C, Fabiani E, Iacono G, D'Agate C, Francavilla R, Biagi F, et al. A prospective, double-blind, placebo-controlled trial to establish a safe gluten threshold for patients with celiac disease. Am J Clin Nutr. 2007;85(1):160–6.
29. Paterson BM, Lammers KM, Arrieta MC, Fasano A, Meddings JB. The safety, tolerance, pharmacokinetic and pharmacodynamic effects of single doses of AT-1001 in coeliac disease subjects: a proof of concept study. Aliment Pharmacol Ther. 2007;26(5):757–66.
30. Spaenij-Dekking L, Kooy-Winkelaar Y, van Veelen P, Drijfhout JW, Jonker H, van Soest L, et al. Natural variation in toxicity of wheat: potential for selection of nontoxic varieties for celiac disease patients. Gastroenterology. 2005;129(3):797–806.
31. Sapone A, Lammers KM, Casolaro V, Cammarota M, Giuliano MT, De Rosa M, et al. Divergence of gut permeability and mucosal immune gene expression in two gluten-associated conditions: celiac disease and gluten sensitivity. BMC Med. 2011;9:23.
32. Biesiekierski JR, Newnham ED, Irving PM, Barrett JS, Haines M, Doecke JD. Gluten causes gastrointestinal symptoms in subjects without celiac disease: a double-blind randomized placebo-controlled trial. Am J Gastroenterol. 2011;106(3):508–14. quiz 515.
33. Carroccio A, Mansueto P, Iacono G, Soresi M, D'Alcamo A, Cavataio F, et al. Non-celiac wheat sensitivity diagnosed by double-blind placebo-controlled challenge: exploring a new clinical entity. Am J Gastroenterol. 2012;107(12):1898–906. quiz 1907.
34. Lundin KE, Alaedini A. Non-celiac gluten sensitivity. Gastrointest Endosc Clin N Am. 2012;22(4):723–34.
35. Sanders DS, Aziz I. Non-celiac wheat sensitivity: separating the wheat from the chat! Am J Gastroenterol. 2012;107(12):1908–12.
36. Cascella NG, Kryszak D, Bhatti B, Gregory P, Kelly DL, Mc Evoy JP, et al. Prevalence of celiac disease and gluten sensitivity in the United States clinical antipsychotic trials of intervention effectiveness study population. Schizophr Bull. 2011;37(1):94–100.
37. Armstrong D, Don-Wauchope AC, Verdu EF. Testing for gluten-related disorders in clinical practice: the role of serology in managing the spectrum of gluten sensitivity. Can J Gastroenterol. 2011;25(4):193–7.
38. Ford AC, Chey WD, Talley NJ, Malhotra A, Spiegel BM, Moayyedi P. Yield of diagnostic tests for celiac disease in individuals with symptoms suggestive of irritable bowel syndrome: systematic review and meta-analysis. Arch Intern Med. 2009;169(7):651–8.
39. Cash BD, Rubenstein JH, Young PE, Gentry A, Nojkov B, Lee D, et al. The prevalence of celiac disease among patients with nonconstipated irritable bowel syndrome is similar to controls. Gastroenterology. 2011;141(4):1187–93.
40. Carroccio A, Mansueto P, Iacono G, Soresi M, D'Alcamo A, Cavataio F, et al. Non-celiac wheat sensitivity diagnosed by double-blind placebo-controlled challenge: exploring a new clinical entity. Clin Gastroenterol Hepatol. 2011;9(11):965–71.
41. Vazquez-Roque MI, Camilleri M, Smyrk T, Murray JA, Marietta E, O'Neill J, et al. A controlled trial of gluten-free diet in patients with irritable bowel syndrome-diarrhea: effects on bowel frequency and intestinal function. Gastroenterology. 2013;144(5):903–11. e903.
42. Arrieta MC, Bistritz L, Meddings JB. Alterations in intestinal permeability. Gut. 2006;55(10):1512–20.
43. Rodgers LS, Beam MT, Anderson JM, Fanning AS. Epithelial barrier assembly requires coordinated activity of multiple domains of the tight junction protein ZO-1. J Cell Sci. 2013;126:1565–75.
44. Furuse M, Fujita K, Hiiragi T, Fujimoto K, Tsukita S. Claudin-1 and −2: novel integral membrane proteins localizing at tight junctions with no sequence similarity to occludin. J Cell Biol. 1998;141(7):1539–50.
45. Madara JL, Pappenheimer JR. Structural basis for physiological regulation of paracellular pathways in intestinal epithelia. J Membr Biol. 1987;100(2):149–64.

46. Tripathi A, Lammers KM, Goldblum S, Shea-Donohue T, Netzel-Arnett S, Buzza MS, et al. Identification of human zonulin, a physiological modulator of tight junctions, as prehaptoglobin-2. Proc Natl Acad Sci USA. 2009;106(39):16799–804.
47. Wang W, Uzzau S, Goldblum SE, Fasano A. Human zonulin, a potential modulator of intestinal tight junctions. J Cell Sci. 2000;113(Pt 24):4435–40.
48. El Asmar R, Panigrahi P, Bamford P, Berti I, Not T, Coppa GV, et al. Host-dependent zonulin secretion causes the impairment of the small intestine barrier function after bacterial exposure. Gastroenterology. 2002;123(5):1607–15.
49. Fasano A, Shea-Donohue T. Mechanisms of disease: the role of intestinal barrier function in the pathogenesis of gastrointestinal autoimmune diseases. Nat Clin Pract Gastroenterol Hepatol. 2005;2(9):416–22.
50. Fasano A, Not T, Wang W, Uzzau S, Berti I, Tommasini A, et al. Zonulin, a newly discovered modulator of intestinal permeability, and its expression in coeliac disease. Lancet. 2000;355(9214):1518–9.
51. Drago S, El Asmar R, Di Pierro M, Grazia Clemente M, Tripathi A, Sapone A, et al. Gliadin, zonulin and gut permeability: effects on celiac and non-celiac intestinal mucosa and intestinal cell lines. Scand J Gastroenterol. 2006;41(4):408–19.
52. Diosdado B, van Bakel H, Strengman E, Franke L, van Oort E, Mulder CJ, et al. Neutrophil recruitment and barrier impairment in celiac disease: a genomic study. Clin Gastroenterol Hepatol. 2007;5(5):574–81.
53. Monsuur AJ, de Bakker PI, Alizadeh BZ, Zhernakova A, Bevova MR, Strengman E, et al. Myosin IXB variant increases the risk of celiac disease and points toward a primary intestinal barrier defect. Nat Genet. 2005;37(12):1341–4.
54. Wapenaar MC, Monsuur AJ, van Bodegraven AA, Weersma RK, Bevova MR, Linskens RK, et al. Associations with tight junction genes PARD3 and MAGI2 in Dutch patients point to a common barrier defect for coeliac disease and ulcerative colitis. Gut. 2008;57(4):463–7.
55. Nilsen EM, Jahnsen FL, Lundin KE, Johansen FE, Fausa O, Sollid LM, et al. Gluten induces an intestinal cytokine response strongly dominated by interferon gamma in patients with celiac disease. Gastroenterology. 1998;115(3):551–63.
56. Nilsen EM, Lundin KE, Krajci P, Scott H, Sollid LM, Brandtzaeg P. Gluten specific, HLA-DQ restricted T cells from coeliac mucosa produce cytokines with Th1 or Th0 profile dominated by interferon gamma. Gut. 1995;37(6):766–76.
57. Kim CY, Quarsten H, Bergseng E, Khosla C, Sollid LM. Structural basis for HLA-DQ2-mediated presentation of gluten epitopes in celiac disease. Proc Natl Acad Sci USA. 2004;101(12):4175–9.
58. Weaver CT, Hatton RD, Mangan PR, Harrington LE. IL-17 family cytokines and the expanding diversity of effector T cell lineages. Annu Rev Immunol. 2007;25:821–52.
59. Castellanos-Rubio A, Santin I, Irastorza I, Castano L, Carlos Vitoria J, Ramon Bilbao J. TH17 (and TH1) signatures of intestinal biopsies of CD patients in response to gliadin. Autoimmunity. 2009;42(1):69–73.
60. Harris KM, Fasano A, Mann DL. Cutting edge: IL-1 controls the IL-23 response induced by gliadin, the etiologic agent in celiac disease. J Immunol. 2008;181(7):4457–60.
61. Sapone A, Lammers KM, Mazzarella G, Mikhailenko I, Carteni M, Casolaro V, et al. Differential mucosal IL-17 expression in two gliadin-induced disorders: gluten sensitivity and the autoimmune enteropathy celiac disease. Int Arch Allergy Immunol. 2010;152(1):75–80.
62. Meresse B, Chen Z, Ciszewski C, Tretiakova M, Bhagat G, Krausz TN, et al. Coordinated induction by IL15 of a TCR-independent NKG2D signaling pathway converts CTL into lymphokine-activated killer cells in celiac disease. Immunity. 2004;21(3):357–66.
63. Granzotto M, dal Bo S, Quaglia S, Tommasini A, Piscianz E, Valencic E, et al. Regulatory T-cell function is impaired in celiac disease. Dig Dis Sci. 2009;54(7):1513–9.
64. Hmida NB, Ben Ahmed M, Moussa A, Rejeb MB, Said Y, Kourda N, et al. Impaired control of effector T cells by regulatory T cells: a clue to loss of oral tolerance and autoimmunity in celiac disease? Am J Gastroenterol. 2012;107(4):604–11.

65. Keet CA, Matsui EC, Dhillon G, Lenehan P, Paterakis M, Wood RA. The natural history of wheat allergy. Ann Allergy Asthma Immunol. 2009;102(5):410–5.
66. Zuidmeer L, Goldhahn K, Rona RJ, Gislason D, Madsen C, Summers C, et al. The prevalence of plant food allergies: a systematic review. J Allergy Clin Immunol. 2008;121(5):1210–8. e1214.
67. Matricardi PM, Bockelbrink A, Beyer K, Keil T, Niggemann B, Gruber C, et al. Primary versus secondary immunoglobulin E sensitization to soy and wheat in the Multi-Centre Allergy Study cohort. Clin Exp Allergy. 2008;38(3):493–500.
68. Ostblom E, Lilja G, Pershagen G, van Hage M, Wickman M. Phenotypes of food hypersensitivity and development of allergic diseases during the first 8 years of life. Clin Exp Allergy. 2008;38(8):1325–32.
69. Inomata N. Wheat allergy. Curr Opin Allergy Clin Immunol. 2009;9(3):238–43.
70. Nakamura A, Tanabe S, Watanabe J, Makino T. Primary screening of relatively less allergenic wheat varieties. J Nutr Sci Vitaminol (Tokyo). 2005;51(3):204–6.
71. Tatham AS, Shewry PR. Allergens to wheat and related cereals. Clin Exp Allergy. 2008;38(11):1712–26.

Chapter 3
Epidemiology of Celiac Disease

Jonas F. Ludvigsson, Federico Biagi, and Gino Roberto Corazza

Celiac disease (CD) is a chronic small intestine immune-mediated enteropathy triggered by exposure to gluten in genetically sensitive individuals (DQ2+ or DQ8+) [1]. Gluten is a protein component found in wheat, barley, and rye but not in oats. The CD-related enteropathy is characterized by small intestinal villous atrophy and crypt hyperplasia. These mucosal aberrations most often resolve on a gluten-free diet (GFD). The GFD is currently the only available treatment for CD, although ongoing pharmacological and vaccine trials promise future alternatives [2].

In this chapter, we review current knowledge about classification and diagnosis of CD, including its prevalence and incidence.

Classification and Diagnosis

Patients with CD differ in their clinical features, with some patients presenting with malabsorption and diarrhea ("classical presentation"), as opposed to "nonclassical" symptoms [1] (e.g., abdominal pain and constipation). In addition, the disease can be asymptomatic, and the threshold for investigation should be low. CD may go undiagnosed for many years, and both doctor's delay and patient's delay are often substantial. Although CD has long been considered to exclusively affect children, it can be diagnosed at any age. In fact, there are data to suggest that the prevalence of CD is highest in older adults [3].

J.F. Ludvigsson, M.D., Ph.D. (✉)
Department of Medical Epidemiology and Biostatistics, Karolinska Institutet, Stockholm 17176, Sweden

Örebro University Hospital, Örebro, Sweden
e-mail: jonasludvigsson@yahoo.com

F. Biagi, M.D. • G.R. Corazza, M.D.
Department of Internal Medicine, IRCCS Policlinico San Matteo, University of Pavia, Pavia, Italy

S.D. Rampertab and G.E. Mullin (eds.), *Celiac Disease*, Clinical Gastroenterology,
DOI 10.1007/978-1-4614-8560-5_3,

The diagnosis usually begins with a clinical consultation followed by serological testing with tissue transglutaminase (TTG2) or endomysium antibodies (EMA) [4]. The umbrella organization for pediatric gastroenterology (European Society of Gastroenterology, Hepatology and Nutrition: ESPGHAN) recently decided that in certain children with high suspicion of CD, an intestinal biopsy may not be necessary to establish the diagnosis of CD. As per ESPGHAN, children with symptoms suggestive of CD, positive genetic tests, 10× the upper limit for normal IgA-TTG2, and positive EMA fall into the category where biopsy does not have to be performed in order to make a diagnosis of CD. Only a small minority of children with CD fulfill all these criteria. There has been some discussion as to what symptoms should be regarded as proof of symptomatic CD since the prevalence of many symptoms in childhood (e.g., constipation, diarrhea, colic, and recurrent abdominal pain) is much higher than the prevalence of CD, and, hence, many symptoms have extremely low positive predictive value for CD [5]. Therefore, biopsy is still a preferred method for those wishing to confirm the diagnosis and to be distinguished from non-celiac gluten-sensitivity [6]. In all other patients (children not fulfilling the above criteria and all adults), a small intestinal biopsy is recommended before diagnosis. HLA-testing has a low positive predictive value (does not rule in CD), but a high negative predictive value (does rule out CD) [7].

Clinical Presentation

The clinical presentation of CD is often described according to the "iceberg model." According to this metaphor, the tip of the iceberg constitutes the diagnosed fraction of CD patients, and the part below the water surface symbolizes those who are still undiagnosed. Many patients with undiagnosed CD have either asymptomatic disease or no symptoms at all (silent CD). Because of this, it becomes very difficult to establish a true prevalence of CD.

Prevalence and Incidence

Traditionally, it has been stated that CD occurs in about 1 % of the Caucasian population [8, 9]. Several studies based on populations in the USA have supported a 1 % prevalence rate. The 1 % assumption holds true for the USA where several recent studies have shown evidence of about 1 % [10]. Rubio-Tapia et al. recently analyzed blood samples from the NHANES study suggesting that 0.71 % of the US population had CD [11]. Most of these individuals were undiagnosed at time of screening. A multicenter study coordinated by the Finnish author Mustalahti and collaborators reported an overall European prevalence of 1 %, with the highest estimates in Finland (2.4 %) and the lowest in Germany (0.3 %) [12]. To our knowledge, the highest reported prevalence of CD are from Finland (2.4 %), but interestingly

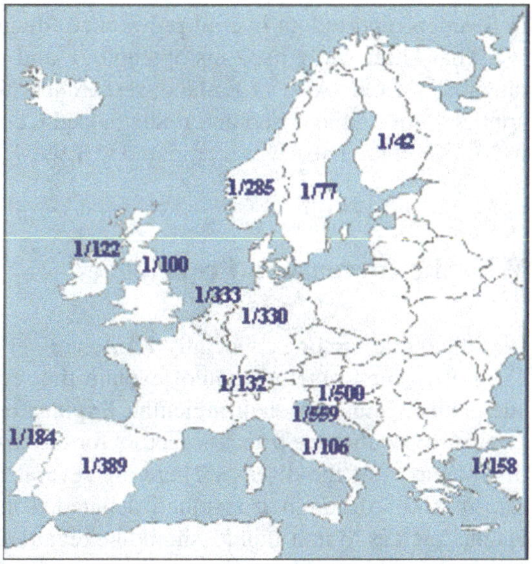

Fig. 3.1 Prevalence of CD in different European countries [8, 12, 13]

enough, these data originate from individuals aged 50 years or older [12]. Until very recently, it was thought that CD was primarily a childhood disease. Figure 3.1 shows the prevalence of CD in the general populations of different European countries.

Other data indicate that the prevalence and incidence of CD have increased in the USA, as well as in Europe, over the last 30 years [3, 14]. When Catassi and collaborators examined the natural history of CD in a community in an American cohort followed since 1974, they reported a prevalence of 1:501 in 1974, which increased to 1:219 in the year 1989 [14]. Murray and collaborators examined the incidence of CD in a well-defined county in Minnesota between 1950 in 2001. The annual age- and gender adjusted incidence rate rose from 0.9 per 100,000 in the 1950s to 3.3 per 100,000 in the 1990s, with an additional threefold further increase up to 9 per 100,000 person-years after 2000 [3]. The rising CD incidence was seen in both sexes and in all age groups except for very young children [3]. In another study, Rubio-Tapia et al. compared age- and calendar-matched cohorts of individuals using historical data from the Warren Air Force Base as baseline [15]. They concluded that during 45 years of follow-up, the prevalence of undiagnosed CD in the USA is likely to have increased fourfold [15].

In the late 1980s Sweden saw a dramatic increase in the incidence of CD, up to 200–240 cases per 100,000 person-years [16]. Only in the mid-1990s did this "epidemic" abate and incidence figures fell to 50–60 individuals per 100,000 person-years. It is not clear why Sweden experienced this peak in CD incidence, but one explanation may be new food introduction recommendations in the 1980s. Reexamining the birth cohort of children from these years, the same research team found a CD prevalence just below 3 % when the participants had reached the age of 12 years [17]. Another Swedish group that studied inhabitants in Northern Kalixanda in Sweden reported an overall prevalence (diagnosed plus undiagnosed) of 1.8 % [9]. That latter study used histopathology and serology in parallel to confirm the diagnosis of CD. Also in Finland, researchers found an increase in CD [18]. This applied both to diagnosed and undiagnosed CD. In total, evidence of CD was seen in 1.05 % in the late 1980s compared to 1.99 % just after the year 2000 [18].

Why the Increase in Prevalence?

While genetic factors, especially HLA, are very important in the pathogenesis of CD [19], genetic factors cannot explain the recent rise in CD incidence. Instead, such causes must be environmental. Explanatory factors can be divided into two groups: those that are true risk factors for the disease, and those that only influence the diagnosis of the disease. There are several factors that influence the diagnosis rate of CD. Although it is much debated, some researchers suggest that minor lesions such as Marsh 1 and 2 should be regarded as CD [20, 21]. Accepting a wider spectrum of histopathology as consistent with CD will naturally increase the CD prevalence.

Some studies have also reported CD prevalence data based solely on serology (see text by Dube et al. [8]). Studies restricted to positive serological testing, without histological confirmation, tend to report higher CD prevalences than those requiring a biopsy for diagnosis [8, 13]. Finally, both healthcare providers as well as the general public have a higher awareness of CD and gluten in the present day as compared to 30 years ago [22]. This, combined with the greater access to serological testing, means that a much larger group of people are currently tested for CD than a generation ago. There are also guidelines stipulating that higher risk groups should undergo testing regularly for CD, further adding to the number of new cases of CD. This has certainly resulted in an increased number of diagnosed CD patients with undeniable benefits for their health. However, in the last few years the number of "false" diagnoses of CD, leading to useless and expensive GFDs, has also considerably increased [23].

High-Risk Groups

There are several high-risk groups for CD. One of these is the first-degree relatives [10, 24]. American researchers screened 344 family members of about 100 CD cases, and discovered that more than 10 % of the family members had CD [24]. Before that, Fasano and collaborators tested first-degree relatives for EMA, and some 4.5 % were positive for CD. This is likely to constitute a relative risk increase of about ten times [10]. Although it is currently clear that first-degree relatives represent a high-risk group and so they need to be tested for CD at least once in their life, it is not clear whether first-degree relatives found to be negative at a first testing need to be further tested in their life. A study performed a few years ago showed an annual incidence of CD of 0.43% among first-degree relatives already found to be EMA-negative in the past [25]. Whether this supports the idea of setting up a serological follow-up in all first-degree relatives and whether this is cost-effective remains to be determined [26].

In addition to first-degree relatives, patients with a number of disorders should undergo testing for CD. One such group is patients with osteoporosis [23, 27–31]. Osteoporosis seems to be more common in CD, both before and after the CD diagnosis [25]. Some data indicate that calcium and 25-vitamin D level are reduced in untreated than in treated patients with CD and volunteers [26]. Another risk group is patients with anemia [32, 33]. Although the prevalence of CD varies greatly in anemic patients, several reports suggest that up to 5 % of patients with iron-deficiency anemia have CD [34].

CD is an immune-mediated disease and given its strong HLA association [35], it is natural that it is associated with several other autoimmune diseases. Among these diseases is type 1 diabetes [36]. A Danish study reported a CD prevalence of 12 % among patients with type 1 diabetes who were screened [37]. A Swedish study found that CD patients are at increased risk also of developing type 1 diabetes [36] later in life, further supporting the association between the two diseases. Autoimmune thyroid disease has been noted in CD patients both before and after diagnosis [38]. Autoimmune thyroid disease occurs in 1:30–1:10 patients with CD. It is therefore reasonable to screen patients with autoimmune thyroid disease [39].

Many physicians regard dermatitis herpetiformis (DH) as a variant of CD [40, 41]. It is an itchy skin condition that responds to a GFD, but the patient's intestinal mucosa may be normal. In contrast to CD, patients with non-celiac DH are at no increased risk of malignancy, osteoporosis, or excess mortality.

Italian data suggest that fatigue and depression are more common in CD [42–44]. Patients with these disorders as well as patients with irritable bowel syndrome (they are at about four times increased risk of CD [45]) may be tested for CD. Finally, CD is associated with pancreatitis [46] and pancreatic insufficiency [47], and patients with GI disorders should undergo screening when there is suspicion of CD.

A number of risk factors may shed light on the pathogenesis and etiology of CD. Females are more often affected by CD [48]. A female predominance is actually seen in most autoimmune diseases [49]. The genetic (HLA) setup is also important. There have so far been very few reports of CD in China and Japan (even though the number of screening studies in these two countries are limited), as opposed to the number of positive reports of CD in Latin America and the Middle East [50–52]. In North America and Europe, research indicates a prevalence around 1 % [12], sometimes lower and sometimes higher (the Saharawi people [53]). Probably, the major staple has a great importance for the risk of CD, and exposure to large amounts of wheat is detrimental for the risk for CD.

Socioeconomic factors seem to play a limited role in CD [54, 55], and when of importance they are likely to mirror other exposures such as smoking (often inversely associated with CD [56, 57], although research findings are contradictory), low body mass index [58], or the likelihood of an individual to go to hospital for testing. However, in many other autoimmune diseases, the so-called hygiene hypothesis has been proposed. This hypothesis stipulates that individuals with an inferior hygiene may have a decreased risk of autoimmunity. To our knowledge, the hygiene hypothesis has not been formally tested with regard to CD.

Pregnancy and Early Childhood

A number of studies have explored the association between intrauterine and perinatal conditions on the risk of CD. One such study reported that being small for gestational age (odds ratio, 1.20) or having a neonatal infection (odds ratio, 1.05) may increase the risk of CD. The role of parental smoking is less clear [59].

Independently of its effect for the future risk of CD [57, 60, 61], smoking should be discouraged for its detrimental effect on general health. A Swedish research group recently published data indicating that elective cesarean section may predispose to CD later in life. However, overall, cesarean section [62] was not associated with CD, and risk increases were moderate in size. Cesarean section may confer other risks in the fetus and in the mother, and the decision to undergo cesarean section should not be based on the future risk in the offspring to develop CD.

Breast-Feeding

Most data suggest that breast-feeding protects against CD [63, 64]. However, so far there are no randomized control trials that can confirm the observation between short breast-feeding duration and CD [65]. In fact, several *prospective* studies argue against breast-feeding having a protective effect against CD [66, 67]. Nevertheless, most observational studies report an inverse relationship between breast-feeding duration and CD, especially in children up to the age of 2 years.

Cesarean Section

Cesarean section could potentially influence the risk of future CD in the offspring through modification of the infant's microflora. A German study of 42 hospitals and academic centers revealed a positive association (OR = 1.8) between cesarean section and later CD [68], while a British study found a negative association between cesarean section and CD [67]. The discrepant results may be explained by small numbers of celiac children and lack of data on potential confounders. One of the co-authors of this chapter (JFL) therefore carried out a nationwide case–control study based on more than 11,000 children with CD [62]. The latter Swedish study found no overall excess risk of CD in children born through cesarean section (OR = 1.06; 95 % CI = 0.99–1.13) but a positive association with elective cesarean section (OR = 1.15; 95 % CI = 1.04–1.26). In contrast with emergency cesarean section, elective cesarean section does not involve contact with the birth canal, and we speculate that the different microflora exposure in children born through elective cesarean section explains their increased risk of CD.

Infection

It is still not clear to what extent various infections influence the risk of CD. Some other immune-mediated disease, notably type 1 diabetes, have been linked to viral infections [69, 70]. Some early seasonal studies [71–75] also suggested that birth in spring or summer (so that the child would be introduced to gluten at the age of 6 months, coinciding with a high exposure of viral infections) is evidence that infectious load can contribute to the etiology of CD. Just recently, a large study of Swedish children found no association whatsoever between birth season and risk of CD [76].

When Welander and collaborators examined risk of CD in a prospective cohort of 9,000 children with breast-feeding in relation to gluten introduction [63], there was a 1.8-fold increased risk of CD among children who were introduced to gluten when having an infection (any kind of infection). The risk estimate (HR = 1.8) was, however, not statistically significant (0.9–3.6). Other studies have found a positive association between high numbers of rotavirus infections and CD [74].

In conclusion, CD is an immune-mediated disease triggered by gluten exposure. It occurs in about 1 % of the population in the Western world, and its incidence seems to be rising.

References

1. Ludvigsson JF, Leffler DA, Bai JC, Biagi F, Fasano A, Green PH, et al. The Oslo definitions for coeliac disease and related terms. Gut. 2013;62(1):43–52.
2. Sollid LM, Khosla C. Novel therapies for coeliac disease. J Intern Med. 2011;269(6):604–13.
3. Murray JA, Van Dyke C, Plevak MF, Dierkhising RA, Zinsmeister AR, Melton 3rd LJ. Trends in the identification and clinical features of celiac disease in a North American community, 1950–2001. Clin Gastroenterol Hepatol. 2003;1(1):19–27.
4. Ludvigsson JF, Green PH. Clinical management of coeliac disease. J Intern Med. 2011;269(6):560–71.
5. van der Windt DA, Jellema P, Mulder CJ, Kneepkens CM, van der Horst HE. Diagnostic testing for celiac disease among patients with abdominal symptoms: a systematic review. JAMA. 2010;303(17):1738–46.
6. Husby S, Koletzko S, Korponay-Szabo IR, Mearin ML, Phillips A, Shamir R, et al. European Society for Pediatric Gastroenterology, Hepatology, and Nutrition guidelines for the diagnosis of coeliac disease. J Pediatr Gastroenterol Nutr. 2012;54(1):136–60.

7. Karell K, Louka AS, Moodie SJ, Ascher H, Clot F, Greco L, et al. HLA types in celiac disease patients not carrying the DQA1*05-DQB1*02 (DQ2) heterodimer: results from the European Genetics Cluster on Celiac Disease. Hum Immunol. 2003;64(4):469–77.
8. Dube C, Rostom A, Sy R, Cranney A, Saloojee N, Garritty C, et al. The prevalence of celiac disease in average-risk and at-risk Western European populations: a systematic review. Gastroenterology. 2005;128(4 Suppl 1):S57–67.
9. Walker MM, Murray JA, Ronkainen J, Aro P, Storskrubb T, D'Amato M, et al. Detection of celiac disease and lymphocytic enteropathy by parallel serology and histopathology in a population-based study. Gastroenterology. 2010;139(1):112–9.
10. Fasano A, Berti I, Gerarduzzi T, Not T, Colletti RB, Drago S, et al. Prevalence of celiac disease in at-risk and not-at-risk groups in the United States: a large multicenter study. Arch Intern Med. 2003;163(3):286–92.
11. Rubio-Tapia A, Ludvigsson JF, Brantner TL, Murray JA, Everhart JE. The prevalence of celiac disease in the United States. Am J Gastroenterol. 2012;107(10):1538–44. quiz 37, 45.
12. Mustalahti K, Catassi C, Reunanen A, Fabiani E, Heier M, McMillan S, et al. The prevalence of celiac disease in Europe: results of a centralized, international mass screening project. Ann Med. 2010;42(8):587–95.
13. Biagi F, Klersy C, Balduzzi D, Corazza GR. Are we not over-estimating the prevalence of coeliac disease in the general population? Ann Med. 2010;42(8):557–61.
14. Catassi C, Kryszak D, Bhatti B, Sturgeon C, Helzlsouer K, Clipp SL, et al. Natural history of celiac disease autoimmunity in a USA cohort followed since 1974. Ann Med. 2010;42(7):530–8.
15. Rubio-Tapia A, Kyle RA, Kaplan EL, Johnson DR, Page W, Erdtmann F, et al. Increased prevalence and mortality in undiagnosed celiac disease. Gastroenterology. 2009;137(1): 88–93.
16. Ivarsson A, Persson LA, Nystrom L, Ascher H, Cavell B, Danielsson L, et al. Epidemic of coeliac disease in Swedish children [see comments]. Acta Paediatr. 2000;89(2):165–71.
17. Myleus A, Ivarsson A, Webb C, Danielsson L, Hernell O, Hogberg L, et al. Celiac disease revealed in 3 % of Swedish 12-year-olds born during an epidemic. J Pediatr Gastroenterol Nutr. 2009;49(2):170–6.
18. Lohi S, Mustalahti K, Kaukinen K, Laurila K, Collin P, Rissanen H, et al. Increasing prevalence of coeliac disease over time. Aliment Pharmacol Ther. 2007;26(9):1217–25.
19. Greco L, Romino R, Coto I, Di Cosmo N, Percopo S, Maglio M, et al. The first large population based twin study of coeliac disease. Gut. 2002;50(5):624–8.
20. Kurppa K, Ashorn M, Iltanen S, Koskinen LL, Saavalainen P, Koskinen O, et al. Celiac disease without villous atrophy in children: a prospective study. J Pediatr. 2010;157(3):373–80. 380. e1.
21. Kaukinen K, Lindfors K, Collin P, Koskinen O, Maki M. Coeliac disease–a diagnostic and therapeutic challenge. Clin Chem Lab Med. 2010;48(9):1205–16.
22. Ludvigsson JF. What a coeliac patient must not eat. Dig Liver Dis. 2002;34(9):682.
23. Stenson WF, Newberry R, Lorenz R, Baldus C, Civitelli R. Increased prevalence of celiac disease and need for routine screening among patients with osteoporosis. Arch Intern Med. 2005;165(4):393–9.
24. Rubio-Tapia A, Van Dyke CT, Lahr BD, Zinsmeister AR, El-Youssef M, Moore SB, et al. Predictors of family risk for celiac disease: a population-based study. Clin Gastroenterol Hepatol. 2008;6(9):983–7.
25. Ludvigsson JF, Michaelsson K, Ekbom A, Montgomery SM. Coeliac disease and the risk of fractures – a general population-based cohort study. Aliment Pharmacol Ther. 2007;25(3):273–85.
26. Hin H, Bird G, Fisher P, Mahy N, Jewell D. Coeliac disease in primary care: case finding study. BMJ. 1999;318(7177):164–7.
27. Corazza GR, Di Sario A, Cecchetti L, Tarozzi C, Corrao G, Bernardi M, et al. Bone mass and metabolism in patients with celiac disease. Gastroenterology. 1995;109(1):122–8.

28. Corazza GR, Di Stefano M, Maurino E, Bai JC. Bones in coeliac disease: diagnosis and treatment. Best Pract Res Clin Gastroenterol. 2005;19(3):453–65.
29. McFarlane XA, Bhalla AK, Reeves DE, Morgan LM, Robertson DA. Osteoporosis in treated adult coeliac disease. Gut. 1995;36(5):710–4.
30. Passananti V, Santonicola A, Bucci C, Andreozzi P, Ranaudo A, Di Giacomo DV, et al. Bone mass in women with celiac disease: role of exercise and gluten-free diet. Dig Liver Dis. 2012;44(5):379–83.
31. Capriles VD, Martini LA, Areas JA. Metabolic osteopathy in celiac disease: importance of a gluten-free diet. Nutr Rev. 2009;67(10):599–606.
32. Halfdanarson TR, Litzow MR, Murray JA. Hematological manifestations of celiac disease. Blood. 2006;109(2):412–21.
33. Howard MR, Turnbull AJ, Morley P, Hollier P, Webb R, Clarke A. A prospective study of the prevalence of undiagnosed coeliac disease in laboratory defined iron and folate deficiency. J Clin Pathol. 2002;55(10):754–7.
34. Sollid LM, Thorsby E. HLA susceptibility genes in celiac disease: genetic mapping and role in pathogenesis. Gastroenterology. 1993;105(3):910–22.
35. Ludvigsson JF, Ludvigsson J, Ekbom A, Montgomery SM. Celiac disease and risk of subsequent type 1 diabetes: a general population cohort study of children and adolescents. Diabetes Care. 2006;29(11):2483–8.
36. Hansen D, Brock-Jacobsen B, Lund E, Bjorn C, Hansen LP, Nielsen C, et al. Clinical benefit of a gluten-free diet in type 1 diabetic children with screening-detected celiac disease: a population-based screening study with 2 years' follow-up. Diabetes Care. 2006;29(11): 2452–6.
37. Elfstrom P, Montgomery SM, Kampe O, Ekbom A, Ludvigsson JF. Risk of thyroid disease in individuals with celiac disease. J Clin Endocrinol Metab. 2008;93(10):3915–21.
38. Catassi C, Kryszak D, Louis-Jacques O, Duerksen DR, Hill I, Crowe SE, et al. Detection of celiac disease in primary care: a multicenter case-finding study in North America. Am J Gastroenterol. 2007;102(7):1454–60.
39. Fry L, Seah PP, Harper PG, Hoffbrand AV, McMinn RM. The small intestine in dermatitis herpetiformis. J Clin Pathol. 1974;27(10):817–24.
40. Seah PP, Fry L, Hoffbrand AV, Holborow EJ. Tissue antibodies in dermatitis herpetiformis and adult coeliac disease. Lancet. 1971;1(7704):834–6.
41. Fera T, Cascio B, Angelini G, Martini S, Guidetti CS. Affective disorders and quality of life in adult coeliac disease patients on a gluten-free diet. Eur J Gastroenterol Hepatol. 2003;15(12):1287–92.
42. Ciacci C, Iavarone A, Mazzacca G, De Rosa A. Depressive symptoms in adult coeliac disease. Scand J Gastroenterol. 1998;33(3):247–50.
43. Siniscalchi M, Iovino P, Tortora R, Forestiero S, Somma A, Capuano L, et al. Fatigue in adult coeliac disease. Aliment Pharmacol Ther. 2005;22(5):489–94.
44. Ford AC, Chey WD, Talley NJ, Malhotra A, Spiegel BM, Moayyedi P. Yield of diagnostic tests for celiac disease in individuals with symptoms suggestive of irritable bowel syndrome: systematic review and meta-analysis. Arch Intern Med. 2009;169(7):651–8.
45. Sadr-Ozadi M, Sanders DS, Murray JA, Ludvigsson JF. Patients with celiac disease have an increased risk for pancreatitis. Clin Gastroenterol Hepatol. 2012;10:1136–42.
46. Leeds JS, Sanders DS. Risk of pancreatitis in patients with celiac disease: is autoimmune pancreatitis a biologically plausible mechanism? Clin Gastroenterol Hepatol. 2008;6(8):951. author reply 51.
47. Ludvigsson JF, Brandt L, Montgomery SM, Granath F, Ekbom A. Validation study of villous atrophy and small intestinal inflammation in Swedish biopsy registers. BMC Gastroenterol. 2009;9(1):19.
48. Jacobson DL, Gange SJ, Rose NR, Graham NM. Epidemiology and estimated population burden of selected autoimmune diseases in the United States. Clin Immunol Immunopathol. 1997;84(3):223–43.

49. Remes-Troche JM, Ramirez-Iglesias MT, Rubio-Tapia A, Alonso-Ramos A, Velazquez A, Uscanga LF. Celiac disease could be a frequent disease in Mexico: prevalence of tissue transglutaminase antibody in healthy blood donors. J Clin Gastroenterol. 2006;40(8):697–700.
50. Gandolfi L, Pratesi R, Cordoba JC, Tauil PL, Gasparin M, Catassi C. Prevalence of celiac disease among blood donors in Brazil. Am J Gastroenterol. 2000;95(3):689–92.
51. Gomez JC, Selvaggio GS, Viola M, Pizarro B, la Motta G, de Barrio S, et al. Prevalence of celiac disease in Argentina: screening of an adult population in the La Plata area. Am J Gastroenterol. 2001;96(9):2700–4.
52. Lionetti P, Favilli T, Chiaravalloti G, Ughi C, Maggiore G. Coeliac disease in Saharawi children in Algerian refugee camps. Lancet. 1999;353(9159):1189–90.
53. Olen O, Bihagen E, Rasmussen F, Ludvigsson JF. Socioeconomic position and education in patients with coeliac disease. Dig Liver Dis. 2012;44(6):471–6.
54. Wingren CJ, Bjorck S, Lynch KF, Ohlsson H, Agardh D, Merlo J. Coeliac disease in children: a social epidemiological study in Sweden. Acta Paediatr. 2012;101(2):185–91.
55. Snook JA, Dwyer L, Lee-Elliott C, Khan S, Wheeler DW, Nicholas DS. Adult coeliac disease and cigarette smoking [see comments]. Gut. 1996;39(1):60–2.
56. West J, Logan RF, Hill PG, Lloyd A, Lewis S, Hubbard R, et al. Seroprevalence, correlates, and characteristics of undetected coeliac disease in England. Gut. 2003;52(7):960–5.
57. Olen O, Montgomery SM, Marcus C, Ekbom A, Ludvigsson JF. Coeliac disease and body mass index: a study of two Swedish general population-based registers. Scand J Gastroenterol. 2009;44(10):1198–206.
58. Ludvigsson JF, Ludvigsson J. Parental smoking and risk of coeliac disease in offspring. Scand J Gastroenterol. 2005;40(3):336–42.
59. Thomason K, West J, Logan RF, Coupland C, Holmes GK. Fracture experience of patients with coeliac disease: a population based survey. Gut. 2003;52(4):518–22.
60. Austin AS, Logan RF, Thomason K, Holmes GK. Cigarette smoking and adult coeliac disease. Scand J Gastroenterol. 2002;37(8):978–82.
61. Marild K, Stephansson O, Montgomery S, Murray JA, Ludvigsson JF. Pregnancy outcome and risk of celiac disease in offspring: a nationwide case–control study. Gastroenterology. 2012;142(1):39–45. e3.
62. Akobeng AK, Ramanan AV, Buchan I, Heller RF. Effect of breast feeding on risk of coeliac disease: a systematic review and meta-analysis of observational studies. Arch Dis Child. 2006;91(1):39–43.
63. Ivarsson A, Hernell O, Stenlund H, Persson LA. Breast-feeding protects against celiac disease. Am J Clin Nutr. 2002;75(5):914–21.
64. Welander A, Tjernberg AR, Montgomery SM, Ludvigsson J, Ludvigsson JF. Infectious disease and risk of later celiac disease in childhood. Pediatrics. 2010;125(3):e530–6.
65. Norris JM, Barriga K, Hoffenberg EJ, Taki I, Miao D, Haas JE, et al. Risk of celiac disease autoimmunity and timing of gluten introduction in the diet of infants at increased risk of disease. JAMA. 2005;293(19):2343–51.
66. Roberts SE, Williams JG, Meddings D, Davidson R, Goldacre MJ. Perinatal risk factors and coeliac disease in children and young adults: a record linkage study. Aliment Pharmacol Ther. 2009;29(2):222–31.
67. Decker E, Engelmann G, Findeisen A, Gerner P, Laass M, Ney D, et al. Cesarean delivery is associated with celiac disease but not inflammatory bowel disease in children. Pediatrics. 2010;125(6):e1433–40.
68. Knip M, Veijola R, Virtanen SM, Hyoty H, Vaarala O, Akerblom HK. Environmental triggers and determinants of type 1 diabetes. Diabetes. 2005;54 Suppl 2:S125–36.
69. Vaarala O, Klemetti P, Juhela S, Simell O, Hyoty H, Ilonen J. Effect of coincident enterovirus infection and cows' milk exposure on immunisation to insulin in early infancy. Diabetologia. 2002;45(4):531–4.
70. Kokkonen J, Simila S, Vuolukka P. The incidence of coeliac disease and pyloric stenosis in children in Northern Finland. Ann Clin Res. 1982;14(3):123–8.

71. Ivarsson A, Hernell O, Nystrom L, Persson LA. Children born in the summer have increased risk for coeliac disease. J Epidemiol Community Health. 2003;57(1):36–9.
72. Season of birth and celiac disease in Massachusetts children. Conference on digestive disease week 2011; Chicago: Gastroenterology; 2011.
73. Stene LC, Honeyman MC, Hoffenberg EJ, Haas JE, Sokol RJ, Emery L, et al. Rotavirus infection frequency and risk of celiac disease autoimmunity in early childhood: a longitudinal study. Am J Gastroenterol. 2006;101(10):2333–40.
74. Lewy H, Meirson H, Laron Z. Seasonality of birth month of children with celiac disease differs from that in the general population and between sexes and is linked to family history and environmental factors. J Pediatr Gastroenterol Nutr. 2009;48(2):181–5.
75. Lebwohl B, Green PH, Murray JA, Ludvigsson JF. Season of birth in a nationwide cohort of coeliac disease patients. Arch Dis Child. 2013;98(1):48–51.
76. Prasad S, Thomas P, Nicholas DS, Sharer NM, Snook JA. Adult endomysial antibody-negative coeliac disease and cigarette smoking. Eur J Gastroenterol Hepatol. 2001;13(6):667–71.

Chapter 4
The Pathophysiology of Celiac Disease

David E. Elliott

Introduction

There are more than 80 recognized autoimmune and immune-mediated inflammatory diseases. Celiac disease (CD) is unique because it shares features of an autoimmune disease (production of self-reactive antibodies) and an inappropriate immune response to an external provocateur. Furthermore, the pathogenesis of CD is better understood than that of any other immune-mediated disease. CD results from a series of cause and effect actions, the first of which is ingestion of gluten.

Gluten as an Antigen

The term "gluten" refers to a broad mixture of storage proteins present in wheat that provide elasticity to dough. Although originally referring to wheat, now gluten is used to connote similar proteins from rye and barley that contain protein sequences that elicit an immune response (i.e., antigens). Oats also contain gluten-type proteins (avenins) that have some of the same peptide sequences, but in much lower amounts. Gluten-type prolamin proteins from other grains mostly lack the peptide sequences that serve as antigens triggering inflammation in patients with CD.

Lymphocytes (B and T cells) each go through a process that involves rearranging gene segments to develop a unique receptor that can recognize specific antigens. Because of this feat, they constitute the "adaptive" immune system. Cells that comprise the "innate" immune system must rely on germline encoded receptors to recognize potential pathogens. Receptors on B cells recognize locations (epitopes) on

D.E. Elliott, M.D., Ph.D. (✉)
Division of Gastroenterology/Hepatology, Department of Internal Medicine,
University of Iowa Carver College of Medicine and Iowa City VAHC, Iowa City, IA, USA
e-mail: david-elliott@uiowa.edu

S.D. Rampertab and G.E. Mullin (eds.), *Celiac Disease*, Clinical Gastroenterology,
DOI 10.1007/978-1-4614-8560-5_4,

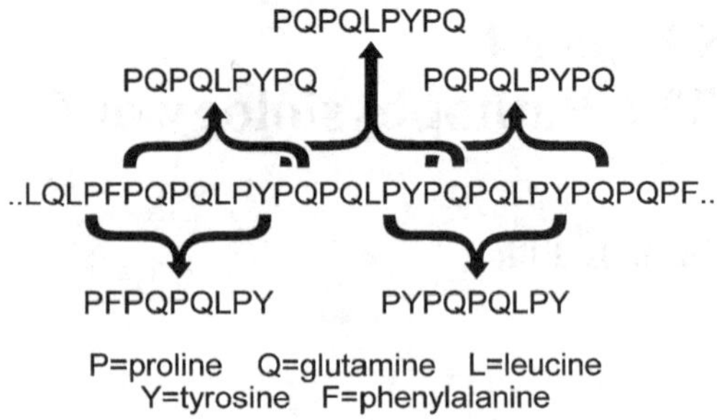

Fig. 4.1 Gluten epitopes. Gliadin contains a 33 amino acid section packed with a peptide sequence (PQPQLPYPQ) that can activate T cells from patients with CD. This sequence is also present in other proteins made by wheat, rye, and barley

native protein antigens, and when stimulated by that antigen, make antibodies. Receptors on helper T cells recognize epitopes on fragments of a protein that are processed and displayed by an antigen-presenting cell (APC). When stimulated by the antigenic epitope and APC, helper T cells make cytokines that direct the behavior of other cells, adaptive and innate, to mount, maintain, and regulate an immune reaction.

Gluten from wheat, rye, and barley is composed of numerous proteins that contain antigenic epitopes for patients with CD. Gluten proteins were originally separated into groups according to their solubility in water, salt solutions, or alcohol. Gliadins are those components from wheat gluten that are soluble in alcohol. Gliadins are further divided into α, β, γ, and ω subtypes. Most of the research into the T-cell antigenicity of gluten has been focused on α-gliadins [1]. Evaluation of these proteins revealed short sequences rich in proline (P) and glutamine (Q) that elicit responses from T cells isolated from patients with CD. These epitopes have sequences similar to PQPQLPYPQ. A section of α2-gliadin contains a 33 amino acid sequence that is resistant to digestion by human gut and pancreatic enzymes. This sequence contains several epitopes that can stimulate CD patient T cells (Fig. 4.1) [2]. Because this polypeptide is resistant to digestion, it remains available to stimulate the immune system. However, many proteins present in wheat, rye, barley, and oats contain potential CD-stimulating epitopes [3].

Gluten Epitopes and Antigen Presentation

Antigen-presenting cells display epitopes to helper T cells on cell surface protein molecules. These antigen-presenting molecules hold epitopes in correct orientation for review by T cells much like picture frames hold paintings for perusal by museum patrons. Any one picture frame can hold different paintings of the right size, but cannot hold paintings of the wrong size. Any one antigen-presenting molecule can hold different epitopes with correctly aligned charge distributions, but cannot hold epitopes with misaligned charges. Therefore, the specific antigen epitopes that can be displayed by a person's APCs depends on the set of antigen-presenting molecules encoded in that person's genome within the human leukocyte antigen (HLA) locus on the short arm of chromosome 6. This section of the genome is highly polymorphic, meaning that many different versions of these genes exist. This wide variation permits a range of responses by different members of a population, ensuring that some will be able to react to a new pathogen.

Antigen presenting molecules that display epitopes to helper T cells are made of an α and β chain, each chain encoded by a different gene. Three sets of these "Class II" antigen-presenting genes are encoded on chromosome 6. The sets are named DP, DQ, and DR. However, the α chain from one chromosome (e.g., paternal) can bind with the β chain of the same set from the other chromosome (e.g., maternal), so four different DQ molecules can be produced. The α and β chains that bind gluten epitopes and contribute to development of CD are encoded by the DQA1*0501 and DQB1*0201 genes [4]. People with this combination have the DQ2.5 molecule. If the DQ2.5 molecule is encoded on one chromosome, the person carries a DR3-DQ2 haplotype. If the DQ2.5 molecule is produced by combining an α and β chain from different chromosomes, the person carries the DR5-DQ7/DR7-DQ2 haplotypes.

As further elaborated in Chap. 5 by de Haas et al., about 95 % of patients with CD express DQ2.5. People who inherit a copy of DQB1*0201 from each parent are at higher risk of developing CD than are those with one copy of DQB1*0201 [5]. Thus, people who are homozygous for DQ2.5 have higher risk than those who are heterozygotes. A very similar set of α and β chains that can bind gluten epitopes are DQA1*0201 and DQB1*0202, which compose the DQ2.2 molecule. Major gluten epitope presentation is not as sustained on DQ2.2 as it is with DQ2.5 [6]. However, other similar gluten epitopes can be stably displayed on DQ2.2 molecules [7]. Moreover, DQ2.5/DQ2.2 heterozygotes have a risk that is higher than a regular DQ2.5 heterozygote. About 5 % of patients with CD lack a DQ2.5 haplotype. Most of these express DQ8, which is composed of the DQB1*0302 and DQA1*0301 chains [8]. There are rare patients with biopsy proven CD that does not express either DQ2 or DQ8 [9]. About one-third of the Caucasian population expresses either DQ2 or DQ8 antigen-presenting molecules. Therefore, the vast majority (97 %) of people with DQ2 or DQ8 antigen presenting molecules will not develop celiac disease.

Intestinal Barrier and Antigen Access

In order to induce inflammation, gluten antigens need to cross from the intestinal lumen into the lamina propria where antigen-presenting cells and lymphocytes reside. Intestinal epithelial cells (IEC) form a polarized sheet that acts as a barrier to luminal contents. Macromolecules like gluten epitopes can cross this barrier through four pathways: (1) by transport through the epithelial cell (transcellular passage), (2) by transport between epithelial cells (paracellular passage), (3) by direct antigen-presenting dendritic cell sampling of luminal contents, and (4) through a break in the epithelium due to some sort of injury (Fig. 4.2).

Intestinal epithelial cells can transport material through the cell from the apical surface to the basal surface. Microfold (M) cells are specialized epithelial cells that

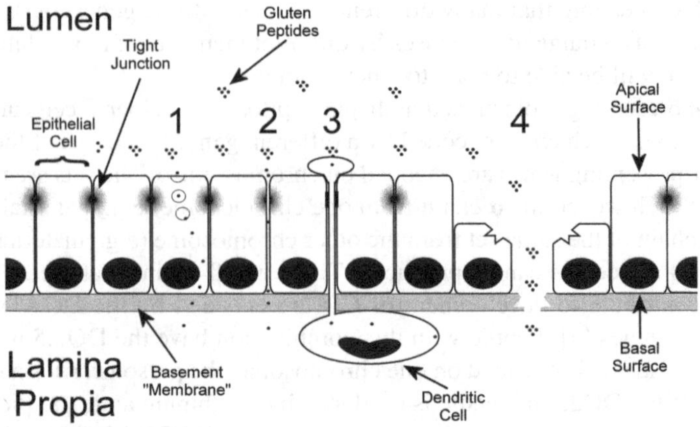

Fig. 4.2 Routes of passage across the epithelial barrier. To initiate inflammation, gluten peptides need to move from the intestinal lumen to the lamina propria, crossing the epithelial cell barrier. Pathways include (1) transcellular passage, (2) paracellular passage, (3) direct sampling by dendritic cells, and (4) passage through an injured area

transport macromolecules and particulate matter (e.g., bacteria) across the cell to underlaying lymphoid follicles for immunologic evaluation. This pathway permits routine sampling of luminal contents and is upregulated in rodents with nonsteroidal anti-inflammatory drug-induced intestinal inflammation [10]. Dietary antigens also are able to pass through normal columnar intestinal epithelial cells. This pathway likely dominates in active CD [11]. One important mechanism is mediated by gluten binding to IgA antibodies in the lumen that then associate with cell surface transferrin receptor (CD71), triggering endocytosis and passage of gluten through the epithelial cell [12]. Apical expression of CD71 increases in active CD as does production of anti-gliadin IgA, creating a potential for progressively worsening inflammation. Other pathways of gluten antigen transport through epithelial cells also exist [13, 14].

Intestinal epithelial cells are bound to each other by a cellular organelle called the "tight junction" or "zonula occludens," which controls passage of ions and macromolecules between cells (paracellular pathway). Tight junction transmembrane, structural, and regulatory proteins form a web that holds adjacent cell membranes in close opposition. The complex is composed of about 30 proteins, including junction adhesion molecule (JAM), claudins, VAP-33, zonula occludens proteins (ZO-1, ZO-2, ZO-3), cingulin, occludin, and regulatory proteins [15]. Tight junction function is regulated by cytokines like interferon-γ (IFN-γ) and tumor necrosis factor-α (TNF-α) in a process that requires occludin [16]. Inflammatory cytokines cause the tight junctions to loosen permitting paracellular transport of macromolecules to the lamina propria for immunologic evaluation and, conversely, rapid egress of fluid and bactericidal molecules to "wash out" offending agents. Zonulin (prehaptoglobin-2) is another human protein that opens tight junctions [17]. Zonulin production is upregulated in active CD, and gliadin stimulates zonulin release from epithelial cells.

Thus, regulation of tight junctions provides another circuit for progressively worsening inflammation. Larazotide acetate (AT-1001) prevents opening of tight channels in response to cytokines or zonulin and was recently tested in clinical trials to determine if the compound would prevent changes in intestinal permeability upon gluten challenge in patients with celiac disease. Larazotide acetate did not appear to be effective in controlling permeability, but the study may have been complicated by high variability in how individual patients respond to gluten challenge [18].

Dendritic cells are the most prodigious antigen-presenting cells and are scattered in the lamina propria beneath the basement membrane [19]. Dendritic cells can send processes up between and even through epithelial cells to sample luminal contents [20]. Dendritic cell sampling can be upregulated by epithelial cell exposure to potentially pathogenic bacteria like salmonella [21]. Small intestinal dysbiosis also may increase antigen presentation by this mechanism [22]. Furthermore, gliadin peptide fragments alone induce maturation of dendritic cells to augment APC function [23]. Regulation of lamina propria dendritic cell function provides another circuit for progressively worsening intestinal inflammation.

Severe injury or inflammation can kill an area of epithelial cells causing an ulcer. Enteric virus infection or medications like aspirin, ibuprofen, and naproxen frequently cause small bowel ulceration. In young children, active CD can present with duodenal ulceration [24]. In adults, ulceration is rare in active CD and suggests ulcerative jejunitis, refractory CD type 2, or enteropathy-associated T-cell lymphoma, which is on the spectrum of aberrant T-cell neoplasms [25]. However the ulcer forms, the break in the epithelial cell lining permits direct access of luminal contents to lamina propria and submucosal APC. Thus, an ulcer due to injury or inflammation can permit ingested gluten peptides to bathe the lamina propria, prompting a reaction that can worsen the ulcer in patients with CD.

It is not surprising that large gluten peptides can cross the epithelial cell barrier and initiate inflammation. Each of the four pathways (see Fig. 4.2) could cause transient or low-grade display of gluten epitopes to T cells by APC. Each of the four pathways is likely active at any given time. Each of the four pathways will increase with worsening inflammation due to active CD, which can cause increase in the other pathways. It is surprising that food allergies are not more common.

Tissue Transglutaminase: A Matchmaker

Tissue transglutaminase (TG2, TTG) is a ubiquitously expressed cellular enzyme that crosslinks proteins through a lysine-glutamine bridge. It can also serve as a deamidase, removing the amide group on the side chain of glutamine and converting it to glutamate. Tissue transglutaminase can deamidate gluten peptides [26]. For example, PQPQLPYPQ is the sequence derived from native 33mer (see Fig. 4.1). If the residue has been deamidated by TTG, the sequence PQPELPYPQ is produced through degradation [3]. This change alters the charge on the polypeptide, which increases its ability to bind in the antigen-presenting groove of DQ2.5. Gluten serves as an ideal substrate for TTG and is quickly and specifically deamidated by the enzyme. The preferred (Q, underlined) glutamine target for TTG is in the sequence QXPF (Y, W, M, L, I, or V) [27], where X is any amino acid. This sequence set is rare or absent in oat avenins [27]. Glutamine can deamidate to glutamate non-enzymatically, but the conversion is slow. It is likely that TTG is central to the process of rendering gluten epitopes highly antigenic by increasing their binding strength (avidity) to CD-associated antigen-presenting molecules. In addition, TTG may also assist in shuttling gluten epitopes through epithelial cells [14].

Lamina Propria T Cells: Stokers of Intestinal Inflammation

We have now set most of the stage for intestinal inflammation. There is an antigen (gluten) that has crossed the epithelial cell barrier and has been acted on by tissue TTG to increase binding to DQ2.5 or DQ8 antigen-presenting molecules on antigen-presenting cells in the lamina propria and draining lymph node. For inflammation to occur, several cell types need to work in concert, communicating by cell surface receptor display and elaboration of signaling molecules called cytokines or interleukins (IL). Appropriate inflammatory reactions are highly regulated and tightly focused. Inappropriate inflammation, like that which occurs in CD, is a result of either excessive pro-inflammatory or ineffective anti-inflammatory (regulatory) communication. At the center of this communication are the T helper lymphocytes.

T helper (Th) cells respond to antigen epitopes displayed on MHC class II (DP,DQ,DR) molecules by a high affinity engagement of a clonally unique T cell receptor complexed to a co-receptor named CD4. The terms "Th cells" and "CD4+ T cells" are functionally synonymous. There are several types of Th identified by the kind of cytokines they make [28]. Major types include Th1 (makers of IFN-γ), Th2 (makers of IL-4), Th17 (makers of IL-17), and T regulatory cells (makers of IL-10, TGF-β, and/or inhibitory cell surface molecules). Each of these Th cell types makes cytokines that amplify development of that type while inhibiting development of the other types. This causes chronic reactions to polarize into a discrete Th type cytokine profile. The cytokines made by Th cells instruct other cells how to respond within an inflammation. Therefore, the mix of T cell types generated in response to an epitope displayed by an APC will determine whether or not an inflammation results and if so, what type of inflammation occurs. This initial decision likely takes place in the mesenteric draining lymph nodes where intestinal dendritic cells have migrated to display captured antigens [29]. Most of the time, the decision produces tolerance (regulatory reaction) toward food antigens and no inflammation occurs. Instead, in CD, the decision is to react. It is likely that several factors conspire to produce a decision to react, such as the strength of epitope/antigen-presenting molecule interaction on an APC [6, 7], the affinity of a randomly generated T cell receptor for that specific gluten epitope, and the coincident mix of

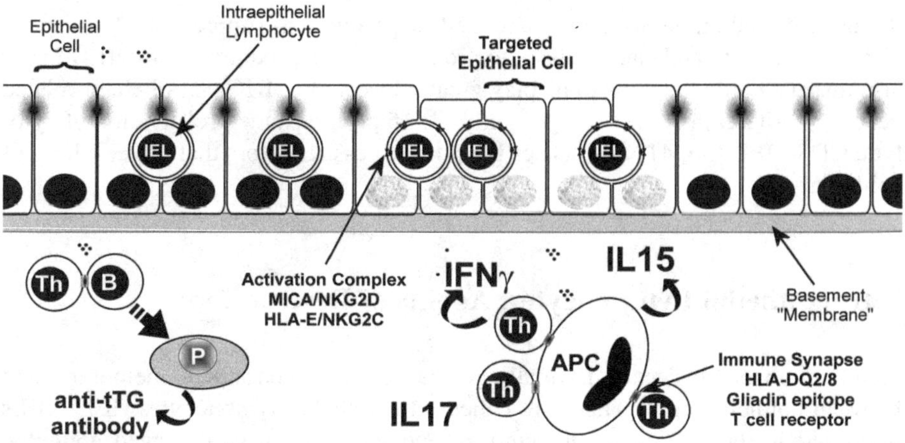

Fig. 4.3 Inflammatory circuits in CD. Multiple cell types are involved in the intestinal inflammation in CD. Anti-deamidated gliadin is taken up by an APC (macrophage or dendritic cell) and is presented to a T cells using a DQ2 or DQ8 antigen-presenting molecule. The activated T cells make IFN-γ and IL-17. The IFN-γ instructs epithelial cells to display HLA-E. The APC also makes IL-15 that causes IEL to proliferate and display NK receptors that recognize HLA and MICA on epithelial cells. The activated IEL then kills the targeted epithelial cells. B cells in the lamina propria also can present antigen to T cells that help the B cells mature into plasma cells that make anti-TTG or anti-deamidated gliadin antibodies

cytokines and co-stimulatory molecules present when that Th cell engages its cognate antigen [28, 30]. In patients with active CD, pro-inflammatory IFN-γ and IL-17 producing (Th1/Th17) cells control the response [31]. These cells leave the draining lymph node and migrate (traffic) back to the intestinal mucosa where, in response to locally displayed gluten epitopes, they help drive the inflammation.

Within the mucosa, several different cell types work together to cause an inflammatory response (Fig. 4.3). Inflammatory Th1/Th17 cells respond to gluten epitopes displayed by lamina propria macrophages and dendritic cells by producing IFN-γ and IL-17. Each of these cytokines has multiple effects on surrounding cells, and both are often found at sites of autoimmune inflammation [32]. IFN-γ feeds back on APC to change their cytokine and cell surface receptor display, enhancing development of more pro-inflammatory T cells. IFN-γ also instructs macrophages to upregulate the ability to kill ingested bacteria. Importantly, IFN-γ instructs epithelial cells to display HLA-E [33], potentially targeting them for injury by intraepithelial lymphocytes (IEL). Th17 cells make IL-17, which increases neutrophil activity and other cytokines like IL-6 and TNF-α, which drive tissue inflammation.

Lamina propria T cell IFN-γ also likely signals APC to make IL-15 [34]. In addition, a specific gliadin peptide (p31-43) can trigger IL-15 production by lamina propria APC [35]. IL-15 is a central cytokine in CD and other immune-mediated inflammatory diseases [36]. Many cell types, including intestinal epithelial cells, can make IL15. Mice engineered to overproduce IL-15 by their intestinal epithelial cells develop inflammation that recapitulates CD [37, 38]. IL-15 has many effects;

it augments inflammatory IFN-γ and TNF-α production, suppresses T regulatory cell function [39], and can feedback to promote its own production [34]. IL-15 may also instruct epithelial cells to display greater levels of "MHC class I chain-related gene A" (MICA) [40]. Most importantly, IL-15 promotes the proliferation of cytolytic CD8+ IEL [36, 41] and causes them to express receptors that target killing of epithelial cells.

Intraepithelial Lymphocytes: Agents of Destruction

Small numbers of T cells normally reside above the basement membrane and between epithelial cells. These are called intraepithelial lymphocytes (IEL). IELs likely aid in the identification, removal, and replacement of damaged epithelial cells. There are few different types of IEL. The majority are CD8+ T cells that utilize a T cell receptor (TCR) generated by recombining gene segments in the α and β TCR loci (CD8+α/β T cells). These cells recognize antigens displayed on Class I MHC molecules. Class I MHC molecules mostly display pieces of proteins that were made by the cell as part of its normal functioning. Cytolytic CD8+ T cells survey this display to find evidence for production of unusual proteins suggesting presence of a mutated or virally infected cell. When discovered, they kill the abnormal cell. Another important group of IEL is CD8+ T cells that utilize a TCR generated by recombining gene segments in the γ and δ TCR loci (CD8+γ/δ T cells). These cells often recognize antigens that can be displayed on "nonclassical" antigen-presenting molecules like CD1 and MICA, which are both expressed by epithelial cells.

In active CD, the number of IELs greatly expands. Indeed, this expansion is a distinctive feature of gluten-induced intestinal inflammation [42]. This expansion is driven by IL1-5 made by lamina propria APC and by stressed epithelial cells [36, 41]. IL-15 also instructs IELs to express a set of receptors normally displayed by "natural killer" (NK) cells. NK cells are similar to CD8+ lymphocytes, but they do not utilize a TCR. Instead, they have a set of germ-line receptors that probe for the absence or presence of abnormal antigen-presenting molecules on a cell's surface [43]. NK cells dispose of virally infected or mutant cells that may not be recognized by CD8+ T cells. IL-15 induces expression of NKG2D [44], which interacts with MICA (and MICB) displayed on epithelial cells. Unlike IEL in normal intestine, IELs in patients with CD also express another NK receptor called CD94/NKG2C [45]. CD94/NKG2C recognizes HLA-E, which is upregulated in epithelial cells in response to IFN-γ [33]. Engagement of NKG2D with MICA/B and CD94/NKG2C with HLA-E activates the IELs without requiring CD8/TCR recognition of an abnormal protein. Acquisition of NKG2D and CD94/NKG2C receptors by IEL and display of MICA/B and HLA-E by epithelial cells target the epithelial cells for destruction.

Thus, the hallmark injury in CD, villous atrophy, results from destruction of intestinal epithelial cells by IEL in response to IL-15 made by intestinal epithelial cells, lamina propria macrophages, and dendritic cells. Epithelial cells are targeted for destruction by cell surface display of MICA/B, induced by cell stress and possibly IL-15, and HLA-E, induced by IFN-γ made by gluten-responsive lamina propria T cells. The cells causing injury are the more numerous CD8+α/β IELs. The CD8+ γ/δ IEL (particularly those expressing inhibitory receptor CD94/NKG2A) may be uninvolved or even protective in CD [42, 46, 47], though γ/δ IEL may also be the cell type that gives rise to enteropathy associated T cell lymphoma (EATL) in refractory CD.

Refractory Celiac Disease: Antigen-Independent Inflammation

The vast majority of patients respond to a gluten-free diet with resolution of their intestinal inflammation and normalization of their serum anti-TTG and anti-deamidated gliadin levels. Rarely, intestinal inflammation remains or returns even though the patient is maintaining a gluten-free lifestyle. Refractory celiac disease (RCD) is defined as persistent or recurrent malabsorptive symptoms and signs, with villous atrophy despite a strict gluten-free diet for more than 12 months [48]. RCD is further broken down into two types based on the absence or presence of abnormal intestinal T cells. Normal T cells express the marker CD3, a component of the TCR complex, on their surface. In RCD I, lamina propria T cells and IEL are surface CD3+ and appear identical to those in untreated active celiac disease. In RCD II, there is development of an aberrant CD4-CD8- γδ T cell clone that expresses intracellular but not surface CD3 and makes up more than 50 % of IEL by immunohistochemistry. These cells also express the integrin CD103+ (αE) common to IEL suggesting they arise from the IEL population [49]. Approximately, 50 % of patients with RCD II develop EATL within 5 years of diagnosis, which is why RCDII has a poor prognosis.

In RCD, intestinal inflammation continues in the absence of known gluten exposure. In RCD I, it is possible that unidentified gluten-like epitopes present in other food are sufficient to maintain the inflammation. In a study of ten patients with RCD I placed on a non-immunogenic elemental diet, eight of the nine patients that completed the study had histologic improvement and seven had a decrease in mucosal IFNγ RNA expression [50]. This suggests that RCD I reflects an ongoing response to an unidentified antigen.

On the other hand, it is possible that RCD results from a self-sustaining inflammation in the absence of Th direction. Epithelial cells are capable of making IL15 [51], and this production is upregulated in active celiac disease [41]. IELs can make IFN-γ, and this production is upregulated in active CD [41, 52]. Thus, epithelial cells can make IL-15 to drive proliferation of IEL that display NKG2D and CD94/NKG2C. These IELs in turn produce IFN-γ that upregulates HLA-E expression by epithelial cells that also display MICA/B. This could create a positive-feedback loop, creating IL-15-dependent inflammation in the absence of specific antigen exposure. Moreover, IL-15 supports the survival proliferation of aberrant T cells in RCD II [53]. Thus, it is easy to hypothesize self-amplifying circuits in RCD. The centrality of IL-15 in these circuits fosters interest in therapeutic trials involving IL-15 blockade [37, 54].

Anti-TTG and Anti-Deamidated Gliadin Antibodies

An important screening tool for CD is testing for high titer (elevated concentration) of antibodies against TTG and deamidated gliadin. However, their role in the pathogenesis of CD is unclear. Anti-gliadin antibodies probably help shuttle gluten peptides transcellularly across the epithelial layer [12]. Antibodies are made by B lymphocytes. B cells differentiate into plasma cells, which secrete copious amounts of antibody. Both cell types are numerous in the intestinal lamina propria. B cells also function as "nonprofessional" APC and can present antigens to T cells. B cells express their clonally unique antibody on their cell surface. Here, the antibody can capture its cognate antigen (gluten or TTG) and cause the B cell to ingest the molecule and process it for presentation to T cells in conjunction with MHC Class 2 molecules like DQ2. T cells that recognize the antigen can secrete growth factors for the B cells to ramp up production of the antibody. In addition, B cells may stimulate T cells to drive inflammation. However, identification of a direct role for celiac-associated antibodies in the pathogenesis of the intestinal inflammation remains elusive [55]. Mice that are engineered to over-express IL15 from intestinal epithelial cells develop celiac-like inflammation with numerous lamina propria B cells and plasma cells and produce elevated serum anti-TTG antibody [38]. This suggests that anti-TTG antibody develops in response to IL-15-driven inflammation rather than causing that inflammation.

Conclusion

CD begins with ingestion of gluten, which finds its way across the epithelial cell barrier to APC. If those APCs utilize DQ2 or DQ8 antigen-presenting molecules, they can display epitopes to Th cells that start to produce IFN-γ and stimulate APC to make IL-15. These cytokines induce IEL to kill epithelial cells and cause the damage that results in celiac disease. Central to the inflammation is IL-15. Antibodies to TTG and anti-deamidated gliadin may increase sensitivity to gluten, but are probably more important as clinical measures of gluten exposure. Although a lot is known, much remains to be discovered.

References

1. Ciccocioppo R, Di Sabatino A, Corazza GR. The immune recognition of gluten in coeliac disease. Clin Exp Immunol. 2005;140(3):408–16.
2. Shan L, Molberg Ø, Parrot I, Hausch F, Filiz F, Gray GM, et al. Structural basis for gluten intolerance in celiac sprue. Science. 2002;297(5590):2275–9.
3. Sollid LM, Qiao SW, Anderson RP, Gianfrani C, Koning F. Nomenclature and listing of celiac disease relevant gluten T-cell epitopes restricted by HLA-DQ molecules. Immunogenetics. 2012;64(6):455–60.
4. Sollid LM, Markussen G, Ek J, Gjerde H, Vartdal F, Thorsby E. Evidence for a primary association of celiac disease to a particular HLA-DQ alpha/beta heterodimer. J Exp Med. 1989;169(1):345–50.
5. Murray JA, Moore SB, Van Dyke CT, Lahr BD, Dierkhising RA, Zinsmeister AR, et al. HLA DQ gene dosage and risk and severity of celiac disease. Clin Gastroenterol Hepatol. 2007;5(12):1406–12.
6. Fallang LE, Bergseng E, Hotta K, Berg-Larsen A, Kim CY, Sollid LM. Differences in the risk of celiac disease associated with HLA-DQ2.5 or HLA-DQ2.2 are related to sustained gluten antigen presentation. Nat Immunol. 2009;10(10):1096–101.
7. Bodd M, Kim CY, Lundin KE, Sollid LM. T-cell response to gluten in patients with HLA-DQ2.2 reveals requirement of peptide-MHC stability in celiac disease. Gastroenterology. 2012;142(3):552–61.
8. Lundin KE, Gjertsen HA, Scott H, Sollid LM, Thorsby E. Function of DQ2 and DQ8 as HLA susceptibility molecules in celiac disease. Hum Immunol. 1994;41(1):24–7.
9. Karell K, Louka AS, Moodie SJ, Ascher H, Clot F, Greco L, et al. HLA types in celiac disease patients not carrying the DQA1*05-DQB1*02 (DQ2) heterodimer: results from the European Genetics Cluster on Celiac Disease. Hum Immunol. 2003;64(4):469–77.
10. Lugering A, Floer M, Lügering N, Cichon C, Schmidt MA, Domschke W, et al. Characterization of M cell formation and associated mononuclear cells during indomethacin-induced intestinal inflammation. Clin Exp Immunol. 2004;136(2):232–8.
11. Heyman M, Abed J, Lebreton C, Cerf-Bensussan N. Intestinal permeability in coeliac disease: insight into mechanisms and relevance to pathogenesis. Gut. 2012;61(9):1355–64.
12. Matysiak-Budnik T, Moura IC, Arcos-Fajardo M, Lebreton C, Ménard S, Candalh C, et al. Secretory IgA mediates retrotranscytosis of intact gliadin peptides via the transferrin receptor in celiac disease. J Exp Med. 2008;205(1):143–54.
13. Berin MC. Mucosal antibodies in the regulation of tolerance and allergy to foods. Semin Immunopathol. 2012;34(5):633–42.
14. Caputo I, Barone MV, Lepretti M, Martucciello S, Nista I, Troncone R, et al. Celiac anti-tissue transglutaminase antibodies interfere with the uptake of alpha gliadin peptide 31-43 but not of peptide 57-68 by epithelial cells. Biochim Biophys Acta. 2010;1802(9):717–27.
15. Anderson JM, Van Itallie CM. Physiology and function of the tight junction. Cold Spring Harb Perspect Biol. 2009;1(2):a002584.
16. Van Itallie CM, Fanning AS, Holmes J, Anderson JM. Occludin is required for cytokine-induced regulation of tight junction barriers. J Cell Sci. 2010;123(Pt 16):2844–52.
17. Fasano A. Zonulin, regulation of tight junctions, and autoimmune diseases. Ann N Y Acad Sci. 2012;1258:25–33.
18. Leffler DA, Kelly CP, Abdallah HZ, Colatrella AM, Harris LA, Leon F, et al. A randomized, double-blind study of larazotide acetate to prevent the activation of celiac disease during gluten challenge. Am J Gastroenterol. 2012;107(10):1554–62.
19. Niess JH, Reinecker HC. Dendritic cells: the commanders-in-chief of mucosal immune defenses. Curr Opin Gastroenterol. 2006;22(4):354–60.
20. Lelouard H, Fallet M, de Bovis B, Méresse S, Gorvel JP et al. Peyer's patch dendritic cells sample antigens by extending dendrites through M cell-specific transcellular pores. Gastroenterology, 2012; 142(3): 592-601 e3.

21. Chieppa M, Rescigno M, Huang AY, Germain RN. Dynamic imaging of dendritic cell extension into the small bowel lumen in response to epithelial cell TLR engagement. J Exp Med. 2006;203(13):2841–52.
22. Wells JM, Rossi O, Meijerink M, van Baarlen P. Epithelial crosstalk at the microbiota-mucosal interface. Proc Natl Acad Sci USA. 2011;108 Suppl 1:4607–14.
23. Palova-Jelinkova L, Rozková D, Pecharová B, Bártová J, Sedivá A, Tlaskalová-Hogenová H, et al. Gliadin fragments induce phenotypic and functional maturation of human dendritic cells. J Immunol. 2005;175(10):7038–45.
24. Mones RL, Mercer GO. Ulcerative duodenitis in a child with celiac disease. J Pediatr. 2011;158(5):857.
25. Rubio-Tapia A, Murray JA. Classification and management of refractory coeliac disease. Gut. 2010;59(4):547–57.
26. Klock C, Diraimondo TR. C. Khosla C. Role of transglutaminase 2 in celiac disease pathogenesis. Semin Immunopathol. 2012;34(4):513–22.
27. Vader LW, de Ru A, van der Wal Y, Kooy YM, Benckhuijsen W, Mearin ML, et al. Specificity of tissue transglutaminase explains cereal toxicity in celiac disease. J Exp Med. 2002;195(5):643–9.
28. Zygmunt B, Veldhoen M. T helper cell differentiation more than just cytokines. Adv Immunol. 2011;109:159–96.
29. Pabst O, Mowat AM. Oral tolerance to food protein. Mucosal Immunol. 2012;5(3):232–9.
30. Vahedi G, C Poholek A, Hand TW, Laurence A, Kanno Y, O'Shea JJ, et al. Helper T-cell identity and evolution of differential transcriptomes and epigenomes. Immunol Rev. 2013;252(1):24–40.
31. Monteleone I, Sarra M, Del Vecchio BG, Paoluzi OA, Franzè E, Fina D, et al. Characterization of IL-17A-producing cells in celiac disease mucosa. J Immunol. 2010;184(4):2211–8.
32. Moudgil KD, Choubey D. Cytokines in autoimmunity: role in induction, regulation, and treatment. J Interferon Cytokine Res. 2011;31(10):695–703.
33. Perera L, Shao L, Patel A, Evans K, Meresse B, Blumberg R, et al. Expression of nonclassical class I molecules by intestinal epithelial cells. Inflamm Bowel Dis. 2007;13(3):298–307.
34. Waldmann TA, Tagaya Y. The multifaceted regulation of interleukin-15 expression and the role of this cytokine in NK cell differentiation and host response to intracellular pathogens. Annu Rev Immunol. 1999;17:19–49.
35. Maiuri L, Ciacci C, Ricciardelli I, Vacca L, Raia V, Auricchio S, et al. Association between innate response to gliadin and activation of pathogenic T cells in coeliac disease. Lancet. 2003;362(9377):30–7.
36. Di Sabatino A, Calarota SA, Vidali F, Macdonald TT, Corazza GR. Role of IL-15 in immune-mediated and infectious diseases. Cytokine Growth Factor Rev. 2011;22(1):19–33.
37. Yokoyama S, Watanabe N, Sato N, Perera PY, Filkoski L, Tanaka T, et al. Antibody-mediated blockade of IL-15 reverses the autoimmune intestinal damage in transgenic mice that overexpress IL-15 in enterocytes. Proc Natl Acad Sci USA. 2009;106(37):15849–54.
38. Yokoyama S, Takada K, Hirasawa M, Perera LP, Hiroi T. Transgenic mice that overexpress human IL-15 in enterocytes recapitulate both B and T cell-mediated pathologic manifestations of celiac disease. J Clin Immunol. 2011;31(6):1038–44.
39. Zanzi D, Stefanile R, Santagata S, Iaffaldano L, Iaquinto G, Giardullo N, et al. IL-15 interferes with suppressive activity of intestinal regulatory T cells expanded in Celiac disease. Am J Gastroenterol. 2011;106(7):1308–17.
40. Zwirner NW, Fuertes MB, Girart MV, Domaica CI, Rossi LE. Immunobiology of the human MHC class I chain-related gene A (MICA): from transplantation immunology to tumor immune escape. Immunologia. 2006;25(1):25–38.
41. Di Sabatino A, Ciccocioppo R, Cupelli F, Cinque B, Millimaggi D, Clarkson MM, et al. Epithelium derived interleukin 15 regulates intraepithelial lymphocyte Th1 cytokine production, cytotoxicity, and survival in coeliac disease. Gut. 2006;55(4):469–77.

42. Abadie V, Discepolo V, Jabri B. Intraepithelial lymphocytes in celiac disease immunopathology. Semin Immunopathol. 2012;34(4):551–66.
43. Rajalingam R. Overview of the killer cell immunoglobulin-like receptor system. Methods Mol Biol. 2012;882:391–414.
44. Meresse B, Chen Z, Ciszewski C, Tretiakova M, Bhagat G, Krausz TN, et al. Coordinated induction by IL15 of a TCR-independent NKG2D signaling pathway converts CTL into lymphokine-activated killer cells in celiac disease. Immunity. 2004;21(3):357–66.
45. Meresse B, Curran SA, Ciszewski C, Orbelyan G, Setty M, Bhagat G, et al. Reprogramming of CTLs into natural killer-like cells in celiac disease. J Exp Med. 2006;203(5):1343–55.
46. Verbeek WH, von Blomberg BM, Scholten PE, Kuik DJ, Mulder CJ, Schreurs MW. The presence of small intestinal intraepithelial gamma/delta T-lymphocytes is inversely correlated with lymphoma development in refractory celiac disease. Am J Gastroenterol. 2008;103(12): 3152–8.
47. Bhagat G, Naiyer AJ, Shah JG, Harper J, Jabri B, Wang TC, et al. Small intestinal CD8+TCRgammadelta+NKG2A+ intraepithelial lymphocytes have attributes of regulatory cells in patients with celiac disease. J Clin Invest. 2008;118(1):281–93.
48. Ludvigsson JF, Leffler DA, Bai JC, Biagi F, Fasano A, Green PH, et al. The Oslo definitions for coeliac disease and related terms. Gut. 2013;62(1):43–52.
49. Malamut G, Meresse B, Cellier C, Cerf-Bensussan N. Refractory celiac disease: from bench to bedside. Semin Immunopathol. 2012;34(4):601–13.
50. Olaussen RW, Løvik A, Tollefsen S, Andresen PA, Vatn MH, De Lange T, et al. Effect of elemental diet on mucosal immunopathology and clinical symptoms in type 1 refractory celiac disease. Clin Gastroenterol Hepatol. 2005;3(9):875–85.
51. Reinecker HC, MacDermott RP, Mirau S, Dignass A, Podolsky DK. Intestinal epithelial cells both express and respond to interleukin 15. Gastroenterology. 1996;111(6):1706–13.
52. Leon F, Sánchez L, Camarero C, Roy G. Cytokine production by intestinal intraepithelial lymphocyte subsets in celiac disease. Dig Dis Sci. 2005;50(3):593–600.
53. Malamut G, El Machhour R, Montcuquet N, Martin-Lannerée S, Dusanter-Fourt I, Verkarre V, et al. IL-15 triggers an antiapoptotic pathway in human intraepithelial lymphocytes that is a potential new target in celiac disease-associated inflammation and lymphomagenesis. J Clin Invest. 2010;120(6):2131–43.
54. Sollid LM, Khosla C. Novel therapies for coeliac disease. J Intern Med. 2011;269(6):604–13.
55. Mesin L, Sollid LM, Di Niro R. The intestinal B-cell response in celiac disease. Front Immunol. 2012;3:313.

Chapter 5
Immunogenetics of Celiac Disease

Esther C. de Haas, Vinod Kumar, and Cisca Wijmenga

Heritability of Celiac Disease

Celiac disease (CD) can be considered as a model for common complex disorders in which the phenotypes result from a combination of environmental triggers, genetic predisposing factors, and their interactions. Although the gliadin fraction of wheat gluten and similar protein fractions of other grains, which are the primary and necessary environmental triggers for CD, have been well defined since the 1950s, the discovery of genetic risk factors is an ongoing process.

In contrast to Mendelian single-gene disorders, CD does not show a clear pattern of inheritance. The importance of genetics is indicated by familial clustering, shown by epidemiological studies comparing the prevalence of CD in related individuals to the prevalence in unrelated individuals. The reported prevalence in first-degree relatives of CD patients ranges from 2.8 to 22.5 %, with the higher prevalences reported in at-risk relatives undergoing routine intestinal biopsy instead of only serological screening [1]. In contrast, the overall prevalence of CD in North America and Western Europe ranges from 0.5 to 2.9 % [1, 2]. The recurrence risk ratio for siblings (λ_s), the prevalence of CD in siblings divided by the prevalence in the general population, has been reported to be as high as 20–60 [3–5]. A large multicenter study in the USA among at-risk and not-at-risk groups found a prevalence of 4.5 % in first-degree relatives and 2.6 % in second-degree relatives, compared to 0.3 % in not-at-risk children and 0.9 % in not-at-risk adults [6].

In order to distinguish the role of genetic factors in familial clustering from environmental factors, twin studies are performed. In a large population-based twin study in Italy, the estimated case-wise concordance, a measure for disease risk if a co-twin is affected, was 83.3 % (95 % confidence interval 70.3–96.4 %) for

E.C. de Haas, M.D. Ph.D. (✉) • V. Kumar, Ph.D. • C. Wijmenga, Ph.D.
Department of Genetics, University Medical Center Groningen, University of Groningen, PO Box 30.001, 9700 RB, Groningen, The Netherlands
e-mail: e.de.haas@umcg.nl

S.D. Rampertab and G.E. Mullin (eds.), *Celiac Disease*, Clinical Gastroenterology, DOI 10.1007/978-1-4614-8560-5_5,

monozygotic twin pairs and 16.7 % (3.6–29.8 %) for dizygotic twin pairs [7]. Since the proportion of affected co-twins in dizygotic twin pairs is in line with the reported prevalence of CD in siblings, the role of shared environmental factors, with the exception of exposure to gluten antigen, is thought to be limited [8]. Assuming a population prevalence between 0.1 and 1.1 %, the variance in CD prevalence attributable to genetic variance, the so-called heritability of CD, is estimated to be 57–87 % (95 % confidence intervals 32–100 %) [7].

The Immunogenetics of Celiac Disease

Identification of Susceptibility Genes for Celiac Disease

The above studies on CD prevalence contribute to estimations of the heritability, but do not provide information on which genes or how many genes are actually involved in disease development. Other approaches are needed to identify susceptibility genes: linkage analysis and genetic association analysis (both candidate genes and genome-wide) (see Text Box 5.1 Genetic Linkage and Association analysis).

The first indentified genetic risk factor for CD, the human leukocyte antigen DQ (HLA-DQ) genotype, is the strongest known genetic risk factor. Since serological studies in the 1970s discovered the association between HLA and CD, many others have confirmed the strong linkage to HLA, specifically to HLA-DQ2 and HLA-DQ8. However, no other genetic associations were consistently found by linkage studies and candidate gene studies. The recent development of genome-wide association studies (GWAS) has led to the discovery of several additional susceptibility genes for CD. So far, GWAS have identified 57 associated single nucleotide polymorphisms (SNPs) located in 39 non-HLA regions, with most of the positional candidate genes having immunological functions.

Association with HLA Genotype

The major HLA class II, also called Major Histocompatibility Complex II (MHC II), molecules DP, DQ, and DR are cell-surface receptors on antigen-presenting cells involved in the presentation of exogenous peptide antigens to T-helper lymphocytes. The encoding genes are part of the 200 genes encompassing 4 Mb HLA-complex on chromosome 6p21. This region corresponds with the *CELIAC1* locus, a region consistently found to be associated with CD in both linkage and association studies.

The first reports on the association with HLA revealed a link between CD and positive serology for HLA class I B8-antigen and later HLA-DR3-antigen [9, 10]. The encoding alleles of the HLA-B gene and HLA-DR genes are strongly linked in the haplotype A1-B8-DR3-DQ2, which is present in approximately 10 % of

Text Box 5.1 Genetic Linkage and Association Analysis

For a long time, the search for genetic risk factors for complex disorders was based on genetic linkage analysis and association studies with candidate genes. In *genetic linkage analysis*, genetic markers are used to identify chromosomal regions that are shared by affected relatives more often than expected by meiotic segregation. Identified regions may contain up to hundreds of genes. Subsequently, fine mapping is needed in order to pinpoint the causal gene. This can be achieved by association analysis.

In *association analysis* the frequencies of genetic variants are compared between patients and healthy control persons. In *candidate gene association studies*, the analyzed genetic variants are often selected for their location in chromosomal regions linked to the disease or because of their hypothesized function in the disease of interest.

The more recent *GWAS* are hypothesis-free and compare large numbers, hundreds to thousands, of patients and healthy control persons for hundreds of thousands to millions of genetic variants, so-called single nucleotide polymorphisms (SNPs), dispersed over the whole genome. An association analysis relies on the strong linkage over short distances between the analyzed SNPs and potential causal genetic variants; this is the so-called linkage disequilibrium (LD). Most disease-associated SNPs are not the causal variant but a marker or tag for a nearby causal variant. GWAS have contributed greatly to identifying genetic risk factors for complex disorders. The use of hundreds of thousands to millions of SNPs means it is possible to achieve a high resolution compared to linkage studies, while the large numbers of analyzed patients and control persons add to the statistical power to detect genetic variants with small or modest effect sizes. Importantly, the hypothesis-free approach has led to the identification of genes and pathways not previously suspected of being involved in the disease of interest.

Northern Europeans [11]. Subsequent studies pinpointed the association of CD to alleles encoding HLA-DQ2 molecules [12, 13].

The HLA-DQ molecule is a heterodimer consisting of an α chain and a β chain, encoded by HLA-DQA1 and HLA-DQB1. Further characterization of the association between HLA-DQ and CD showed that especially homozygosity for the HLA-DQ2.5 heterodimer (encoded by the alleles DQA1*0501 and DQB1*0201) and, to a lesser degree, heterozygosity for the HLA-DQ2.5 heterodimer combined with the HLA-DQ2.2 heterodimer (encoded by the alleles DQA1*0201 and DQB1*0202) were associated with a strongly increased susceptibility for CD [14, 15] (Fig. 5.1). Assuming a CD prevalence of 1 % in the general population, the absolute risk for CD is estimated at >7 % for this high-risk group [16].

Heterozygosity for the HLA-DQ2.5 heterodimer combined with another HLA-DQ heterodimer, or homozygosity or heterozygosity for the HLA-DQ8

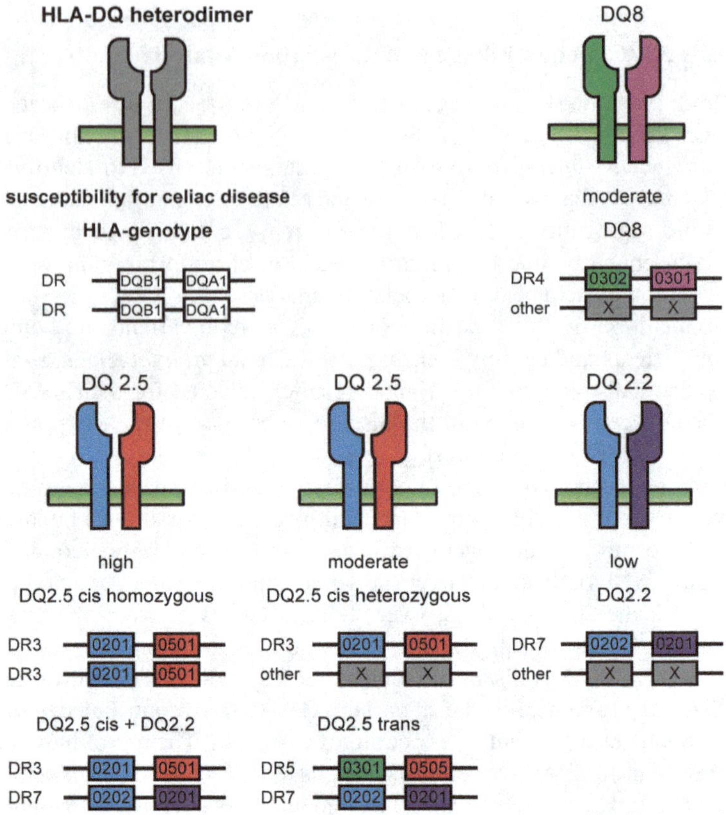

Fig. 5.1 HLA-DQ heterodimers with coding HLA-genotypes and corresponding susceptibility for CD

heterodimer (encoded by the alleles DQA1*0301 and DQB1*0302), confers a more moderately increased risk for CD, with an absolute risk for CD estimated at 0.1–7 % [16]. Functional studies showed that these HLA-DQ2 molecules and, to a lesser degree, HLA-DQ8 molecules have a high affinity for gluten peptides and that gluten-reactive T lymphocytes from the small intestinal mucosa of CD patients preferentially recognize gluten peptides when presented by HLA-DQ2 or HLA-DQ8 [17–20]. Approximately, 95 % of the CD patients carry the HLA-DQ2.5 genotype, and many of the other 5 % carry HLA-DQ8 [13, 21, 22]. There is a significant worldwide correlation between the combination of wheat consumption and frequency of HLA-DQ2 and HLA-DQ8, on the one hand, and the incidence of CD, on the other hand (estimated correlation coefficient $R^2=0.4$) [23]. This observation is in line with a CD model of genetically susceptible individuals in whom dietary gluten triggers intestinal inflammation.

Although the presence of either HLA-DQ2 or HLA-DQ8 can be considered necessary for the development of CD, neither is sufficient, since only some 3 % of the approximately 40 % of Caucasians who carry either HLA-DQ2 or HLA-DQ8 will actually develop CD [24]. This suggests that, in addition to wheat gluten consumption and HLA genotype, other environmental and genetic factors must be involved in CD etiology. A recent study on the HLA-complex in CD showed that this region, with its many genes in strong linkage disequilibrium (LD), might contain more susceptibility genes for CD [25].

Based on the assumption of a multiplicative model of genetic risk and an estimated recurrence risk for siblings stratified for HLA genotype (λ_{sHLA}) of 2.3–5.3, the contribution of HLA to the heritability of celiac disease is estimated at between 21 and 44 % [4, 5].

Association with non-HLA Genes

With the completion of the human genome sequence, millions of SNPs have been identified. Using these SNPs as genetic markers, called tag SNPs, GWAS have helped to identify thousands of susceptibility variants for hundreds of complex diseases.

Two GWAS on CD and their follow-up studies revealed 26 non-HLA regions to be associated with CD [26–29]. Denser genotyping with the Immunochip, a custom-made array that covers common variants from 186 GWAS loci associated with 12 immune-mediated diseases, identified 13 additional non-HLA regions [30].

Thus, in addition to HLA, there are now 39 known non-HLA regions associated with CD, of which 36 have been genotyped with a high variant density. These regions contain 57 independently associated SNPs [30] (Fig. 5.2). The association signal can be refined to a single candidate gene for 19 of the regions (see Text Box 5.2. "From Genetic Markers to Candidate Genes and Pathways"). However, only three of the associated SNPs are linked to protein-altering variants located in exonic regions, and eight additional SNPs are localized upstream around the transcription start site (5′ untranslated region) of a specific gene or downstream around the 3′ untranslated region [30]. Although most SNPs are localized in nonprotein coding intergenic and intronic regions, the regions associated with CD are greatly enriched with regions involved in regulating the expression of one or more genes, so-called expression Quantitative Trait Loci (eQTLs) [29].

The candidate genes for CD identified by GWAS provide important clues to the disease pathogenesis, including the pathways that are deregulated in CD. Pathway enrichment analyses using susceptibility genes have shown that most susceptibility genes for celiac disease are involved in immune processes. These pathways concern both the adaptive immune response and the innate immune response. The adaptive immune response includes T-lymphocyte maturation and differentiation (e.g., the *RUNX3*, *ETS1*, *IL2*, *IL21*, *IL12A*, *IL18R1*, and *IL18RAP* genes), T- and B-lymphocyte activation and immune cell signaling (e.g., the *CD28*, *CTLA4*, *ICOS*, *ICOSLG*, *PTPN2*, *SOCS1*, SH2B3, *UBASH3A*, and *FASLG* genes), and chemokine-induced cell migration (e.g., the *CCR1-3* and *CCR4* genes). The innate immune response

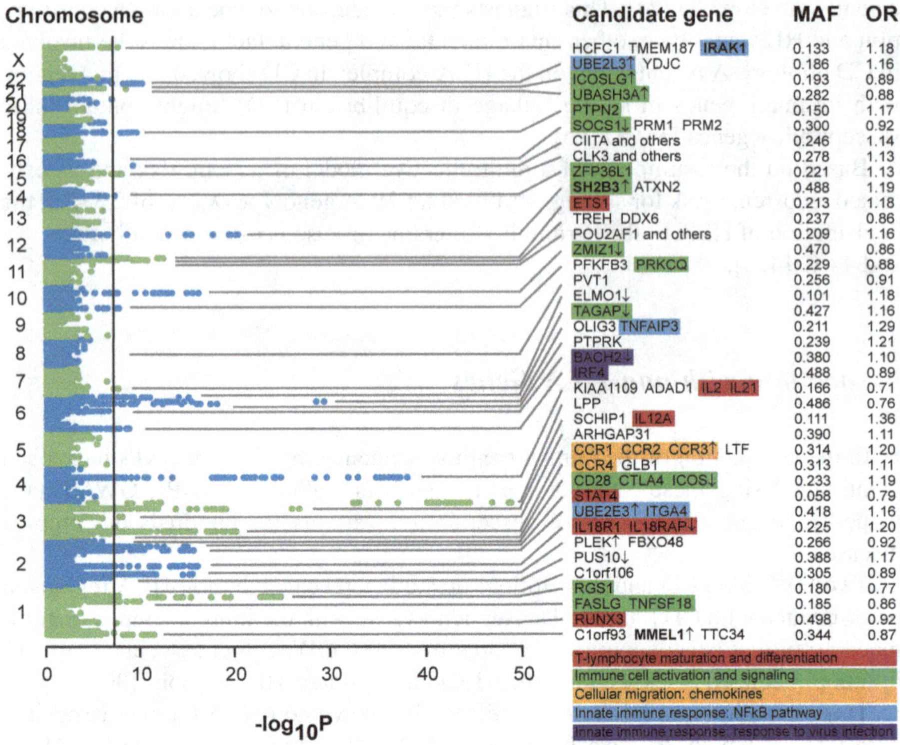

Fig. 5.2 Manhattan plot of the 39 non-HLA regions associated with CD and identified by Immunochip analysis. The *vertical line* represents the genome-wide significance threshold at $P=5\times10^{-8}$. For each associated region the candidate genes are shown with the minor allele frequency (MAF) in the European control population and the odds ratio (OR) for the most significantly associated single nucleotide polymorphism (SNP) of each region. In three regions, the most significantly associated SNP is linked to a protein-altering variant (IRAK1, SH2B3, and MMEL1, in *bold*). Several SNPs are associated with a change in expression of one or more genes: ↑ for increased expression and ↓ for decreased expression (Kumar V et al., unpublished data). Candidate genes known to be involved in immunological pathways are highlighted

includes the NFκB-pathway (e.g., the *UBE2E3* and *TNFAIP3* genes) and the response to viral infections (e.g., the *BACH2* and *IRF4* genes) [29, 31] (see Fig. 5.2).

These results do indeed suggest that CD is a T lymphocyte-mediated immune disorder. Furthermore, enrichment of genes involved in natural killer (NK) cell-activation and interferon-gamma production compared to other autoimmune diseases indicates involvement of this pathway in CD [23]. Altogether, celiac susceptibility genes appear to be involved in both the adaptive as well as innate immunity. It has been suggested that the interplay between innate and adaptive immunity on exposure to environmental triggers is a main pathogenic factor in CD [32]. In addition to gluten, various infectious agents have been proposed as triggering environmental factors in genetically predisposed individuals. Moreover, it has been hypothesized that gut microbiota may play a role in CD pathogenesis

Text Box 5.2 From Genetic Markers to Candidate Genes and Pathways

Since the associated SNPs in GWAS will in most cases not be the causal variant but a tag for a nearby causal variant, additional analyses can help to pinpoint the best candidate genes. *Denser genotyping* with the analysis of multiple SNPs located within the same LD block as the tag SNP may help identify SNPs with a stronger association to the disease of interest and narrow down the genetic region to study. *Sequencing* of regions of interest may help to identify less common variants with a potential biological effect. In *eQTL analysis*, the associated SNPs are tested for their correlation with the expression levels of nearby genes (*cis*-eQTL) or genes some distance away (*trans-eQTL*). The result may suggest a functional role for the genes whose expression correlates with the disease-associated SNPs. *Annotation catalogues*, containing information on the functions of genes and genetic variants, and *gene co-expression networks* can further contribute to identifying genes and pathways that may have a function in the disease of interest.

(as discussed in depth in Chap. 7) [33, 34]. Hence, it might be relevant to analyze CD susceptibility genes in the context of interactions between microbes and the host immune response.

Current Challenges in the Search for Genetic Susceptibility Factors

Although GWAS have identified 57 independently associated non-HLA SNPs to CD, the exact causal variant in each region is still unknown. This can be explained by the fact that the analyzed SNPs are in fact tag SNPs, which are in linkage with more than one variant within a so-called LD block. Molecular functional analyses will be necessary to delineate the true causal variants and to understand the mechanism of how these variants affect CD. In addition, most of the associated SNPs are common and associated with a modest increase in CD risk (median odds ratio 1.17, range 1.10–1.70) or a modest decrease in risk (median odds ratio 0.88, range 0.71–0.91) [30]. Since the associated SNPs are tag SNPs, the true effect sizes of the causal variants may be underestimated.

The known non-HLA susceptibility regions, together with HLA, explain approximately 54 % of the heritability of CD [35]. So nearly 50 % of the heritability still needs to be explained. It is not clear whether this hidden heritability is due to thousands of common variants with smaller effect sizes or to individual mutations with strong effect sizes. Future studies performing whole genome sequencing in CD patients may provide answers to this question [36].

From the ENCODE project, it is now apparent that most of the human genome is transcribed to not only protein-coding transcripts but also to large numbers of noncoding RNA molecules of different size [37]. These noncoding RNAs include short noncoding RNAs such as microRNAs (miRNAs), small interfering RNAs (siRNAs), and piwi-interacting RNAs (piRNAs), as well as a new class of long noncoding RNAs (lncRNAs), which are larger than 200 nucleotides [38]. Interestingly, several CD-associated SNPs map to lncRNA regions [39], and it has been shown that disease-associated SNPs can alter lncRNA expression [40]. Hence, the identification of genetic variants associated with CD and that map to noncoding transcripts could help us not only to explain the hidden heritability of CD but also to better understand the disease mechanism.

Shared Immunogenetics with Immune-Related Diseases

CD is associated with several other autoimmune diseases and immune-mediated diseases. Patients with type 1 diabetes mellitus and autoimmune thyroiditis (Graves' disease and Hashimoto's disease) belong to the high-risk populations for CD, with estimated prevalences of 3–6 % in type 1 diabetes patients [1] and 3–8 % in autoimmune thyroiditis patients [41]. In addition, the prevalence of immune-related diseases, including type 1 diabetes and autoimmune thyroiditis, is increased in CD patients compared to the general population [42–45]. In different cohorts of CD patients, the overall prevalence of autoimmune diseases, excluding dermatitis herpetiformis, was approximately 20 %, compared to approximately 11 % in control groups [44–46]. In a retrospective study of CD patients, their cumulative risk for autoimmune disease increased from 8 % at 15 years of age to 33 % at 50 years of age. Type 1 diabetes comprised 29 % of the reported cases and autoimmune thyroiditis 26 %, while other diseases such as psoriasis (8 %), inflammatory bowel disease (7 %), and rheumatoid arthritis (3 %) were reported in fewer patients [45].

Risk factors for the development of another autoimmune disease were a positive family history for autoimmune disease (hazard ratio 2.4, 95 % confidence interval 1.7–3.3) and a diagnosis of CD before 36 years of age (hazard ratio 2.7, 95 % confidence interval 1.8–3.9). In contrast, a positive family history for CD was not associated with an increased risk for other autoimmune diseases in CD patients [45]. This suggests that some susceptibility genes for CD may be shared with other immune-related diseases.

Many immune-related diseases have been linked to the HLA region. The CD HLA risk haplotypes containing HLA-DQ2.5 and HLA-DQ8 also belong to the most susceptible HLA haplotypes for type 1 diabetes [47]. It is estimated that approximately one-third of the type 1 diabetes patients who are homozygous for HLA-DQ2.5 have CD-associated transglutaminase autoantibodies, compared to 1 % of the patients without HLA-DQ2 or HLA-DQ8. It is therefore likely that CD and type 1 diabetes share more risk factors [48].

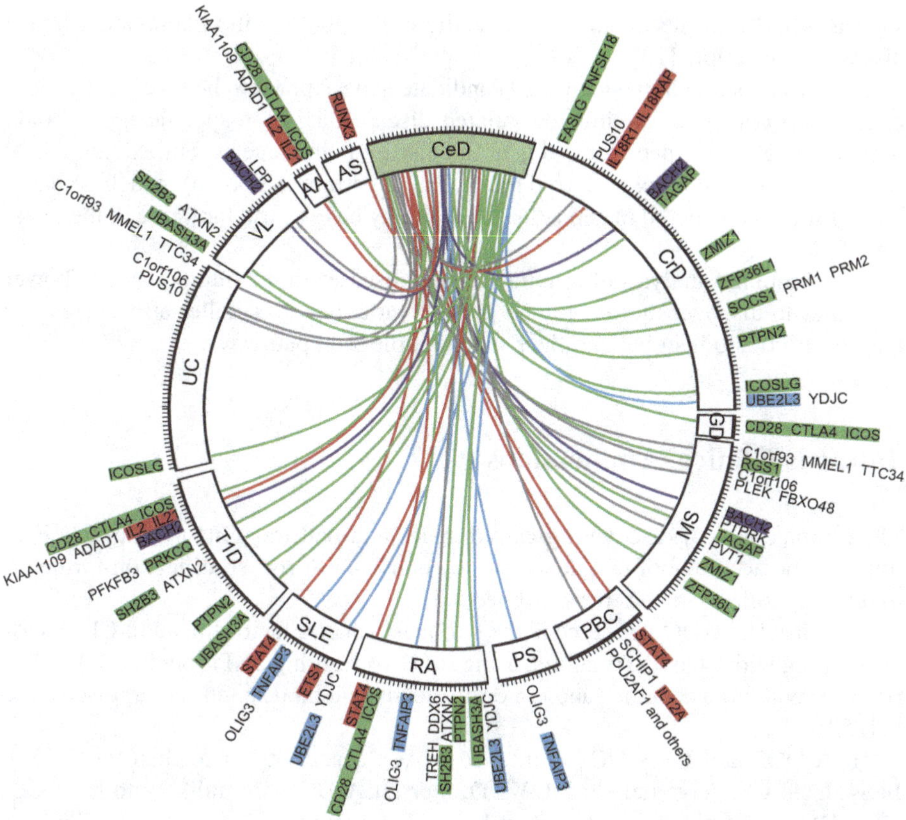

Fig. 5.3 Non-HLA susceptibility regions shared between celiac disease (CeD) and the following immune-related diseases (using a genome-wide significance threshold at $P = 5 \times 10^{-8}$): *CrD* Crohn's disease, *GD* Graves' disease, *MS* multiple sclerosis, *PBC* primary biliary cirrhosis, *PS* psoriasis, *RA* rheumatoid arthritis, *SLE* systemic lupus erythematosus, *T1D* type 1 diabetes mellitus, *UC* ulcerative colitis, *VL* vitiligo, *AA* alopecia areata, *AS* ankylosing spondylitis. Adapted from [59]

A meta-analysis on genetic susceptibility regions discovered by GWAS for immune-related diseases (including CD and type 1 diabetes) showed that 44 % of the regions were associated with more than one immune-related disease. This confirms a widespread sharing of non-HLA susceptibility regions between immune-related diseases [49]. Of the non-HLA susceptibility regions for celiac disease, 30/39 (80 %) have been associated with other immune-related diseases (Fig. 5.3).

Analysis of pathways shared by candidate genes directly associated with two or more immune-related diseases showed that there are three major immunological pathways involved: T-lymphocyte differentiation, immune cell signaling, and the innate immune response [50]. CD susceptibility genes appear to be linked to pathways that are strongly involved in T lymphocyte-mediated autoimmune diseases, such as type 1 diabetes and autoimmune thyroiditis, but not in inflammatory bowel disease, for example [23].

In addition, some of the identified candidate genes appear to be specifically associated with one or a few immune-related diseases. Disease-specific genes could provide insight into specific aspects of the disease pathogenesis. For example, LPP (LIM domain-containing preferred translocation partner in lipoma), which is shared with vitiligo, is involved in cell adhesion and may have a structural role in the intestine [50].

The combined analysis of immune-related diseases in the future may add power to studies to discover more common genetic variants with smaller effect sizes and may contribute to insights into their shared etiological pathways.

Towards Clinical Applications

The ultimate aim of discovering causal genes and pathways involved in CD is to improve the accuracy of diagnosis and to contribute to risk stratification for determining the follow-up and treatment needed.

Thus far, HLA-DQ genotype is the strongest genetic factor linked to CD. HLA-genotyping with a tag SNP method, using six HLA-tagging SNPs, predicts HLA-DQ risk type with high accuracy and is a cost-effective method suited for large-scale use [51, 52].

HLA-DQ2 and HLA-DQ8 combined have a sensitivity of median 96 % [53]. Individuals who have neither HLA-DQ2 nor HLA-DQ8 are unlikely to have CD. HLA-DQ genotyping could therefore be used to exclude CD or make it unlikely in patients with an uncertain diagnosis. In addition, genotyping could be used as a first-line test in the screening of asymptomatic individuals with an increased risk for CD, for example, patients with type 1 diabetes or autoimmune thyroiditis, and the first-degree relatives of CD patients [53, 54]. For example, in siblings of children with CD, who have an overall risk for CD of 10 %, HLA-DQ genotyping was used to stratify ~40 % of the siblings into a group with a small residual risk of <1 % and another ~30 % into a group with a residual risk of 1–10 % [55].

In contrast, the specificity of HLA-DQ genotyping is rather low, with a combined median specificity for HLA-DQ2 and HLA-DQ8 of 54 % [53]. The presence of HLA-DQ2 or HLA-DQ8, in combination with the presence of CD-specific antibodies, could strengthen the diagnosis in patients in whom CD is clinically strongly suspected but in whom no intestinal biopsy will be performed [53]. However, even at a relatively high a priori chance for CD, the proportion of individuals with false-positive results is rather high. Thus, because of the low positive predictive value of HLA-DQ genotyping, a combination with additional risk factors may lead to better prediction of CD risk. A two-step approach could be applied: first excluding individuals without HLA-DQ2 and HLA-DQ8, and second classifying the remaining individuals into different risk groups based on their non-HLA genetic risk factors [16].

In a genetic risk model based on HLA-DQ genotype and ten non-HLA susceptibility SNPs, the presence of 13 or more risk alleles in an individual implied an odds ratio of 6.2 (95 % confidence interval 4.1–9.3) for CD, compared to individuals with 5 or fewer risk alleles [56]. An intermediate HLA-genotype risk combined with 13 non-HLA risk alleles led to an increased risk for CD (odds ratio 6.1) comparable to a high HLA-genotype risk combined with no non-HLA risk alleles (odds ratio 6.2) [56].

The combination of HLA-DQ genotype and the 57 known non-HLA susceptibility SNPs in a genetic risk score leads to a further increase in accuracy of the genetic risk score, with 11 % of the individuals being reclassified to a more accurate risk group. This combination shows a moderate discriminative accuracy with an area under the receiver operating characteristic (ROC) curve of 0.854, corresponding with a chance of 85 % to classify a random CD patient correctly as having a higher risk for the disease than a random individual without CD (J. Romanos et al. unpublished data). However, there is still a large overlap in genetic risk scores between CD patients and healthy individuals, as shown by the percentage of patients and healthy controls classified at intermediate risk: 51 % of the patients and 40 % of the healthy controls. The high-risk category, consisting of the top 25 % of genetic risk scores, has a sensitivity of 43 % and a specificity of 93 %. The positive predictive value for the high-risk category is estimated to be 6 % at a CD prevalence of 1 % and 43 % for a high-risk population with an a priori risk of 10 %. In both situations, the negative predictive value is expected to be higher than 99 %. With a prospective cohort study, the positive and negative predictive values of a genetic prediction model can be estimated more accurately. For example, the PreventCD Study encompasses a European multicenter study among high-risk CD families, in which approximately 1000 newborns who tested positive for HLA-DQ2, and/or HLA-DQ8 will be genotyped in more detail [57].

New insights into genetic risk factors, including their interaction with environmental factors, may contribute to further refining of the prediction models. Genetic data will probably need to be combined with other biomarkers in order to identify subgroups that can usefully guide follow-up and treatment [58].

An important aspect of genetic studies remains the discovery of causal genetic variants and new pathways, including the pathways shared with other immune-related diseases. These may eventually contribute to the identification of new therapeutic targets.

Acknowledgments We thank Jackie Senior for editing the manuscript.

Funding

Work in the Wijmenga group is supported by grants from the Celiac Disease Consortium (an innovative cluster approved by the Netherlands Genomics Initiative and partly funded by the Dutch Government (grant BSIK03009 to CW)) and the Dutch Digestive Disease Foundation (MLDS WO11-30 to CW).

References

1. Dubé C, Rostom A, Sy R, Cranney A, Saloojee N, Garritty C, et al. The prevalence of celiac disease in average-risk and at-risk Western European populations: a systematic review. Gastroenterology. 2005;128:S57–67.
2. Myléus A, Ivarsson A, Webb C, Danielsson L, Hernell O, Högberg L, et al. Celiac disease revealed in 3 % of Swedish 12-year-olds born during an epidemic. J Pediatr Gastroenterol Nutr. 2009;49:170–6.
3. Risch N. Assessing the role of HLA-linked and unlinked determinants of disease. Am J Hum Genet. 1987;40:1–14.
4. Petronzelli F, Bonamico M, Ferrante P, Grillo R, Mora B, Mariani P, et al. Genetic contribution of the HLA region to the familial clustering of coeliac disease. Ann Hum Genet. 1997;61:307–17.
5. Bevan S, Popat S, Braegger CP, Busch A, O'Donoghue D, Falth-Magnusson K, et al. Contribution of the MHC region to the familial risk of coeliac disease. J Med Genet. 1999;36:687–90.
6. Fasano A, Berti I, Gerarduzzi T, Not T, Colletti RB, Drago S, et al. Prevalence of celiac disease in at-risk and not-at-risk groups in the United States: a large multicenter study. Arch Intern Med. 2003;163:286–92.
7. Nisticò L, Fagnani C, Coto I, Percopo S, Cotichini R, Limongelli MG, et al. Concordance, disease progression, and heritability of coeliac disease in Italian twins. Gut. 2006;55:803–8.
8. Greco L, Romino R, Coto I, Di Cosmo N, Percopo S, Maglio M, et al. The first large population based twin study of coeliac disease. Gut. 2002;50:624–8.
9. Falchuk ZM, Rogentine GN, Strober W. Predominance of histocompatibility antigen HL-A8 in patients with gluten-sensitive enteropathy. J Clin Invest. 1972;51:1602–5.
10. Keuning JJ, Peña AS, van Leeuwen A, van Hooff JP, van Rood JJ. HLA-DW3 associated with coeliac disease. Lancet. 1976;1(7958):506–8.
11. Price P, Witt C, Allcock R, Sayer D, Garlepp M, Kok CC, et al. The genetic basis for the association of the 8.1 ancestral haplotype (A1, B8, DR3) with multiple immunopathological diseases. Immunol Rev. 1999;167:257–74.
12. Tosi R, Vismara D, Tanigaki N, Ferrara GB, Cicimarra F, Buffolano W, et al. Evidence that celiac disease is primarily associated with a DC locus allelic specificity. Clin Immunol Immunopathol. 1983;28:395–404.
13. Sollid LM, Markussen G, Ek J, Gjerde H, Vartdal F, Thorsby E. Evidence for a primary association of celiac disease to a particular HLA-DQ α/β heterodimer. J Exp Med. 1989;169:345–50.
14. Van Belzen MJ, Koeleman BP, Crusius JB, Meijer JW, Bardoel AF, Pearson PL, et al. Defining the contribution of the HLA region to cis DQ2-positive coeliac disease patients. Genes Immun. 2004;5:215–20.
15. Vader W, Stepniak D, Kooy Y, Mearin L, Thompson A, van Rood JJ, et al. The HLA-DQ2 gene dose effect in celiac disease is directly related to the magnitude and breadth of gluten-specific T cell responses. Proc Natl Acad Sci USA. 2003;100:12390–5.
16. Romanos J, Wijmenga C. Predicting susceptibility to celiac disease by genetic risk profiling. Ann Gastroenterol Hepatol. 2010;1:11–8.
17. Lundin KE, Scott H, Hansen T, Paulsen G, Halstensen TS, Fausa O, et al. Gliadin-specific, HLA-DQ(α1*0501, β1*0201) restricted T cells isolated from the small intestinal mucosa of celiac disease patients. J Exp Med. 1993;178:187–96.
18. Lundin KE, Scott H, Fausa O, Thorsby E, Sollid LM. T cells from the small intestinal mucosa of a DR4, DQ7/DR4, DQ8 celiac disease patient preferentially recognize gliadin when presented by DQ8. Hum Immunol. 1994;41:285–91.
19. Kim CY, Quarsten H, Bergseng E, Khosla C, Sollid LM. Structural basis for HLA-DQ2-mediated presentation of gluten epitopes in celiac disease. Proc Natl Acad Sci USA. 2004;101:4175–9.

20. Henderson KN, Tye-Din JA, Reid HH, Chen Z, Borg NA, Beissbarth T, et al. A structural and immunological basis for the role of human leukocyte antigen DQ8 in celiac disease. Immunity. 2007;27:23–34.
21. Spurkland A, Sollid LM, Polanco I, Vartdal F, Thorsby E. HLA-DR and -DQ genotypes of celiac disease patients serologically typed to be non-DR3 or non-DR5/7. Hum Immunol. 1992;35:188–92.
22. Louka AS, Sollid LM. HLA in coeliac disease: unravelling the complex genetics of a complex disorder. Tissue Antigens. 2003;61:105–17.
23. Abadie V, Sollid LM, Barreiro LB, Jabri B. Integration of genetic and immunological insights into a model of celiac disease pathogenesis. Annu Rev Immunol. 2011;29:493–525.
24. Liu E, Rewers M, Eisenbarth GS. Genetic testing: who should do the testing and what is the role of genetic testing in the setting of celiac disease? Gastroenterology. 2005;128:S33–7.
25. Ahn R, Ding YC, Murray J, Fasano A, Green PH, Neuhausen SL, et al. Association analysis of the extended MHC region in celiac disease implicates multiple independent susceptibility loci. PLoS One. 2012;7:e36926.
26. Van Heel DA, Franke L, Hunt KA, Gwilliam R, Zhernakova A, Inouye M, et al. A genome-wide association study for celiac disease identifies risk variants in the region harboring IL2 and IL21. Nat Genet. 2007;39:827–9.
27. Hunt KA, Zhernakova A, Turner G, Heap GA, Franke L, Bruinenberg M, et al. Newly identified genetic risk variants for celiac disease related to the immune response. Nat Genet. 2008;40:395–402.
28. Trynka G, Zhernakova A, Romanos J, Franke L, Hunt KA, Turner G, et al. Coeliac disease-associated risk variants in TNFAIP3 and REL implicate altered NF-κB signalling. Gut. 2009;58:1078–83.
29. Dubois PC, Trynka G, Franke L, Hunt KA, Romanos J, Curtotti A, et al. Multiple common variants for celiac disease influencing immune gene expression. Nat Genet. 2010;42:295–302.
30. Trynka G, Hunt KA, Bockett NA, Romanos J, Mistry V, Szperl A, et al. Dense genotyping identifies and localizes multiple common and rare variant association signals in celiac disease. Nat Genet. 2011;43:1193–201.
31. Trynka G, Wijmenga C, van Heel DA. A genetic perspective on coeliac disease. Trends Mol Med. 2010;16:537–50.
32. Fasano A, Shea-Donohue T. Mechanisms of disease: the role of intestinal barrier function in the pathogenesis of gastrointestinal autoimmune diseases. Nat Clin Pract Gastroenterol Hepatol. 2005;2:416–22.
33. Forsberg G, Fahlgren A, Hörstedt P, Hammarström S, Hernell O, Hammarström ML. Presence of bacteria and innate immunity of intestinal epithelium in childhood celiac disease. Am J Gastroenterol. 2004;99:894–904.
34. Collado MC, Donat E, Ribes-Koninckx C, Calabuig M, Sanz Y. Specific duodenal and faecal bacterial groups associated with paediatric coeliac disease. J Clin Pathol. 2009;62:264–9.
35. Kumar V, Wijmenga C, Withoff S. From genome-wide association studies to disease mechanisms: celiac disease as a model for autoimmune diseases. Semin Immunopathol. 2012;34:567–80.
36. Gibson G. Rare and common variants: twenty arguments. Nat Rev Genet. 2012;13:135–45.
37. The ENCODE Project Consortium. Identification and analysis of functional elements in 1 % of the human genome by the ENCODE pilot project. Nature. 2007;447:799–816.
38. Derrien T, Johnson R, Bussotti G, Tanzer A, Djebali S, Tilgner H, et al. The GENCODE v7 catalog of human long noncoding RNAs: analysis of their gene structure, evolution, and expression. Genome Res. 2012;22:1775–89.
39. Cabili MN, Trapnell C, Goff L, Koziol M, Tazon-Vega B, Regev A, et al. Integrative annotation of human large intergenic noncoding RNAs reveals global properties and specific subclasses. Genes Dev. 2011;25:1915–27.
40. Kumar V, Westra H, Karjalainen J, Zhernakova DV, Esko T, Hrdlickova B, et al. Human disease-associated genetic variation impacts large intergenic non-coding RNA expression. PLoS Genet. 2013;9:e1003201.

41. Hadithi M, de Boer H, Meijer JW, Willekens F, Kerckhaert JA, Heijmans R, et al. Coeliac disease in Dutch patients with Hashimoto's thyroiditis and vice versa. World J Gastroenterol. 2007;13:1715–22.
42. Collin P, Reunala T, Pukkala E, Laippala P, Keyriläinen O, Pasternack A. Coeliac disease-associated disorders and survival. Gut. 1994;35:1215–8.
43. Ventura A, Magazzù G, Greco L. Duration of exposure to gluten and risk for autoimmune disorders in patients with celiac disease. SIGEP Study Group for Autoimmune Disorders in Celiac Disease. Gastroenterology. 1999;117:297–303.
44. Sategna Guidetti C, Solerio E, Scaglione N, Aimo G, Mengozzi G. Duration of gluten exposure in adult coeliac disease does not correlate with the risk for autoimmune disorders. Gut. 2001;49:502–5.
45. Cosnes J, Cellier C, Viola S, Colombel JF, Michaud L, Sarles J, et al. Incidence of autoimmune diseases in celiac disease: protective effect of the gluten-free diet. Clin Gastroenterol Hepatol. 2008;6:753–8.
46. Viljamaa M, Kaukinen K, Huhtala H, Kyrönpalo S, Rasmussen M, Collin P. Coeliac disease, autoimmune diseases and gluten exposure. Scand J Gastroenterol. 2005;40:437–43.
47. Erlich H, Valdes AM, Noble J, Carlson JA, Varney M, Concannon P, et al. HLA DR-DQ haplotypes and genotypes and type 1 diabetes risk: analysis of the type 1 diabetes genetics consortium families. Diabetes. 2008;57:1084–92.
48. Bao F, Yu L, Babu S, Wang T, Hoffenberg EJ, Rewers M, et al. One third of HLA DQ2 homozygous patients with type 1 diabetes express celiac disease-associated transglutaminase autoantibodies. J Autoimmun. 1999;13:143–8.
49. Cotsapas C, Voight BF, Rossin E, Lage K, Neale BM, Wallace C, et al. Pervasive sharing of genetic effects in autoimmune disease. PLoS Genet. 2011;7:e1002254.
50. Zhernakova A, van Diemen CC, Wijmenga C. Detecting shared pathogenesis from the shared genetics of immune-related diseases. Nat Rev Genet. 2009;10:43–55.
51. Monsuur AJ, de Bakker PI, Zhernakova A, Pinto D, Verduijn W, Romanos J, et al. Effective detection of human leukocyte antigen risk alleles in celiac disease using tag single nucleotide polymorphisms. PLoS One. 2008;3:e2270.
52. Koskinen L, Romanos J, Kaukinen K, Mustalahti K, Korponay-Szabó I, Barisani D, et al. Cost-effective HLA typing with tagging SNPs predicts celiac disease risk haplotypes in the Finnish, Hungarian, and Italian populations. Immunogenetics. 2009;61:247–56.
53. Husby S, Koletzko S, Korponay-Szabó IR, Mearin ML, Phillips A, Shamir R, et al. European Society for Pediatric Gastroenterology, Hepatology, and Nutrition guidelines for the diagnosis of coeliac disease. J Pediatr Gastroenterol Nutr. 2012;54:136–60.
54. Hill ID, Dirks MH, Liptak GS, Colletti RB, Fasano A, Guandalini S, et al. Guideline for the diagnosis and treatment of celiac disease in children: recommendations of the North American Society for Pediatric Gastroenterology, Hepatology and Nutrition. J Pediatr Gastroenterol Nutr. 2005;40:1–19.
55. Bourgey M, Calcagno G, Tinto N, Gennarelli D, Margaritte-Jeannin P, Greco L, et al. HLA related genetic risk for coeliac disease. Gut. 2007;56:1054–9.
56. Romanos J, van Diemen CC, Nolte IM, Trynka G, Zhernakova A, Fu J, et al. Analysis of HLA and non-HLA alleles can identify individuals at high risk for celiac disease. Gastroenterology. 2009;137:834–40.
57. Hogen Esch CE, Rosén A, Auricchio R, Romanos J, Chmielewska A, Putter H, et al. The Prevent CD Study design: towards new strategies for the prevention of coeliac disease. Eur J Gastroenterol Hepatol. 2010;22:1424–30.
58. Cho JH, Gregersen PK. Genomics and the multifactorial nature of human autoimmune disease. N Engl J Med. 2011;365:1612–23.
59. Hindorff LA, MacArthur J (European Bioinformatics Institute), Morales J (European Bioinformatics Institute), Junkins HA, Hall PN, Klemm AK, and Manolio TA. A catalog of published genome-wide association studies. Available at: http://www.genome.gov/gwastudies. Accessed 01/15, 2013.

Chapter 6
Using Animal Models of Celiac Disease to Understand the Role of MHC II

Eric V. Marietta, Alberto Rubio-Tapia, and Joseph A. Murray

Untreated CD patients develop increased numbers of intraepithelial lymphocytes, inflammatory infiltration of the lamina propria, intestinal permeability, and in a majority of cases, total or subtotal villous atrophy [1]. The trigger for the development of CD is gluten, typically derived from wheat, barley, and rye [2]. Gluten is a group of storage proteins found in wheat, rye, and barley. In wheat, gluten consists of two smaller subgroups of proteins, gliadins, and glutenins. In established CD patients, gliadin-specific T cells are more prevalent than glutenin-specific T cells [3]; however, there may be an initial stage of development for all CD patients in which their T cells respond to a greater number of epitopes [4]. A focusing phenomenon occurs later in which T cells in well-established CD patients are predominantly specific for epitopes that are a result of deamidation of gliadin by tissue transglutaminase [5]. CD is also strongly associated with HLA-DQ2 and HLA-DQ8, wherein 95 % are DQ2+ and most of the remaining are DQ8+ [6]. This contribution of MHC II is only 40 % of the familial risk, though, leaving 60 % of the genetic risk due to non-HLA genes [7]. This latter point is of great interest to the researchers that use animal models of CD for a number of reasons.

The first reason is that none of the spontaneous animal models seem to have a clear association with specific MHC II alleles, as is seen in human CD [8]. This may be interpreted in a number of ways. One interpretation is that MHC II does not play a vital role in the development of gluten-dependent enteropathy; however, years of clinical research have shown that the HLA molecules are necessary, though not sufficient, for CD to occur [9]. Indeed, crucial information has come from T-cell lines derived from the jejunum of CD patients. Studies with these in vitro models using DQ2 and/or DQ8 restricted T cells determined that these intestinally derived T cells

E.V. Marietta, Ph.D. • A. Rubio-Tapia, M.D.
Division of Gastroenterology and Hepatology, Mayo Clinic, Rochester, MN, USA

J.A. Murray, M.D. (✉)
Division of Gastroenterology and Hepatology, Mayo Clinic, 200 1st Street SW, Rochester, MN 55906, USA
e-mail: Murray.Joseph@mayo.edu

S.D. Rampertab and G.E. Mullin (eds.), *Celiac Disease*, Clinical Gastroenterology,
DOI 10.1007/978-1-4614-8560-5_6,

are responsive to specific epitopes and that the process of deamidation causes some of these epitopes to be more immunogenic [10]. Therefore, one has to conclude that MHC II is necessary, but insufficient by itself to develop gluten-dependent enteropathy. This chapter will therefore highlight what we have learned from animal models of celiac disease about the interplay between MHC II molecules and non-MHC II molecules that results in gluten-dependent enteropathy.

Non-transgenic Animal Models

Spontaneous

Of the non-transgenic animal models there are two categories, spontaneous and induced. All of the spontaneous animal models are large animals and include non-human primates, dogs, and horses [11–18]. Of these three models, the role of MHC II has been clearly defined in only the dog model, and Polvi et al. determined that the gluten-dependent enteropathy in the Irish Setter pups was not associated with specific MHC II alleles [16]. The role of MHC II in the rhesus macaque (nonhuman primate) model of CD is not clear. In the first two publications on the rhesus model of CD, the authors stated that "the two gluten-sensitive macaques studied extensively herein and in the accompanying report, FH09 and FH45, are of genotype DRB1*0303(12), DRB*1007 at the Mamu class II DRB(1) locus" [11, 12]. This statement suggests that there may be an association of the gluten-dependent enteropathy in the rhesus macaques, but in their third publication, no reference was made to MHC II [13]. Therefore, it is still possible that specific MHC II alleles may be associated with the gluten-dependent enteropathy in the monkey model, but with time this possibility becomes less likely. The recent publication that characterized a single horse association with MHC is uncertain [18]. Of the three spontaneous animal models, then, MHC II molecules may be necessary for the development of gluten-dependent enteropathy, but specific alleles that exclusively contribute to the development of inflammatory gluten-responsive T cells do not appear to be present as is found in CD (humans).

Induced

The induction of enteropathy has been done with the rodent models of CD, but not the large animal models of CD. In one rat model, gliadin is administered by gavage immediately after birth to germ-free Wistar AVN rats, resulting in shortened villi, crypt hyperplasia, and increased numbers of intestinal CD8$\alpha\beta$+IELs [19]. A similar model was developed in 2012 using Balb/c mice [20]. In this model, Balb/c mice were fed a gluten-free chow for three generations, and then the third-generation mice were fed a gluten-containing chow [20]. The gluten-challenged mice (G+) developed increased IELs, villous atrophy, and crypt hyperplasia as compared to untreated mice [G–].

There is also a mouse model of induction that uses the transfer of $CD4^{+}CD25^{-}$ $CD45RB^{lo}$ cells from gliadin-sensitized mice to recipient Rag 1–/– mice [21]. The recipient Rag1–/– mice developed infiltration of the basal lamina propria, cryptitis, crypt abscesses, lymphocytic infiltration of the lamina propria, crypt hyperplasia, and villous atrophy.

Transgenic Animal Models

MHC II Molecules

Transgenic animal models have been used extensively to address specific questions about the pathogenesis of CD. So far, the large-animal models, especially the rhesus macaque model, have recreated most of the disease, but is lacking in the tight association of specific alleles of MHC II with the development of gluten-dependent enteropathy. Thus, transgenic mice have been used to determine the role of MHC II in the development of CD.

Transgenic mice that express HLA-DQ8 were the first HLA transgenic mice to be evaluated for gluten sensitivity [22]. These mice did not spontaneously develop gluten-dependent enteropathy, but did generate a strong T-cell response to gluten after intraperitoneal injection of gluten with Complete Freund's Adjuvant [22]. In another study, sensitization of these mice to DQ8-α-I, a gliadin-derived epitope that is DQ8-restricted, demonstrated that the T-cell receptor (TCR) repertoire induced by sensitization with native peptides had a heteroclitic (stronger) response to deamidated peptides [4]. This result suggested that the focusing of the immune response in CD over time against deamidated gliadin epitopes may be a consequence of the T-cell response to gliadin-derived peptides that are presented by DQ8 and presumably DQ2. These DQ8 transgenic mice also did not develop enteropathy after gliadin sensitization [4].

In a later study, these mice were sensitized parenterally to gliadin and later administered gliadin orally; they subsequently developed increased numbers of intra-epithelial cell numbers (IELs) [23]. This would demonstrate that DQ8 is necessary for the development of gluten-specific T cells, as well as generating T-cell responses against deamidated gliadin, but is not sufficient for the development of gluten-dependent enteropathy. Indeed, the sensitization protocols demonstrated that environmental factors have to also contribute in order for the development of mild enteropathy (increased IELs, villous shortening) to occur.

Other studies with transgenic mice that express DQ2 and DR3 provided the same results [24–26]. Therefore, initial studies with HLA transgenic mice demonstrated that CD is the result of a combination of contributing factors, including (but not exclusive to) predisposing HLA genes, environmental factors, and non-HLA genes. Other studies reinforced the conclusion that strong T-cell responses to gluten or gliadin were not sufficient to generate gluten-dependent enteropathy and, in fact, further demonstrated that environmental and/or non-HLA genes are significant contributing factors. In one study, a transgenic mouse was designed to express a TCR that was specific for HLA-DQ2 presenting an immunodominant epitope of gliadin, and then this was bred with HLA-DQ2/DR3 mice [26]. Even these mice did not develop gluten (gliadin)-dependent enteropathy after gliadin sensitization and oral feeding of gliadin [26].

Since the above HLA transgenic models did not fully develop gluten-dependent enteropathy, a number of studies induced enteropathy through the administration of drugs or chemicals. This method does have precedence in the human system. Indomethacin, a nonsteroidal anti-inflammatory drug (NSAID), causes enteropathy in humans, resulting in increased intestinal permeability and increased numbers of IELs [27]. Other drugs and chemicals have been used to induce enteropathy in the different mouse models described above to address the interaction of gluten-specific T cells with the IELs that mediate enteropathy.

Reagents used to induce mild enteropathy in rodents include polyinosinic/polycytidylic acid (poly I:C), indomethacin, and methotrexate. Cholera toxin is also used, but it breaks oral tolerance, as opposed to generating enteropathy [28]. Poly I:C has been used in a number of rodent studies of CD. The first instance was where (CBA×BALB/c)F1 mice were injected intraperitoneally with poly I:C diluted in 0.01 M NaOH. These mice developed significant villous atrophy and crypt hyperplasia by 1 day postinjection that began to resolve 3 days postinjection [29]. Because poly I:C induces the production of IFN-α/β in vivo, poly I:C administration also resulted in a significant increase in natural killer (NK) cell activation [29]. A later study found that the intestinal epithelial cells treated with poly I:C expressed higher levels of IL-15, allowing for the expansion of cytotoxic IELs (CD8$\alpha\alpha$+) that express NK1.1 [30]. A different study found that the increased IL-15 production by poly I:C treated epithelial cells induced the expression of NKG2D by CD8$\alpha\alpha$ IELs [31].

NSAIDs include diclofenac and indomethacin, both of which increase intestinal permeability in rats [32]. So far, the only NSAID used in the mouse models of CD has been indomethacin. In two studies, intestinal paracellular permeability was found to increase with the administration of indomethacin to HLA-DQ8 transgenic mice [33, 34]. Sensitization to gluten, consisting of an injection of gluten intraperitoneally, followed by gavage with gluten, in addition to indomethacin treatment, resulted in increased intestinal permeability [33].

In a different study, HLA-DQ8 transgenic mice were administered indomethacin orally for 13 days after oral sensitization to gliadin using cholera toxin [35]. Villous height was decreased in the mice that were sensitized to gliadin and injected with indomethacin, but was not when the mice were only injected with indomethacin or only sensitized to gliadin. IFN-γ production was also increased with the combined treatment of indomethacin and gliadin sensitization.

Methotrexate, which is an anti-folate drug, induces mucositis for 3–5 days after treatment [36]. This intestinal inflammation is characterized by increased production of the inflammatory cytokines TNF-α and IFN-γ, by lamina propria lymphocytes in the absence of any shortening of villi. A later study used methotrexate in combination with gliadin feeding of DQ2 transgenic mice [37]; however, no gliadin-specific T cells were generated using this protocol, suggesting that methotrexate treatment does not break oral tolerance established for gliadin in these mice.

Non-MHC II Molecules

There have been a number of GWAS studies that have identified non-HLA genes as contributing to the development of CD [38, 39]. None of these genes have been evaluated in animal models of CD. Instead, genes encoding other molecules that have been demonstrated to play a role in the development of CD have been used in animal models. These include TTG and IL-15.

Tissue transglutaminase type 2 (TTG) is the self-protein to which there is a clear autoimmune response in CD [40]. However, it is unclear as to whether it has a pathogenic role or is simply a marker of enteropathy [41]. One study determined that CD patients do have anti-TTG antibodies depositing in the small intestine of untreated celiac patients [42]. To determine if anti-TTG antibodies by themselves can mediate damage to the small intestine, a number of studies utilizing mice have addressed the roles of TTG and anti-TTG antibodies. Our group observed that significant increases in anti-TTG IgA developed with age, but that this did not result in significant changes in enteropathy (Fig. 6.1 and unpublished data).

One group analyzed the pathogenicity of anti-TTG antibodies by overexpressing in mice anti-TTG antibodies that had been isolated from intestinal lymphocytes of a CD patient [43]. To do this, they used recombinant adeno-associated virus (rAAV) and a sequence for an antihuman TTG antibody identified with a phage display library. The final miniantibody (MB) replaced the human Fc domains with those of mouse, and 10^{10} anti-TTG MB rAAV virions were injected into C57BL6 mice [44]. Four weeks after injection, anti-TTG antibodies were detected in the sera, and deposits were found in the muscle tissue that was injected; however, no deposits were detected in the intestine and no increases in intestinal permeability were detected. These results demonstrated that anti-TTG antibodies by themselves cannot mediate the development of enteropathy.

Two other studies used mice that had TTG knocked out [45, 46]. The untreated TTG−/− mouse had no major developmental abnormalities [45]. A later study using the same line of mice and poly I:C treatment demonstrated that the temporary enteropathy (villous atrophy) induced by poly I:C still developed in the TTG knockout construct [46]. This latter result further supports the hypothesis that anti-TTG antibodies are not a cause of, but are instead a consequence of, enteropathy.

In in vitro studies, gliadin has been found to generate the production of cytokines by cell types other than T cells. The monocyte is one of these cell types, although the receptor is not fully elucidated [47]. In this in vitro study, THP cells, a monocytic cell line, produced IL-8 and TNF-α in response to stimulation with

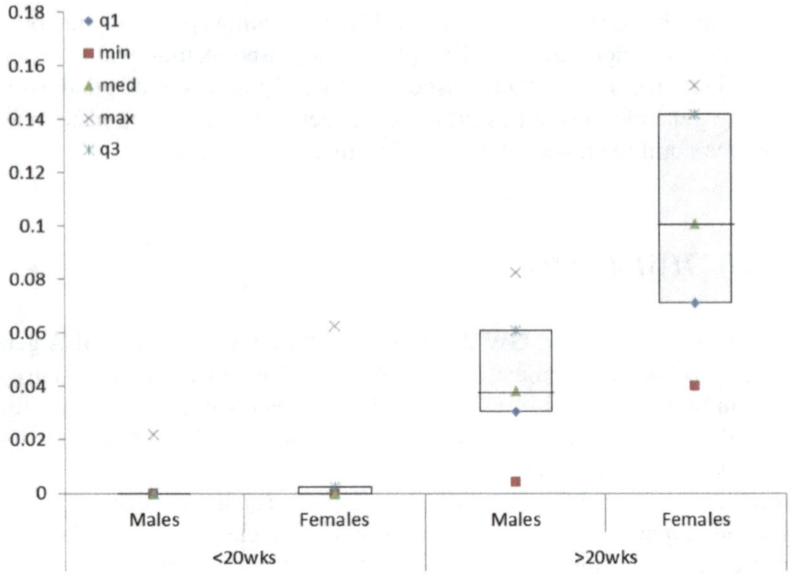

Fig. 6.1 Effect of age upon anti-TTG IgA serum levels in NOD Abo DQ8 mice. Forty-four NOD Abo DQ8 mice were evaluated for serum anti-TTG IgA using a guinea pig TTG-based ELISA. The units on the *y*-axis are Optical Density (OD) values

pepsin-digested gliadin in a manner that was independent of CD14 [47]. Our own studies have shown that gliadin-treated THP cells also express CXCL10 (T-cell recruiting chemokine) transcripts 2 h after stimulation with a peptic tryptic digest of gliadin, but not CXCL11 (Fig. 6.2a). This results in a significantly increased secretion of CXCL10 protein 24 h after stimulation with PTD gliadin (Fig. 6.2b).

Another cytokine, IL-15, has also been shown to play a significant role in the development of CD. CD patients have a higher expression of IL-15 by epithelial cells than normal controls [48]. This aberrant expression of IL-15 is thought to contribute to the expansion of cytotoxic CD8+ IELs that subsequently kill enterocytes [49]. To prove this, transgenic mice that overexpress IL-15 were used. So far, two different lines of IL-15 transgenic mice have been generated by two different groups [50, 51]. With the first IL-15 transgenic mouse that was generated, the mouse IL-15 gene was placed behind the promoter of a minimal MHC class I D^d gene (D gene of H-2^d haplotype) for expression throughout the mouse [51]. For the second IL-15 transgenic mouse generated, human IL-15 was placed behind an enterocyte-specific promoter (T3b) [50]. The phenotype of the D^d-IL-15 mouse without sensitization was the expansion of NK cells and memory CD8+ cells that resulted in a fatal leukemia that had an NK T-cell phenotype [50]. The T3b-IL-15 mouse developed increased numbers of CD8+ cells that infiltrated the small intestine as well as the development of anti-TTG IgA [52]. Neither of these models proved to develop enteropathy in a gluten-dependent manner; albeit they did develop enteropathy similar to that found in CD [53].

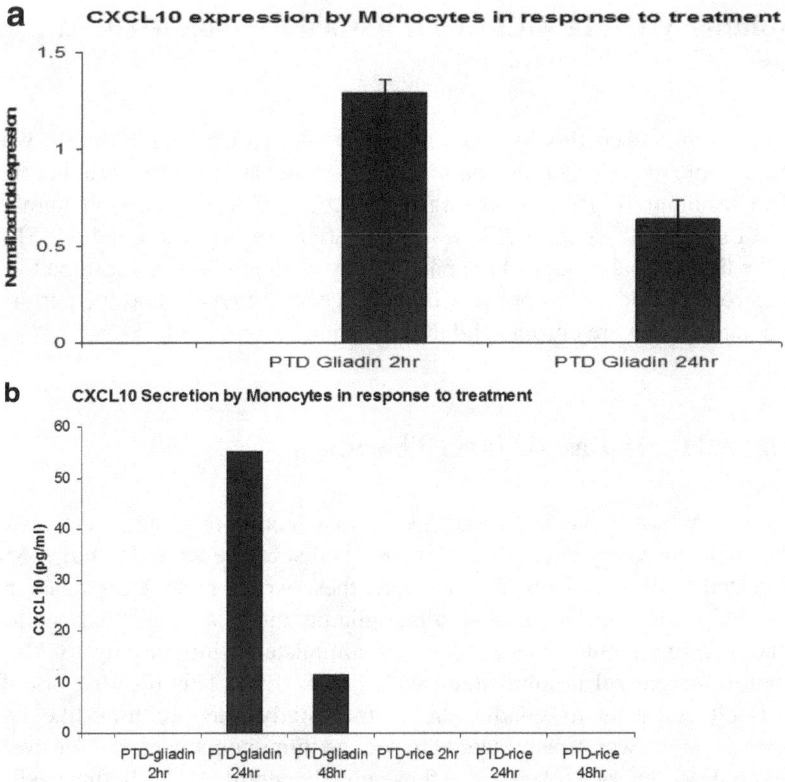

Fig. 6.2 CXCL10 expression and secretion. (**a**) CXCL 10 mRNA transcripts were present at 2 h post-gliadin treatment and significantly decreased 24 h after treatment with gliadin. (**b**) A significant increase in CXCL10 secretion occurred 24 h after THP monocytes were treated with a peptic tryptic digest of gliadin. Treatment with PTD rice did not result in detectable levels of secreted CXCL10

The above two IL-15 transgenic animal models demonstrate, then, that alterations to certain innate immune pathways, such as the expansion of activated IELs via IL-15, can by itself lead to autoimmune enteropathy. Indeed, autoimmune enteropathy in humans has many features that are similar with gluten-induced enteropathy (CD). These include almost exclusive small bowel involvement, villous blunting, and atrophy. Differences, though, are that only CD has increased numbers of IELs, and that only CD has a clear association with MHC II [54]. This, therefore, demonstrates that CD is a unique intertwining between gluten (gliadin)-reactive T cells and alterations to the innate immune system that lead to the development of enteropathy. For a true animal model of CD, these two phenomena need to not only be intertwined but essentially propagate each other.

Combining MHC II with Celiac Associated Non-MHC II Genes

One study approached this by crossing the D^d -IL-15 transgenic mouse with the DQ8 transgenic mouse, thereby combining gluten sensitivity with chronic enteropathy. The resultant IL-15 DQ8 transgenic mice developed increased numbers of CD3+ IELs in the absence of villous atrophy after feeding with gliadin [55]. Thus, this is the first animal model where enteropathy is gluten dependent (albeit without villous atrophy), and that is because both the genetic element and the perturbation to the innate system are chronic and not transient.

Testing MHC II-Based Novel Therapies

Because HLA transgenic mice are models that incorporate the celiac-associated MHC II molecules, any novel therapies for CD that are generated to target MHC II can be tested in these models. For example, these would include therapies that are based upon generating tolerance to alpha-gliadin and gliadin-derived peptides. In one study, recombinant alpha-gliadin was administered intranasally to Abo DQ8 mice before parenteral immunization with gliadin [56]. This resulted in a diminished T-cell response to gliadin. In another study, the probiotic-like bacteria *Lactococcus lactis* was bioengineered to secrete immunogenic gliadin-derived peptides in order to generate tolerance to those gliadin peptides [57]. In this study, DQ8 transgenic mice that were given these bacteria had a diminished delayed type hypersensitivity (DTH) response to the gliadin peptides but not control peptides, demonstrating that the administration of these bioengineered bacteria did suppress the immune response to the gliadin peptides in an antigen-specific manner.

Not Yet Evaluated by Animal Models

Although the animal models described above have provided extensive knowledge as to the pathogenesis of CD, there are some fundamental gaps that have not been addressed with animal models. These would include the roles of other molecules that have not been identified with GWAS studies but have been shown with in vitro models to clearly be playing a role in the pathogenesis of CD.

Probably, the most important set of molecules not yet addressed by animal models is zonulin and CXCR3. In a number of in vitro model studies, zonulin has been shown to be released by epithelial cells in response to gliadin binding to CXCR3, and that in turn loosens the tight junction proteins between the epithelial cells [58, 59]. This increased permeability then allows for the paracellular passage of even more gluten-derived peptides to enter the lamina propria and further propagate the

T-cell response to gluten-derived epitopes. The one animal model that has come the closest to addressing the roles of zonulin and CXCR3 in CD is the rhesus macaque model, in which gluten-dependent intestinal permeability was shown to be increased in the monkeys that developed celiac-like symptoms and was not seen in the monkeys that did not develop anti-TTG antibodies [11]. As of yet, no animal model has been generated that either overexpresses zonulin or knocks it out. There is a knockout construct of CXCR3, though [60, 61]. In a model of lung inflammation (short-term exposure to cigarette smoke), the numbers of infiltrating cytotoxic CD8+ cells were significantly decreased in the CXCR3 knockout mice as compared to the wild-type mice that were subjected to smoking [61]. The intestines of these mice were used in *ex vivo* experiments to determine that CXCR3 is the receptor for gliadin [59]. Neither paper explicitly addressed the architecture of the small intestines of the CXCR3–/– mice, so presumably these would have displayed normal villous height, etc. No models of overexpression of CXCR3 systemically or in the intestine have yet been generated.

Another molecule that has been shown to play a crucial role in the development of CD using in vitro models is CD71. This molecule is the receptor for transferrin and also binds to IgA antibodies at the cell surface. Once bound, it then transports the IgA with any bound ligand across the epithelial barrier into the lamina propria (transcellular transport). Previous studies have shown that gliadin-specific and/or TTG-specific antibodies bound to gliadin or TTG can then be transported to the lamina propria, where the proteins are then phagocytosed and presented to T cells by phagocytic antigen presenting cells. In the Balb/c model of gluten-dependent enteropathy, the CD71/IgA/gluten/tTG transcellular pathway was determined to be active [20]. In the Balb/c third-generation mice that were fed a gluten-containing chow (G+), CD71 expression was increased on the enterocytes as compared to the enterocytes of the (G–) mice, and IgA+ cells were increased in the lamina propria of the G+ mice as compared to the (G–) mice. No determination of the specificity of the IgA bound to the lamina propria cells was done, but CD71 and IgA did co-localize at both the apical and basal poles of the epithelial cells. This latter result strongly suggests that transcellular transport of IgA and bound proteins is occurring in the G+ mice. Because CD71 plays such a crucial role in the transport of iron, CD71 knockout constructs are embryonic lethal [62]. Still, constructs that overexpress CD71, especially a conditional expression, could provide more insight into the pathogenic role of this pathway in gluten-dependent enteropathy.

Conclusion

All of the animal models of CD have provided results that support the theory that the generation of gluten-specific T cells can arise independently of enteropathy (Table 6.1). The results from all of the animal models also suggest that there are a number of different MHC II alleles in all the species evaluated (dog, monkey, horse, rat, mouse) that can recognize gliadin-derived epitopes, but that in humans, only two,

Table 6.1 Animal Models of Celiac Disease

Animal models	Original characterization as celiac model
Horse	Van der Kolk, Vet Q, 2012
Dog	Batt, Res Vet Sci, 1984
Primate	Bethune et al., Plos One, 2008
Germ-free Wistar AVN rat	Stepankova, Scand J. Gastroenterol, 1996
Balb/c mice	Papista, Laboratory Investigation, 2012
Rag1−/− mice and cell transfer	Freitag, Gut, 2009
HLA-DQ2 transgenic mice	DeKauwe, J Immunol, 2009
HLA-DQ8 transgenic mice	Black, J Immunol, 2002
TTG mini antibody mice	Di Niro, Molecular Immunol, 2008
TTG −/− mice	De Laurenzi, Mol Cell Biol, 2001
IL-15 transgenic mice	Yokoyama, J Clin Immunol, 2011
IL-15-DQ8+ transgenic mice	DePaolo, Nature, 2012

DQ2 and DQ8, can give rise to inflammatory T cells that respond to deamidated gliadin epitopes. The animal models have also demonstrated that CD is a unique intertwining of the adaptive and innate immune responses to gliadin that gives rise to a self-propagating immune response in the presence of gliadin. What needs to be further examined (and determined) in CD using animal models is what factors are necessary for this intertwining. The need to use poly I:C, indomethacin, methotrexate, and cholera toxin in the animal models to induce intestinal inflammation along with gluten-specific T cells to generate enteropathy similar to CD, all point towards environmental factors as triggers of this intertwining. It should be noted that although CD is the autoimmune disease that is most closely associated with specific MHC class II alleles (DQ2 and DQ8), only 3–4 % of the DQ2+ population actually develops CD [63]; therefore, a relatively rare combination of genetics and environmental factors are required to develop well-established CD in DQ2+ and/or DQ8+ individuals.

Acknowledgment This work was supported in part by NIH grant DK071003 and Mayo Foundation for Medical Education and Research.

Conflicts of Interest

The authors have no conflicts of interest to disclose.

References

1. Jabri B, Sollid LM. Mechanisms of disease: immunopathogenesis of celiac disease. Nat Clin Pract Gastroenterol Hepatol. 2006;3(9):516–25 [Research Support, N.I.H., Extramural Research Support, Non-U.S. Gov't Review].
2. Green PH, Jabri B. Celiac disease. Annu Rev Med. 2006;57:207–21.

3. Dissanayake AS, Jerrome DW, Offord RE, Truelove SC, Whitehead R. Identifying toxic fractions of wheat gluten and their effect on the jejunal mucosa in coeliac disease. Gut. 1974;15(12):931–46.
4. Hovhannisyan Z, Weiss A, Martin A, Wiesner M, Tollefsen S, Yoshida K, et al. The role of HLA-DQ8 beta57 polymorphism in the anti-gluten T-cell response in coeliac disease. Nature. 2008;456(7221):534–8 [Research Support, N.I.H., Extramural Research Support, Non-U.S. Gov't].
5. Sollid LM, Jabri B. Celiac disease and transglutaminase 2: a model for posttranslational modification of antigens and HLA association in the pathogenesis of autoimmune disorders. Curr Opin Immunol. 2011;23(6):732–8 [Research Support, N.I.H., Extramural Research Support, Non-U.S. Gov't Review].
6. Spurkland A, Ingvarsson G, Falk ES, Knutsen I, Sollid LM, Thorsby E. Dermatitis herpetiformis and celiac disease are both primarily associated with the HLA-DQ (alpha 1*0501, beta 1*02) or the HLA-DQ (alpha 1*03, beta 1*0302) heterodimers. Tissue Antigens. 1997;49(1):29–34 [Research Support, Non-U.S. Gov't].
7. Kagnoff MF. Celiac disease: pathogenesis of a model immunogenetic disease. J Clin Invest. 2007;117(1):41–9.
8. Marietta EV, Murray JA. Animal models to study gluten sensitivity. Semin Immunopathol. 2012;34(4):497–511 [Research Support, N.I.H., Extramural Research Support, Non-U.S. Gov't Review].
9. Marietta EV, Schuppan D, Murray JA. In vitro and in vivo models of celiac disease. Expert Opin Drug Discov. 2009;4(11):1113–23.
10. Molberg O, McAdam SN, Korner R, Quarsten H, Kristiansen C, Madsen L, et al. Tissue transglutaminase selectively modifies gliadin peptides that are recognized by gut-derived T cells in celiac disease. Nat Med. 1998;4(6):713–7 [Research Support, Non-U.S. Gov't].
11. Bethune MT, Ribka E, Khosla C, Sestak K. Transepithelial transport and enzymatic detoxification of gluten in gluten-sensitive rhesus macaques. PLoS One. 2008;3(3):e1857 [Research Support, N.I.H., Extramural].
12. Bethune MT, Borda JT, Ribka E, Liu MX, Phillippi-Falkenstein K, Jandacek RJ, et al. A non-human primate model for gluten sensitivity. PLoS One. 2008;3(2):e1614 [Research Support, N.I.H., Extramural].
13. Sestak K, Mazumdar K, Midkiff CC, Dufour J, Borda JT, Alvarez X. Recognition of epidermal transglutaminase by IgA and tissue transglutaminase 2 antibodies in a rare case of Rhesus dermatitis. J Vis Exp. 2011;58:Pii: 3154 [Research Support, N.I.H., Extramural Video-Audio Media].
14. Batt RM, Carter MW, McLean L. Morphological and biochemical studies of a naturally occurring enteropathy in the Irish setter dog: a comparison with coeliac disease in man. Res Vet Sci. 1984;37(3):339–46 [Comparative Study Research Support, Non-U.S. Gov't].
15. Hall EJ, Batt RM. Dietary modulation of gluten sensitivity in a naturally occurring enteropathy of Irish setter dogs. Gut. 1992;33(2):198–205 [Research Support, Non-U.S. Gov't].
16. Polvi A, Garden OA, Houlston RS, Maki M, Batt RM, Partanen J. Genetic susceptibility to gluten sensitive enteropathy in Irish setter dogs is not linked to the major histocompatibility complex. Tissue Antigens. 1998;52(6):543–9 [Research Support, Non-U.S. Gov't].
17. Hall EJ, Carter SD, Barnes A, Batt RM. Immune responses to dietary antigens in gluten-sensitive enteropathy of Irish setters. Res Vet Sci. 1992;53(3):293–9 [Research Support, Non--U.S. Gov't].
18. van der Kolk JH, van Putten LA, Mulder CJ, Grinwis GC, Reijm M, Butler CM, et al. Gluten-dependent antibodies in horses with inflammatory small bowel disease (ISBD). Vet Q. 2012;32(1):3–11.
19. Stepankova R, Tlaskalova-Hogenova H, Sinkora J, Jodl J, Fric P. Changes in jejunal mucosa after long-term feeding of germfree rats with gluten. Scand J Gastroenterol. 1996;31(6):551–7 [Research Support, Non-U.S. Gov't].

20. Papista C, Gerakopoulos V, Kourelis A, Sounidaki M, Kontana A, Berthelot L, et al. Gluten induces coeliac-like disease in sensitised mice involving IgA, CD71 and transglutaminase 2 interactions that are prevented by probiotics. Lab Invest. 2012;92(4):625–35 [Research Support, Non-U.S. Gov't].
21. Freitag TL, Rietdijk S, Junker Y, Popov Y, Bhan AK, Kelly CP, et al. Gliadin-primed CD4+CD45RBlowCD25- T cells drive gluten-dependent small intestinal damage after adoptive transfer into lymphopenic mice. Gut. 2009;58(12):1597–605 [Research Support, N.I.H., Extramural].
22. Black KE, Murray JA, David CS. HLA-DQ determines the response to exogenous wheat proteins: a model of gluten sensitivity in transgenic knockout mice. J Immunol. 2002;169(10):5595–600 [Research Support, U.S. Gov't, P.H.S.].
23. Verdu EF, Huang X, Natividad J, Lu J, Blennerhassett PA, David CS, et al. Gliadin-dependent neuromuscular and epithelial secretory responses in gluten-sensitive HLA-DQ8 transgenic mice. Am J Physiol Gastrointest Liver Physiol. 2008;294(1):G217–25 [Research Support, N.I.H., Extramural Research Support, Non-U.S. Gov't].
24. Chen Z, Dudek N, Wijburg O, Strugnell R, Brown L, Deliyannis G, et al. A 320-kilobase artificial chromosome encoding the human HLA DR3-DQ2 MHC haplotype confers HLA restriction in transgenic mice. J Immunol. 2002;168(6):3050–6 [Research Support, Non-U.S. Gov't].
25. Chen D, Ueda R, Harding F, Patil N, Mao Y, Kurahara C, et al. Characterization of HLA DR3/DQ2 transgenic mice: a potential humanized animal model for autoimmune disease studies. Eur J Immunol. 2003;33(1):172–82 [Research Support, U.S. Gov't, Non-P.H.S.].
26. de Kauwe AL, Chen Z, Anderson RP, Keech CL, Price JD, Wijburg O, et al. Resistance to celiac disease in humanized HLA-DR3-DQ2-transgenic mice expressing specific anti-gliadin CD4+ T cells. J Immunol. 2009;182(12):7440–50 [Research Support, Non-U.S. Gov't].
27. Bjarnason I, Takeuchi K. Intestinal permeability in the pathogenesis of NSAID-induced enteropathy. J Gastroenterol. 2009;44 Suppl 19:23–9.
28. Pierre P, Denis O, Bazin H, Mbongolo Mbella E, Vaerman JP. Modulation of oral tolerance to ovalbumin by cholera toxin and its B subunit. Eur J Immunol. 1992;22(12):3179–82 [Research Support, Non-U.S. Gov't].
29. Garside P, Felstein MV, Green EA, Mowat AM. The role of interferon alpha/beta in the induction of intestinal pathology in mice. Immunology. 1991;74(2):279–83 [Research Support, Non-U.S. Gov't].
30. Zhou R, Wei H, Sun R, Tian Z. Recognition of double-stranded RNA by TLR3 induces severe small intestinal injury in mice. J Immunol. 2007;178(7):4548–56 [Research Support, Non--U.S. Gov't].
31. Zhou R, Wei H, Sun R, Zhang J, Tian Z. NKG2D recognition mediates Toll-like receptor 3 signaling-induced breakdown of epithelial homeostasis in the small intestines of mice. Proc Natl Acad Sci USA. 2007;104(18):7512–5 [Research Support, Non-U.S. Gov't].
32. Reuter BK, Davies NM, Wallace JL. Nonsteroidal anti-inflammatory drug enteropathy in rats: role of permeability, bacteria, and enterohepatic circulation. Gastroenterology. 1997;112(1):109–17 [Research Support, Non-U.S. Gov't].
33. Natividad JM, Huang X, Slack E, Jury J, Sanz Y, David C, et al. Host responses to intestinal microbial antigens in gluten-sensitive mice. PLoS One. 2009;4(7):e6472 [Research Support, N.I.H., Extramural Research Support, Non-U.S. Gov't].
34. Silva MA, Jury J, Sanz Y, Wiepjes M, Huang X, Murray JA, et al. Increased bacterial translocation in gluten-sensitive mice is independent of small intestinal paracellular permeability defect. Dig Dis Sci. 2012;57(1):38–47 [Research Support, N.I.H., Extramural Research Support, Non-U.S. Gov't].
35. D'Arienzo R, Stefanile R, Maurano F, Luongo D, Bergamo P, Mazzarella G, et al. A deregulated immune response to gliadin causes a decreased villus height in DQ8 transgenic mice. Eur J Immunol. 2009;39(12):3552–61 [Research Support, Non-U.S. Gov't].
36. de Koning BA, van Dieren JM, Lindenbergh-Kortleve DJ, van der Sluis M, Matsumoto T, Yamaguchi K, et al. Contributions of mucosal immune cells to methotrexate-induced mucositis. Int Immunol. 2006;18(6):941–9 [Comparative Study Research Support, Non-U.S. Gov't].

37. Du Pre MF, Kozijn AE, van Berkel LA, ter Borg MN, Lindenbergh-Kortleve D, Jensen LT, et al. Tolerance to ingested deamidated gliadin in mice is maintained by splenic, type 1 regulatory T cells. Gastroenterology. 2011;141(2):610–20. 20.e1-2 [Research Support, Non-U.S. Gov't].
38. Izzo V, Pinelli M, Tinto N, Esposito MV, Cola A, Sperandeo MP, et al. Improving the estimation of celiac disease sibling risk by non-HLA genes. PLoS One. 2011;6(11):e26920 [Research Support, Non-U.S. Gov't].
39. Dubois PC, Trynka G, Franke L, Hunt KA, Romanos J, Curtotti A, et al. Multiple common variants for celiac disease influencing immune gene expression. Nat Genet. 2010;42(4):295–302 [Research Support, N.I.H., Extramural Research Support, Non-U.S. Gov't].
40. Gianfrani C, Troncone R, La Cava A. Autoimmunity and celiac disease. Mini Rev Med Chem. 2008;8(2):129–34 [Research Support, N.I.H., Extramural Review].
41. Stamnaes J, Fleckenstein B, Sollid LM. The propensity for deamidation and transamidation of peptides by transglutaminase 2 is dependent on substrate affinity and reaction conditions. Biochim Biophys Acta. 2008;1784(11):1804–11 [Research Support, N.I.H., Extramural Research Support, Non-U.S. Gov't].
42. Korponay-Szabo IR, Halttunen T, Szalai Z, Laurila K, Kiraly R, Kovacs JB, et al. In vivo targeting of intestinal and extraintestinal transglutaminase 2 by coeliac autoantibodies. Gut. 2004;53(5):641–8 [Research Support, Non-U.S. Gov't].
43. Di Niro R, Ziller F, Florian F, Crovella S, Stebel M, Bestagno M, et al. Construction of miniantibodies for the in vivo study of human autoimmune diseases in animal models. BMC Biotechnol. 2007;7:46 [Research Support, Non-U.S. Gov't].
44. Di Niro R, Sblattero D, Florian F, Stebel M, Zentilin L, Giacca M, et al. Anti-idiotypic response in mice expressing human autoantibodies. Mol Immunol. 2008;45(6):1782–91 [Research Support, Non-U.S. Gov't].
45. De Laurenzi V, Melino G. Gene disruption of tissue transglutaminase. Mol Cell Biol. 2001;21(1):148–55 [Research Support, Non-U.S. Gov't].
46. Dafik L, Albertelli M, Stamnaes J, Sollid LM, Khosla C. Activation and inhibition of transglutaminase 2 in mice. PLoS One. 2012;7(2):e30642 [Research Support, N.I.H., Extramural Research Support, Non-U.S. Gov't].
47. Jelinkova L, Tuckova L, Cinova J, Flegelova Z, Tlaskalova-Hogenova H. Gliadin stimulates human monocytes to production of IL-8 and TNF-alpha through a mechanism involving NF-kappaB. FEBS Lett. 2004;571(1–3):81–5 [Research Support, Non-U.S. Gov't].
48. Di Sabatino A, Ciccocioppo R, Cupelli F, Cinque B, Millimaggi D, Clarkson MM, et al. Epithelium derived interleukin 15 regulates intraepithelial lymphocyte Th1 cytokine production, cytotoxicity, and survival in coeliac disease. Gut. 2006;55(4):469–77.
49. Meresse B, Malamut G, Cerf-Bensussan N. Celiac disease: an immunological jigsaw. Immunity. 2012;36(6):907–19 [Research Support, Non-U.S. Gov't Review].
50. Ohta N, Hiroi T, Kweon MN, Kinoshita N, Jang MH, Mashimo T, et al. IL-15-dependent activation-induced cell death-resistant Th1 type CD8 alpha beta+NK1.1+ T cells for the development of small intestinal inflammation. J Immunol. 2002;169(1):460–8 [Research Support, Non-U.S. Gov't].
51. Fehniger TA, Suzuki K, Ponnappan A, VanDeusen JB, Cooper MA, Florea SM, et al. Fatal leukemia in interleukin 15 transgenic mice follows early expansions in natural killer and memory phenotype CD8+ T cells. J Exp Med. 2001;193(2):219–31 [Research Support, Non-U.S. Gov't Research Support, U.S. Gov't, P.H.S.].
52. Yokoyama S, Takada K, Hirasawa M, Perera LP, Hiroi T. Transgenic mice that overexpress human IL-15 in enterocytes recapitulate both B and T cell-mediated pathologic manifestations of celiac disease. J Clin Immunol. 2011;31(6):1038–44 [Research Support, Non-U.S. Gov't].
53. Yokoyama S, Perera PY, Waldmann TA, Hiroi T, Perera LP. Tofacitinib, a janus kinase inhibitor demonstrates efficacy in an IL-15 transgenic mouse model that recapitulates pathologic manifestations of celiac disease. J Clin Immunol. 2013;33(3):586–94.
54. Gentile NM, Murray JA, Pardi DS. Autoimmune enteropathy: a review and update of clinical management. Curr Gastroenterol Rep. 2012;14(5):380–5 [Research Support, N.I.H., Extramural Research Support, Non-U.S. Gov't Review].

55. DePaolo RW, Abadie V, Tang F, Fehlner-Peach H, Hall JA, Wang W, et al. Co-adjuvant effects of retinoic acid and IL-15 induce inflammatory immunity to dietary antigens. Nature. 2011;471(7337):220–4 [Research Support, N.I.H., Extramural Research Support, Non-U.S. Gov't].
56. Senger S, Luongo D, Maurano F, Mazzeo MF, Siciliano RA, Gianfrani C, et al. Intranasal administration of a recombinant alpha-gliadin down-regulates the immune response to wheat gliadin in DQ8 transgenic mice. Immunol Lett. 2003;88(2):127–34.
57. Huibregtse IL, Marietta EV, Rashtak S, Koning F, Rottiers P, David CS, et al. Induction of antigen-specific tolerance by oral administration of Lactococcus lactis delivered immunodominant DQ8-restricted gliadin peptide in sensitized nonobese diabetic Abo Dq8 transgenic mice. J Immunol. 2009;183(4):2390–6 [Research Support, N.I.H., Extramural].
58. El Asmar R, Panigrahi P, Bamford P, Berti I, Not T, Coppa GV, et al. Host-dependent zonulin secretion causes the impairment of the small intestine barrier function after bacterial exposure. Gastroenterology. 2002;123(5):1607–15 [In Vitro Research Support, Non-U.S. Gov't Research Support, U.S. Gov't, P.H.S.].
59. Lammers KM, Lu R, Brownley J, Lu B, Gerard C, Thomas K, et al. Gliadin induces an increase in intestinal permeability and zonulin release by binding to the chemokine receptor CXCR3. Gastroenterology. 2008;135(1):194–204. e3 [Research Support, N.I.H., Extramural].
60. Hancock WW, Lu B, Gao W, Csizmadia V, Faia K, King JA, et al. Requirement of the chemokine receptor CXCR3 for acute allograft rejection. J Exp Med. 2000;192(10):1515–20 [Research Support, U.S. Gov't, P.H.S.].
61. Nie L, Xiang RL, Liu Y, Zhou WX, Jiang L, Lu B, et al. Acute pulmonary inflammation is inhibited in CXCR3 knockout mice after short-term cigarette smoke exposure. Acta Pharmacol Sin. 2008;29(12):1432–9 [Research Support, Non-U.S. Gov't].
62. Levy JE, Jin O, Fujiwara Y, Kuo F, Andrews NC. Transferrin receptor is necessary for development of erythrocytes and the nervous system. Nat Genet. 1999;21(4):396–9 [Comparative Study Research Support, Non-U.S. Gov't Research Support, U.S. Gov't, P.H.S.].
63. Megiorni F, Mora B, Bonamico M, Barbato M, Nenna R, Maiella G, et al. HLA-DQ and risk gradient for celiac disease. Hum Immunol. 2009;70(1):55–9.

Chapter 7
Role of Gut Microbes in Celiac Disease Risk and Pathogenesis

José Moisés Laparra, Marta Olivares, and Yolanda Sanz

Introduction

Celiac disease (CD) is a chronic enteropathy triggered by wheat gluten (e.g., gliadins) and other cereal-related proteins in genetically predisposed individuals. Typical cases of CD often appear in early childhood soon after the first exposure to dietary gluten, but the disease is also being increasingly diagnosed in late adulthood, suggesting that gluten intake is not the only triggering factor [1, 2].

The etiology and pathogenesis of the disease is strongly associated with Human Leukocyte Antigen (HLA) genes, encoding the HLA-DQ2 (HLA-DQ2.5 and HLA-DQ2.2) and HLA-DQ8 heterodimers, involved in antigen presentation and T-cell activation. These genetic factors are necessary for the disease to develop but not sufficient, since they are also present in ~35% of the general population and only a small percentage (3–5 %) develops the disease [3, 4].

To date, gluten is the only known environmental factor to play a direct causal role in CD. As discussed by Ludvigsson et al. in Chap. 3 and elsewhere in this book, epidemiological studies report that mode of delivery at birth, milk-feeding type and incidence of infections and antibiotic intake, which may also influence the gut ecosystem, are some other factors influencing the risk of developing CD [5–8]. In early stages of life, interactions between gut microbiota and innate and adaptive immunity play a crucial role in influencing T effector- and regulatory-cell balance and the development of tolerance towards dietary antigens [9, 10]. In this context, the

J.M. Laparra, Ph.D. • M. Olivares
Microbial Ecology, Nutrition and Health, Institute of Agrochemistry and Food Technology, National Research Council (IATA-CSIC), Paterna, Valencia, Spain

Y. Sanz, Ph.D. (✉)
Microbial Ecology, Nutrition and Health, Institute of Agrochemistry and Food Technology, National Research Council (IATA-CSIC), Av. Agustín Escardino 7, Paterna, Valencia 46980, Spain
e-mail: yolsanz@iata.csic.es

S.D. Rampertab and G.E. Mullin (eds.), *Celiac Disease*, Clinical Gastroenterology,
DOI 10.1007/978-1-4614-8560-5_7, © Springer Science+Business Media New York 2014

incidence of gastrointestinal viral infections, which generate Th1-protective responses, has been investigated as a possible factor contributing to CD risk [11]. Prospective studies in infants at risk of CD are also underway to find out possible relationships between their gut colonization pattern and CD onset [6, 12]. In addition, observational studies in children and adults have revealed alterations in the gut microbiota composition of subjects with active CD (symptomatic and untreated) and non-active CD (non-symptomatic after following a gluten-free diet) compared to that of control subjects, which could contribute to the disease pathogenesis [5].

Currently, CD is among the most prevalent chronic digestive disorders, but the only effective therapy for CD patients is life-long adherence to a strict gluten-free diet. Complying with this dietary recommendation is difficult because gluten is present in most processed food, and patients are continuously exposed to gluten. Also, a small proportion of patients (~5 %) do not experience improved clinical symptoms on a gluten-free diet and can be diagnosed with refractory CD [13–15]. Therefore, there is a need to identify modifiable factors that contribute to CD risk and pathogenesis in order to make progress in the identification of complementary strategies to improve the quality of life of patients and to prevent the disease from developing in populations at risk.

Influence of Milk-Feeding Type in Gut Microbiota and Risk of CD Development

Dietary influences are particularly relevant at early stages of development, when the infant's gut and immune system are immature, because of their possible contribution to either the development of oral tolerance to innocuous antigens and commensal bacteria or to increasing overreactions and disease risk. Colonization of the intestine starts immediately after birth and represents the main environmental stimulus for immune system maturation. This process depends, among other factors, on the type of delivery, type of milk-feeding, and, possibly, host genotype (Fig. 7.1) [16].

Breast-feeding is an environmental factor that seems to protect or at least delay CD development; this effect can be due to its immune and other biologically active components [17], as well as to its effect on the intestinal microbiota composition [18]. Breast-fed children exhibit higher prevalence of bifidobacteria; meanwhile, formula-feeding favors the colonization of a more heterogeneous microbiota that is more similar to that identified in the adult population [19, 20].

Studies using real-time PCR and denaturing gradient gel electrophoresis (DGGE) in a cohort of 164 infants at risk of developing CD have also demonstrated that both milk-feeding type and HLA-DQ genotype influence the intestinal microbiota [6, 12]. The microbiota of infants at high risk of developing CD showed reduced numbers of *Bifidobacterium* spp. and, particularly, of *B. longum*. Although breast-feeding reduced the genotype-related bifidobacterial alterations, these were not

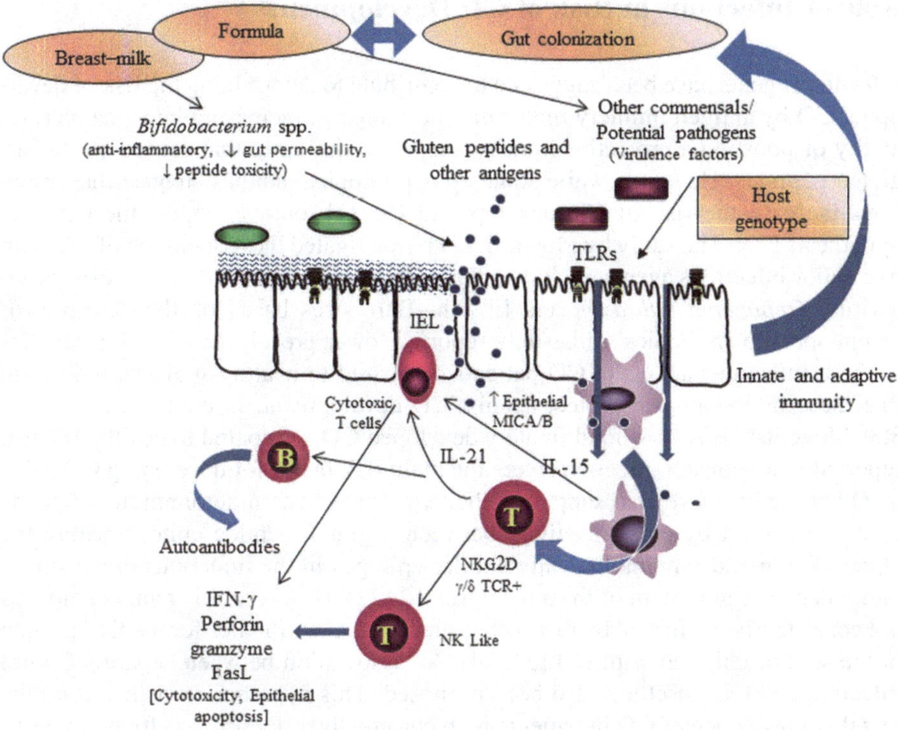

Fig. 7.1 Schematic representation of different factors influencing gut microbiota composition and its possible role in CD pathogenesis and risk of developing CD

completely normalized, suggesting that both factors (milk-feeding type and HLA-DQ genotype) influence the composition and numbers of *Bifidobacterium* spp. [6]. Formula-fed infants at high genetic risk of developing CD also showed increased numbers of the *Bacteroides fragilis* group but not breast-fed infants, suggesting that the effect of breast-feeding on colonization of this bacterial group is stronger than the possible effect of the CD genotype [6].

In infants at high risk of developing CD, numbers of *Staphylococcus* spp. were increased in both breast- and formula-fed groups, suggesting a major role of the HLA-DQ genotype in defining the colonization of this bacterial group [6]. In another study with a subgroup of infants [12] from this cohort and using DGGE, increased *B. vulgatus* prevalence was associated with the high-risk genotype, while increased *B. uniformis* prevalence was associated with both the low-risk genotype and breast-feeding. Overall, breast-feeding seems to attenuate the differences in microbiota related to the HLA-DQ genotype, which could partly explain its protective effect against CD development reported in previous epidemiological studies.

Role of Infections in Risk of CD Development

Infectious agents have been suggested to contribute to determining the risk of developing CD by antigen mimicry molecular mechanisms, increasing intestinal permeability or boosting a protective immune response similar to that caused by dietary gluten peptides. However, while some epidemiological studies suggest that infections increase the risk of CD development [9, 21], others support the opposite hypothesis [22]. The study by Plot et al. [21] investigated the association of CD with five major infectious agents, including *Toxoplasma gondii*, rubella virus, cytomegalovirus, *Treponema pallidum,* and Epstein–Barr virus based on the detection of serum-specific antibodies. This study reported lower prevalence of IgG antibodies to these infectious agents in CD patients compared to healthy subjects, indicating that these infections can protect against CD development. In contrast, a study in 3,392 Swedish infants, who ultimately developed CD, compared to healthy infants, reported that neonatal infections were the main risk factor for developing CD [9].

Other studies have also supported the hypothesis that an autoimmune response could be caused by cross-reactivity between a gluten peptide epitope within the alpha-gliadin and immunologically similar epitopes in the infectious organism, in particular the Elb protein of the adenovirus 12 [22]. However, this relationship was not consistently confirmed by measuring specific IgG antibodies for the E1d protein in the sera of children with CD [23, 24]. An association between hepatitis C viral infection and CD onset has also been proposed. This hypothesis was based on the fact that prevalence of CD in patients with chronic liver disease was found to be 15 times higher than in the general population [25], and that 5 % of autoimmune diseases diagnosed in these subjects was CD [26]. Nevertheless, other studies have not reported an increased prevalence of CD in patients suffering hepatitis C [27]. Increased incidence of rotavirus infection has also been linked to increased risk of CD autoimmunity in a prospective study including 1,931 children carrying CD HLA risk alleles [11]. In some particular cases, gastrointestinal infections caused by *Campylobacter jejuni* [11] or *Giardia lamblia* [28] have also been associated to CD onset based on their simultaneous diagnosis.

Intestinal Dysbiosis and CD Pathogenesis

CD has been associated with alterations in the intestinal microbiota composition (intestinal dysbiosis) in several observational human studies in children and adults (Table 7.1). The microbiota of CD children showed an increased ratio of Gram-negative to Gram-positive bacteria. In particular, CD patients showed reduced numbers of *Bifidobacterium* spp. and *B. longum* and increased numbers of *Bacteroides* spp. in stools and duodenal biopsies, analyzed by molecular quantitative methods (e.g., FISH and real-time PCR), compared to controls [29, 30]. Enterobacteria and staphylococci numbers were also higher in untreated CD patients than in controls,

Table 7.1 Summary of studies reporting associations between gut microbiota composition and celiac disease

Study group	Sample	Technique	Results	References
Children with active CD and non-active CD[a]	Duodenal biopsy	FISH coupled with flow cytometry	↑ Total and Gram-negative bacteria in patients with active CD ↑ *Bacteroides-Prevotella* and *E. coli* in patients with active CD ↓ *Lactobacillus* + *Bifidobacterim*/*Bacteroides-Prevotella* + *E. coli* in patients with active and non-active CD	[29]
Children with active CD and non-active CD	Feces and duodenal biopsies	Real-time PCR	↑ *Bacteroides* and *Clostridium leptum* groups in feces and biopsies of patients with active and non-active CD ↑ *E. coli* and *Staphylococcus* spp. in feces and biopsies of patients with active CD ↑ *Bifidobacterium* spp. and *B. longum* in feces of both groups of CD patients and in biopsies of patients with active CD	[30]
Children with active CD and non-active CD	Duodenal biopsy	TTGE	↑ Diversity (number of bands) in patients (with active plus non-active CD) ↑ *Bacteroides vulgatus* and *E. coli* in patients (with active plus non-active CD)	[31]
Children with active CD (newly diagnosed and challenged with gluten) and non-active CD	Jejunal biopsies	SEM	↑ Rod-shaped bacteria in patients with active and non-active CD than in controls	[32]
Children with active CD (newly diagnosed and challenged with gluten) and non-active CD	Distal duodenum/proximal jejunum biopsies	SEM 16S rRNA gene sequencing	No differences by SME in samples collected from 2004 to 2007 ↑ *Haemophilus* spp. and ↓ *Neisseria polysaccharea* in patients (with active plus non-active CD) than in controls in samples collected from 2004 to 2007 ↑ Unclassified *Clostridiales, Actinomyces graevenitzii, Prevotella spp., Bacteroidetes, Firmicutes* and *Fusobacteria* in SME + biopsies than in SME-biopsies collected in the Swedish CD epidemic (1985–1996)	[33]

(continued)

Table 7.1 (continued)

Study group	Sample	Technique	Results	References
Adults patients with active and non-active CD	Fecal samples	DGGE	↓ Diversity *Lactobacillus* and *Bifidobacterium* species in patients with non-active CD ↑ *Bifidobacterium bifidum* patients with active CD than in healthy adults	[34]
Children with non-active CD	Duodenal biopsy and fecal samples	DGGE Plate counts	↑ Diversity of Eubacteria in duodenal samples of CD patients and differences in DGGE profiles compared with controls ↓ *Lactobacillus, Enterococcus*, and *Bifidobacterium* plate counts in fecal samples of CD patients than in controls ↑ *Bacteroides, Staphylococcus, Salmonella, Shigella*, and *Klebsiella* plate counts in CD than in controls	[35]
Healthy adults before and after GFD	Fecal samples	FISH Real-time PCR	↓ *Bifidobacterium, Clostridium lituseburense*, and *Faecalibacterium prausnitzii* proportions after GFD by FISH ↓ *Bifidobacterium, Lactobacillus*, and *Bifidobacterium longum* and ↑ *Enterobacteriaceae* and *E. coli* after GFD by real-time PCR	[36]
Children with active CD, adults with non-active CD	Small intestinal biopsy	Real-time PCR	No differences in numbers or prevalence of groups analyzed (*Bifidobacterium, Bacteroides-Prevotella, Bacteroides, Streptococcus*, and *Lactobacillus*)	[37]
Children with active CD	Small intestinal biopsy	IS-pro, 16S-23S interspacer region-based profiling	No differences in diversity and composition	[38]
Adults with active CD with different symptomatology	Duodenal biopsy	DGGE	↓ Diversity in CD patients with gastrointestinal symptoms and anemia than those with dermatitis herpetiformis (DH) ↑ Proteobacteria in CD patients with gastrointestinal symptoms in comparison with those with DH and controls	[39]

[a]Patients with active CD were newly diagnosed cases on a normal gluten-containing diet (or in a few cases challenged with gluten) and patients with non-active CD were symptomatic-free treated with a gluten-free diet

but the differences were restored in CD subjects on a long-term gluten-free diet [30]. Another research group also analyzed the mucosa-associated microbiota of children with CD, before and after following a gluten-free diet, by temporal temperature gradient gel electrophoresis (TTGE) reporting that prevalence of *Bacteroides vulgatus* and *Escherichia coli* in CD patients was higher than in controls [31], partially in agreement with previous studies [30]. In adults it was reported that rod-shaped bacteria were frequently associated with the mucosa of CD patients (both active and treated with a gluten-free diet), but not with controls, as determined by scanning electron microscopy [32].

A further retrospective study of the biopsy samples of these CD patients by 16S rDNA sequencing identified *Clostridium* spp., *Prevotella* spp., and *Actinomyces* spp. as the main components of the small intestinal microbiota of children born during the Swedish CD epidemic in 2004–2007, concluding that these microbial groups could have been risk factors contributing to the increased disease incidence [33]. Nevertheless, these bacteria have not been found in new CD cases, suggesting that initial associations were casual, while causality between specific intestinal bacteria and CD onset has yet to be proven. Additional studies of the microbiota of adult CD patients by DGGE clustered the dominant microbial communities of healthy individuals together and separated from those of untreated CD patients [34]. Adult CD patients treated with a gluten-free diet also showed different DNA profiles and/or reduced diversity of *Lactobacillus* spp. and *Bifidobacterium* spp. [34, 35]. In agreement, quantitative analyses of the microbiota of healthy subjects under a gluten-free diet indicate that the diet per se reduced the numbers of *Lactobacillus* spp. and *Bifidobacterium* spp. and is partly responsible for the differences found between treated CD patients and controls [36]. The analysis of metabolites derived from intestinal microbiota activity has also revealed significant differences between treated CD patients and healthy adults, suggesting metabolic signatures of CD [34, 35]. In the most recent study, the duodenal microbiota of CD patients, stratified according to the disease manifestation for the first time, has been analyzed by DGGE [39]. The findings indicate that patients with gastrointestinal symptoms have differences in the microbiota structure (dominated by Proteobacteria) in comparison with those that have dermatitis herpetiformis and controls, suggesting that intestinal microbiota play a role in the manifestation of CD [39].

The isolation and identification of clones belonging to some bacterial groups associated with CD and characterization of their virulence-related genes have recently led to the identification of more specific differences between CD patients, with active and non-active disease, and controls [40, 41; Table 7.2]. *E. coli* clones belonging to virulent phylogenetic groups (B2 and D) isolated from untreated and treated CD patients carried a higher number of virulence genes encoding P fimbriae, capsule K5, and hemolysin than those isolated from healthy controls [40]. The isolation and identification of clones belonging to the genus *Staphylococcus* also revealed that *S. epidermidis* carrying methicillin-resistant genes (*mecA*) was more abundant in both treated and untreated CD patients than in controls [42]. Of the *Bacteroides* spp. isolated and identified from stools, *B. fragilis* carrying genes

Table 7.2 Summary of pathogenic features identified in gut bacteria isolated from celiac disease patients

Pathogenic bacteria	Virulence factor (gene) analyzed	Results	References
Escherichia coli	Phylogenetic classification in commensal (A + B1) and virulent (B2 + D) groups	The four phylogenetic groups were equally distributed in healthy control children.	[40]
	Type 1 fimbriae (*fimA*), P fimbriae (*papC*), S fimbriae (*sfaD/E*), Dr haemagglutinin (*draA*), haemolysin (*hlyA*), capsule K I (*neuB*), capsule k5 (*KfiC*), aerobactin (*iutA*)	↑ Virulent group B2 in patients with active CD ↑ Virulent group D in patients with non-active CD ↑ Carriage of genes coding for P fimbriae, capsule k5 and haemolysin in patients with active and non-active CD	
Bacteroides spp.	Metalloproteases (*bft* and *mpII*)	↑ *B. fragilis* isolates carrying genes coding for metalloproteases in patients with active and non-active CD	[41]
Staphylococcus spp.	Adhesion (*atlE* and *fbe*), cell aggregation (*icaD*), global regulatory (*agr* and *sar*), and methicillin-resistant (*mecA*)	↑ *Staphylococcus epidermidis* coding for the *mecA* gene and simultaneously for both the *mecA* and *atlE* genes in patients with active and non-active CD	[42]

encoding metalloproteases was more abundant in CD patients (treated with a gluten-free diet and untreated) than in healthy controls [41]. Taken together, these studies demonstrate that imbalances in gut microbiota of CD patients do not occur as a consequence of inflammatory processes associated with active phases of CD alone, and could primarily contribute to disease onset and pathological manifestations, although effects of the gluten-free diet cannot be ruled out [41].

In contrast, two other studies reported that the duodenal mucosa-associated microbiota was similar in untreated CD patients and controls by using a DNA profiling method based on amplification of the 16S-23S interspacer gene region [38] and quantitative reverse transcription PCR [37], which contradicts evidence supported by the majority of studies. The question of whether small intestine bacterial overgrowth (SIBO) is more prevalent in CD or when present is a contributor to refractory sprue was addressed in only one study reported by Chang and Green who found no benefit for the use of Rifaximin in CD patients with SIBO having poorly responsive disease [43].

Several mechanisms by which intestinal dysbiosis may influence pathogenesis of CD have been proposed, including the generation of toxic and immunogenic peptides from gliadins by their proteolytic activities [41], alteration of the gut barrier function and the composition of the glycocalix modifying bacterial adhesion and possible peptide translocation [44, 45], and activation of inflammatory cytokine production [46].

Defects in intestinal barrier function favor the access of gliadins to the lamina propria and its interaction with infiltrated lymphocytes and antigen presenting cells. Gliadins impair intestinal integrity through alterations of proteins (zonulin, occludin, cadherin, and claudins) involved in tight junctions between intestinal cells [47, 48]. This response occurs in parallel with the production of pro-inflammatory cytokines such as TNF-α and IL-1 β, exerting a negative feedback and increasing intestinal permeability [49, 50].

Patients with CD present increased production of type 2 mucin (MUC2), in comparison to patients on a gluten-free diet [32], associated with metaplasia of goblet cells and intestinal mucosal atrophy. Recent data from animal trials using intestinal loops also demonstrated the ability of potentially harmful enterobacteria (*E. coli* CBL2) and pathogens (*Shigella*) to reduce the number of goblet cells producing mucus and to increase intestinal permeability, leading to gliadin translocation to the lamina propria [46]. These enterobacteria also exert negative effects by reducing the production of a tissue inhibitor of a metalloprotease (TIMP-1) and increasing the secretion of vascular endothelial growth factor in intestinal loops [46]. In vitro studies in peripheral blood mononuclear cells (PBMCs) have indicated that these enterobacteria induce the production of IL-12 and/or interferon-γ, associated with increased expression of molecules HLA-DR and CD40, which could boost the adverse response to gluten [51]. In contrast, none of the effects described above have been observed for *Bifidobacterium bifidum* CECT 7365 and *Bifidobacterium longum* ATCC 15707 [46, 51]. *B. bifidum* CECT 7365 and *B. longum* CECT 7347 have also shown to exert positive effects increasing IL-10 and decreasing interferon-γ production by PBMCs [52].

Activation of toll-like receptors (TLRs), whose response may be enhanced by MHC-II molecules [53], play an important role in the recognition of microbial and other antigens, activation of different signaling pathways, expression of genes, and production of cytokines [54] regulating innate immunity (Fig. 7.1). Analyses of biopsies from CD patients have reported an increased expression of TLR2-sensing bacterial lipopeptides [37, 55–57] and TLR9-sensing bacterial DNA [37]; meanwhile, opposite results concerning TLR4 expression-sensing lipopolisaccharide from Gram-negative bacteria have been published [37, 55–57]. It can be hypothesized that increased expression of TLRs in the CD mucosa could amplify signaling through interactions with intestinal bacterial antigens and act together with gluten to immune activation. Activation of TLR3, for example, by virus, is known to induce cytokine production through a signaling pathway dependent on MyD88, which activates production of molecules related to type 1-like interferons that could contribute to insaturation of autoimmune diseases such as CD [58]. Moreover, wheat components such as the alpha-amylase/trypsin inhibitors like CM3 and 0.19, present in the globulin fraction of cereal grains, have also been identified as strong activators of TLR4 in monocytes, macrophages, and dendritic cells [59].

Potential Role of Probiotics in CD

The associations between CD and intestinal dysbiosis and the role attributed to some probiotics in the regulation of the gut barrier function and immunity in several inflammatory disease models have motivated investigations into the potential protective role of specific intestinal bacteria in CD [60, 61]. It has been suggested that these bacteria could contribute to reducing the risk and severity of the disease by their immunomodulatory features, capacity to eliminate immunogenic peptides from gluten, and improvement of intestinal permeability and restoration of the intestinal ecosystem (see Fig. 7.1).

In vitro studies have demonstrated the ability of different bifidobacteria (especially *B. longum* CECT 7347) to hydrolyze gliadin peptides, thereby generating products with lower inflammatory potential and cytotoxicity than those generated during simulated gastrointestinal digestion in absence of bifidobacteria [62]. Some other components of the *Rothia* genus from the oral cavity have also proved their proteolytic capacity on gluten peptides, cleaving down immunogenic epitopes, and reducing their inflammatory potential [63]. In addition, a strain of *Bifidobacterium lactis* positively counteracted harmful effects of toxic gliadin on intestinal epithelial cell culture integrity, reducing membrane ruffle formation [64].

Diverse studies indicate that specific probiotic strains can play a role in the production of chemokines and cytokines, determining Th1/Th2-cell balance and regulating oral tolerance to innocuous antigens [65]. Specific probiotic strains can also influence innate immune responses via their interaction with TLRs and antigen presenting cells, although most evidence comes from animal studies. Data from transgenic mice expressing HLA-DQ8 molecules demonstrate that maturation of dendritic cells, isolated from bone marrow of these animals, is favored by incubation with the different lactobacilli (*L. paracasei* IMPC2.1, *L. fermentum* BIO-DRL36, and *L. casei* ATCC 9595) showing strain-specific effects on TNFα production [66]. Moreover, the simultaneous administration of gliadins and *L. casei* ATCC 9595 to animals sensitized with indomethacin also boosted immune response of T (CD4+)-cells against gliadins in these transgenic mice [67]. The authors of the aforementioned study suggested the potential use of this strain as coadjutant in vaccines, favoring adaptive immunity against gluten antigens. Another study evaluated the influence of *B. longum* CECT 7347 orally administered to weanling Wistar rats, sensitized with interferon-γ, and fed gliadin to partially reproduce CD [61]. In this model, animals fed with this *Bifidobacterium* stain had lower numbers of peripheral T CD4+ and T regulatory (Treg) CD4+/Foxp3+ (forkhead transcription factor 3) cells and increased IL-10 production in jejunal sections compared to animals fed with placebo. However, human studies are required to confirm that CD patients and populations at risk of CD benefit from bifidobacteria and lactobacilli intake, evaluated preclinically to date.

In summary, scientific evidence from most human observational studies demonstrates that CD is associated with shifts in the assembly of intestinal microbiota to a state of dysbiosis that involves overgrowth of potentially pathogenic bacteria.

Although these perturbations are partially restored after adherence to a gluten-free diet and could be considered as a secondary consequence of the disease, they may alter the host-microbe crosstalk and contribute to CD pathogenesis. Furthermore, healthy infants at risk of developing CD also show alterations in the intestinal colonization pattern early in life, which suggest a primary role for the intestinal microbiota in this disorder. Altogether, findings indicate that gut microbiota and the impact of host and environmental perturbations on it could be part of the puzzling features of CD and its investigation could help to understand the disease onset and identify preventive strategies targeting the gut ecosystem.

Acknowledgments This work was supported by grants AGL2011-25169 and Consolider Fun-*C*-Food CSD2007-00063 from the Spanish Ministry of Economy and Competitiveness. The scholarship to M. Olivares and the postdoctoral contract to J.M. Laparra from CSIC are fully acknowledged.

References

1. Schuppan D, Junker Y, Barisani D. Celiac disease: from pathogenesis to novel therapies. Gastroenterology. 2009;137(6):1912–33.
2. Ludvigsson J, Lebwohl B, Kämpe O, Murray J, Green PH, Ekbom A. Risk of thyroid cancer in a nationwide cohort of patients with biopsy-verified celiac disease. Thyroid. 2013. doi:10.1089/thy.2012.0306.
3. Greco L, Romino R, Coto I, Di Cosmo N, Percopo S, Maglio M, Paparo F, et al. The first large population based twin study of coeliac disease. Gut. 2002;50:624–8.
4. Bahia M, Penna FJ, Del Castillo DM, Hassegawa MG, Vieira AC, Orlando VR. Discrepancy of celiac disease presentation in monozygotic twins. Arq Gastroenterol. 2010;47(1):56–60.
5. Sanz Y, De Palma G, Laparra M. Unraveling the ties between celiac disease and intestinal microbiota. Int Rev Immunol. 2011;30(4):207–18.
6. De Palma G, Capilla A, Nova E, Castillejo G, Varea V, Pozo T, Garrote JA, et al. Influence of milk-feeding type and genetic risk of developing coeliac disease on intestinal microbiota of infants: the PROFICEL study. PLoS One. 2012;7(2):e30791.
7. Pozo-Rubio T, Capilla A, Mujico JR, De Palma G, Marcos A, Sanz Y, et al. Influence of breast-feeding versus formula feeding on lymphocyte subsets in infants at risk of coeliac disease: the PROFICEL study. Eur J Nutr. 2012. doi:10.1007/s00394-012-0367-8.
8. Mårild K, Stephansson O, Montgomery S, Murray JA, Ludvigsson JF. Pregnancy outcome and risk of celiac disease in offspring: a nationwide case–control study. Gastroenterology. 2012;142(1):39–45.
9. Sandberg-Bennich S, Dahlquist G, Källén B. Coeliac disease is associated with intrauterine growth and neonatal infections. Acta Paediatr. 2002;91(1):30–3.
10. Jabri B, Sollid LM. Tissue-mediated control of immunopathology in coeliac disease. Nat Rev Immunol. 2009;9(12):858–70.
11. Stene LC, Honeyman MC, Hoffenberg EJ, Haas JE, Sokol RJ, Emery L, et al. Rotavirus infection frequency and risk of celiac disease autoimmunity in early childhood: a longitudinal study. Am J Gastroenterol. 2006;101(10):2333–40.
12. Sánchez E, De Palma G, Capilla A, Nova E, Pozo T, Castillejo G, et al. Influence of environmental and genetic factors linked to celiac disease risk on infant gut colonization by Bacteroides species. Appl Environ Microbiol. 2011;77(15):5316–23.
13. Daum S, Cellier C, Mulder CJ. Refractory coeliac disease. Best Pract Res Clin Gastroenterol. 2005;19(3):413–24.

14. Mooney PD, Evans KE, Singh S, Sanders DS. Treatment failure in coeliac disease: a practical guide to investigation and treatment of non-responsive and refractory coeliac disease. J Gastrointestin Liver Dis. 2012;21(2):197–203.
15. Malamut G, Murray JA, Cellier C. Refractory celiac disease. Gastrointest Endosc Clin N Am. 2012 Oct;22(4):759–72.
16. Toivanen P, Vaahtovuo J, Eerola E. Influence of major histocompatibility complex on bacterial composition of fecal flora. Infect Immun. 2001;69(4):2372–7.
17. Fernández L, Langa S, Martín V, Maldonado A, Jiménez E, Martín R, et al. The human milk microbiota: origin and potential roles in health and disease. Pharmacol Res. 2013;69(1):1–10.
18. Penders J, Thijs C, Vink C, Stelma FF, Snijders B, Kummeling I, et al. Factors influencing the composition of the intestinal microbiota in early infancy. Pediatrics. 2006;118(2):511–21.
19. Salminen S, Isolauri E. Intestinal colonization, microbiota, and prebiotics. J Pediatr. 2006;149:S115–20.
20. Bezirtzoglou E, Tsiotsias A, Welling GW. Microbiota profile in feces of breast- and formula-fed newborns by using fluorescence in situ hybridization (FISH). Anaerobe. 2011;17(6): 478–82.
21. Plot L, Amital H, Barzilai O, Ram M, Nicola B, Shoenfeld Y. Infections may have a protective role in the etiopathogenesis of celiac disease. Ann N Y Acad Sci. 2009;1173:670–84.
22. Kagnoff MF, Paterson YJ, Kumar PJ, Kasarda DD, Carbone FR, Unsworth DJ, et al. Evidence for the role of a human intestinal adenovirus in the pathogenesis of coeliac disease. Gut. 1987;28(8):995–1001.
23. Lähdeaho ML, Lehtinen M, Rissa HR, Hyöty H, Reunala T, Mäki M. Antipeptide antibodies to adenovirus E1b protein indicate enhanced risk of celiac disease and dermatitis herpetiformis. Int Arch Allergy Immunol. 1993;101(3):272–86.
24. Howdle PD, Blair Zajdel ME, Smart CJ, Trejdosiewicz LK, Blair GE, Losowky MS. Lack of a serologic response to an E1B protein of adenovirus 12 in coeliac disease. Scand J Gastroenterol. 1989;24(3):282–96.
25. Lindgren S, Sjöberg K, Eriksson S. Unsuspected coeliac disease in chronic cryptogenic liver disease. Scand J Gastroenterol. 1994;29(7):661–74.
26. Volta U, De Franceschi L, Molinaro N, Cassani F, Muratori L, Lenzi M, et al. Frequency and significance of anti-gliadin and anti-endomysial antibodies in autoimmune hepatitis. Dig Dis Sci. 1998;43(10):2190–5.
27. Hernández L, Johnson TC, Naiyer AJ, Kryszak D, Ciaccio EJ, Min A, et al. Chronic hepatitis C virus and celiac disease, is there an association? Dig Dis Sci. 2008;53(1):256–61.
28. Verdú EF, Mauro M, Bourgeois J, Armstrong D. Clinical onset of celiac disease after an episode of Campylobacter jejuni enteritis. Can J Gastroenterol. 2007;21(7):453–65.
29. Nadal I, Donat E, Ribes-Koninckx C, Calabuig M, Sanz Y. Imbalance in the composition of the duodenal microbiota of children with coeliac disease. J Med Microbiol. 2007;56:1669–74.
30. Collado MC, Donat E, Ribes-Koninckx C, Calabuig M, Sanz Y. Specific duodenal and faecal bacterial groups associated with paediatric coeliac disease. J Clin Pathol. 2009;62(3):264–9.
31. Schippa S, Iebba V, Barbato M, Di Nardo G, Totino V, Checchi MP, et al. A distinctive 'microbial signature' in celiac pediatric patients. BMC Microbiol. 2010;10:175.
32. Forsberg G, Fahlgren A, Hörstedt P, Hammarström S, Hernell O, Hammarström ML. Presence of bacteria and innate immunity of intestinal epithelium in childhood celiac disease. Am J Gastroenterol. 2004;99(5):894–904.
33. Ou G, Hedberg M, Hörstedt P, Baranov V, Forsberg G, Drobni M, et al. Proximal small intestinal microbiota and identification of rod-shaped bacteria associated with childhood celiac disease. Am J Gastroenterol. 2009;104(12):3058–67.
34. Nistal E, Caminero A, Vivas S, de Morales JM R, de Miera LE S, Rodríguez-Aparicio LB, et al. Differences in faecal bacteria populations and faecal bacteria metabolism in healthy adults and celiac disease patients. Biochimie. 2012;94(8):1724–9.
35. Di Cagno R, De Angelis M, De Pasquale I, Ndagijimana M, Vernocchi P, Ricciuti P, et al. Duodenal and faecal microbiota of celiac children: molecular, phenotype and metabolome characterization. BMC Microbiol. 2011;11:219.

36. De Palma G, Nadal I, Collado MC, Sanz Y. Effects of a gluten-free diet on gut microbiota and immune function in healthy adult human subjects. Br J Nutr. 2009;102(8):1154–60.
37. Kalliomäki M, Satokari R, Lähteenoja H, Vähämiko S, Grönlund J, Routi T, Salminen S. Expression of microbiota, Toll-like receptors, and their regulators in the small intestinal mucosa in celiac disease. J Pediatr Gastroenterol Nutr. 2012;54(6):727–32.
38. de Meij TG, Budding AE, Grasman ME, Kneepkens CM, Savelkoul PH, Mearin ML. Composition and diversity of the duodenal mucosa-associated microbiome in children with untreated coeliac disease. Scand J Gastroenterol. 2013;48(5):530–6.
39. Wacklin P, Kaukinen K, Tuovinen E, Collin P, Lindfors K, Partanen J, et al. The duodenal microbiota composition of adult celiac disease patients is associated with the clinical manifestation of the disease. Inflamm Bowel Dis. 2013;19(5):934–41.
40. Sánchez E, Nadal I, Donat E, Ribes-Koninckx C, Calabuig M, Sanz Y. Reduced diversity and increased virulence-gene carriage in intestinal enterobacteria of coeliac children. BMC Gastroenterol. 2008;8:50.
41. Sánchez E, Laparra JM, Sanz Y. Discerning the role of *Bacteroides fragilis* in celiac disease pathogenesis. Appl Environ Microbiol. 2012;78(18):6507–15.
42. Sánchez E, Ribes-Koninckx C, Calabuig M, Sanz Y. Intestinal Staphylococcus spp. and virulent features associated with coeliac disease. J Clin Pathol. 2012;65(9):830–4.
43. Chang MS, Green PH. A review of rifaximin and bacterial overgrowth in poorly responsive celiac disease. Therap Adv Gastroenterol. 2012;5(1):31–6.
44. Koropatkin NM, Cameron EA, Martens EC. How glycan metabolism shapes the human gut microbiota. Nat Rev Microbiol. 2012;10(5):323–35.
45. Vecchi M, Torgano G, Tronconi S, Agape D, Ronchi G. Evidence of altered structural and secretory glycoconjugates in the jejunalmucosa of patients with gluten sensitive enteropathy and subtotal villous atrophy. Gut. 1989;30:804–10.
46. Cinova J, De Palma G, Stepankova R, Kofronova O, Kverka M, Sanz Y, et al. Role of intestinal bacteria in gliadin-induced changes in intestinal mucosa: study in germ-free rats. PLoS One. 2011;6(1):e16169.
47. Clemente MG, Virgiliis S, Kang JS, Macatagney R, Musu MP, Di Pierro MR, et al. Early effects of gliadin on enterocyte intracellular signalling involved in intestinal barrier function. Gut. 2003;52(2):218–23.
48. Lammers KM, Lu R, Brownley J, Lu B, Gerard C, Thomas K, et al. Gliadin induces an increase in intestinal permeability and zonulin release by binding to the chemokine receptor CXCR3. Gastroenterology. 2008;135(1):194–204. e3.
49. Ma D, Forsythe P, Bienenstock J. Live lactobacillus reuteri is essential for the inhibitory effect on tumor necrosis factor alpha-induced interleukin-8 expression. Infect Immun. 2004;72(9): 5308–14.
50. Victoni T, Coelho FR, Soares AL, de Freitas A, Secher T, Guabiraba R, et al. Local and remote tissue injury upon intestinal ischemia and reperfusion depends on the TLR/MyD88 signaling pathway. Med Microbiol Immunol. 2010;199(1):35–42.
51. De Palma G, Cinova J, Stepankova R, Tuckova L, Sanz Y. Pivotal advance: bifidobacteria and gram negative bacteria differentially influence immune responses in the proinflammatory milieu of celiac disease. J Leuko Biol. 2010;87:765–78.
52. Medina M, De Palma G, Ribes-Koninckx C, Calabuig M, Sanz Y. Bifidobacterium strains suppress in vitro the pro-inflammatory milieu triggered by the large intestinal microbiota of coeliac patients. J Inflamm. 2008;5:19.
53. Frei R, Steinle J, Birchler T, Loeliger S, Roduit C, Steinhoff D, et al. MHC class II molecules enhance Toll-like receptor mediated innate immune responses. PLoS One. 2010;5(1):e8808.
54. Medzhitov R. Toll-like receptors and innate immunity. Nat Rev Immunol. 2001;1:135–45.
55. Szebeni B, Veres G, Dezsofi A, Rusai K, Vannay A, Bokodi G, et al. Increased mucosal expression of Toll-like receptor (TLR)2 and TLR4 in coeliac disease. J Pediatr Gastroenterol Nutr. 2007;45(2):187–93.
56. Cseh Á, Vásárhelyi B, Szalay B, Molnár K, Nagy-Szakál D, Treszl A, et al. Immune phenotype of children with newly diagnosed and gluten-free diet-treated celiac disease. Dig Dis Sci. 2011;56(3):792–8.

57. Eiró N, González-Reyes S, González L, González LO, Altadill A, Andicoechea A, et al. Duodenal expression of Toll-like receptors and interleukins are increased in both children and adult celiac patients. Dig Dis Sci. 2012;57(9):2278–85.
58. Alexopoulou L, Holt AC, Medzhitov R, Flavell RA. Recognition of double-stranded RNA and activation of NF-kappaB by Toll-like receptor 3. Nature. 2001;413:732–8.
59. Junker Y, Zeissig S, Kim SJ, Barisani D, Wieser H, Leffler DA, et al. Wheat amylase trypsin inhibitors drive intestinal inflammation via activation of toll-like receptor 4. J Exp Med. 2012;209(13):2395–408.
60. D'Arienzo R, Stefanile R, Maurano F, Mazzarella G, Ricca E, Troncone R, et al. Immunomodulatory effects of *Lactobacillus casei* administration in a mouse model of gliadin-sensitive enteropathy. Scand J Immunol. 2011;74(4):335–41.
61. Laparra JM, Olivares M, Gallina O, Sanz Y. Bifidobacterium longum CECT 7347 modulates immune responses in a gliadin-induced enteropathy animal model. PLoS One. 2012;7(2): e30744.
62. Laparra JM, Sanz Y. Bifidobacteria inhibit the inflammatory response induced by gliadins in intestinal epithelial cells via modifications of toxic peptide generation during digestion. J Cell Biochem. 2010;109(4):801–7.
63. Zamakhchari M, Wei G, Dewhirst F, Lee J, Schuppan D, Oppenheim FG, et al. Identification of Rothia bacteria as gluten-degrading natural colonizers of the upper gastro-intestinal tract. PLoS One. 2011;6(9):e24455.
64. Lindfors K, Blomqvist T, Juuti-Uusitalo K, Stenman S, Venäläinen J, Mäki M, et al. Live probiotic Bifidobacterium lactis bacteria inhibit the toxic effects induced by wheat gliadin in epithelial cell culture. Clin Exp Immunol. 2008;152(3):552–8.
65. Isolauri E, Sütas Y, Kankaanpää P, Arvilommi H, Salminen S. Probiotics: effects on immunity. Am J Clin Nutr. 2001;73:444S–50.
66. D'Arienzo R, Maurano F, Lavermicocca P, Ricca E, Rossi M. Modulation of the immune response by probiotic strains in a mouse model of gluten sensitivity. Cytokines. 2009;48: 254–9.
67. D'Arienzo R, Maurano F, Luongo D, Mazzarella G, Stefanile R, Troncone R, et al. Adjuvant effect of *Lactobacillus casei* in a mouse model of gluten sensitivity. Immunol Lett. 2008;119: 78–83.

Chapter 8
Presentation of Celiac Disease in Children and Adults

Norelle Rizkalla Reilly and Peter H.R. Green

Celiac disease (CD) is common; however, the vast majority of people with CD are undiagnosed [1, 2]. Originally considered a malabsorptive condition of childhood [3–5], it is now diagnosed at any age [6–8]. The wide spectrum of presenting symptoms of affected individuals makes the condition challenging to diagnose in some. Symptoms vary significantly from childhood to adulthood, and, even among children, distinct trends in presentations may be seen according to age.

Terminology and Definitions

There have been several terms used to classify the presentations of CD in both childhood and adulthood. Such terms as "typical," "atypical," "classical," "nonclassical," "silent," "asymptomatic," "latent," and "potential celiac disease" have added confusion to the topic. Recently, consensus documents have attempted to bring clarity to the field [9]. When used to describe the presentation of CD, the terms "typical" and "atypical" are particularly perplexing, as they suggest the opposite of what they are intended to reflect. "Typical" symptoms are now far less common than the "atypical." In this regard the terms "classical" and "nonclassical" are preferable since they refer to the historical perception of the nature of disease presentations while not alluding to their frequency. Additionally, the term "asymptomatic" is preferred to "silent" in referring to those with CD without symptoms.

N.R. Reilly, M.D.
Division of Pediatric Gastroenterology, Columbia University Medical Center, Celiac Disease Center at Columbia University, New York, NY, USA

P.H.R. Green, M.D. (✉)
Department of Medicine, Columbia University Medical Center, Celiac Disease Center at Columbia University, 180 Fort Washington Avenue, Suite 936, New York, NY 10032, USA
e-mail: pg11@columbia.edu

S.D. Rampertab and G.E. Mullin (eds.), *Celiac Disease*, Clinical Gastroenterology,
DOI 10.1007/978-1-4614-8560-5_8,

Presenting Symptoms of Celiac Disease in Children and Adults

The majority of children with CD tend to present in one of three ways: with abdominal pain or distension, with growth issues, or through an asymptomatic presentation brought about by serological screening performed due to an associated condition or family history of CD [10–14].

Very young children commonly present with "classical," usually diarrheal, symptoms [15–18]. However, in our recent experience and as described by other authors, the classical presentation of childhood CD is no longer the most common. Children presenting with diarrhea are currently among the minority when all patients with CD are considered; only 9 % of our pediatric patients presented this way, suggesting that diarrhea and malabsorption are no longer the characteristic manifestations of this disease among young patients [10, 19, 20]. Moreover, the bulk of children with diarrheal presentations are below 2 years of age [10, 21]. In contrast, older children and adolescents more often present with nonclassical or "atypical" gastrointestinal complaints such as abdominal pain, vomiting, and constipation and extraintestinal symptoms such as arthritis, neurologic symptoms, or anemia. Some may have asymptomatic disease, diagnosed upon serological screening [11, 17] (Fig. 8.1). Screening was the mode of presentation of about 25 % of children seen in our center [19] and includes family members of adults and children previously diagnosed with CD, many of whom were asymptomatic, as well as those with associated autoimmune conditions [10].

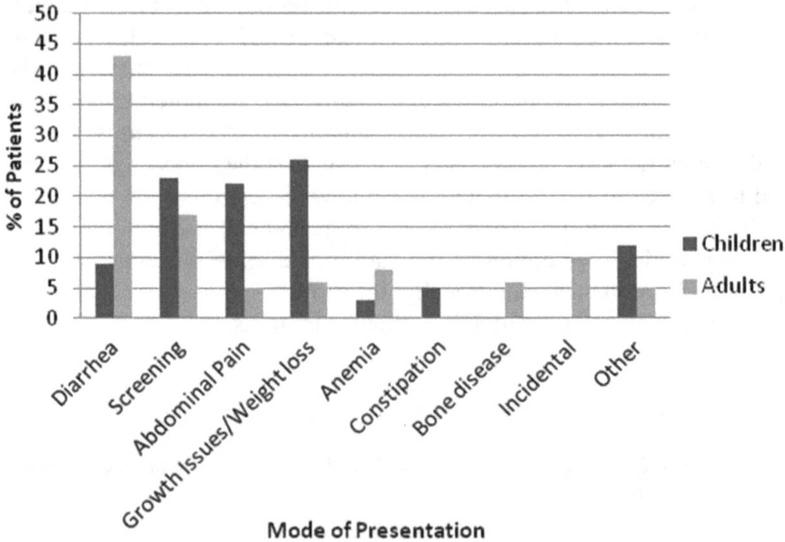

Fig. 8.1 Presenting symptoms of children and adults with CD. Adults $n = 1{,}499$, children $n = 318$

Among adults, the major mode of presentation is diarrhea, comprising about 50 % of patients [22, 23]. One potential explanation for the increase in diarrheal presentations in this group is the relative infrequency with which young adults present for routine medical care, resulting in missed opportunities to unearth subtle symptoms of CD. Diarrheal symptoms may drive many such patients to seek medical attention early. However, the elderly had a similar rate of diarrhea presentations as young adults in one study [23].

Serological screening of at-risk groups, responsible for increased detection of CD in children, is an important mode of presentation among adults as well [24]. About 10 % of those adults recently diagnosed with CD at our center presented through screening of at-risk groups (see Fig. 8.1). However, not all of those individuals detected by screening are in fact asymptomatic [25, 26].

Anemia is more frequently seen at presentation in adults compared to children [27]. Anemia as a presenting symptom of CD is mainly due to iron deficiency, though anemia due to nutritional factors and chronic disease may also be present at diagnosis of CD [28, 29].

Osteoporosis is another presentation of CD in adults. Reduced bone density is common in patients with CD [30, 31], and there is increased fracture risk [32, 33]. Bone mineral density correlated inversely with the duodenal Marsh stage in one study of Spanish adults with CD, though differences in parathyroid hormone and IGF-1 among patients with and without villous atrophy were not observed [34]. A study from the United States demonstrated an increased prevalence of CD among osteoporotic patients [35], though this was not seen in other studies from France and among postmenopausal women in Turkey [36, 37]. Low bone mineral density is commonly seen in children with CD at the time of diagnosis, and some reversal is seen upon dietary treatment [38, 39]. However, this is not typically a presenting symptom of CD in children, and this finding appears to be unrelated to other symptoms at diagnosis [40]. Early diagnosis of children with CD and early management of existing metabolic bone disease may be an important factor in preventing adult osteoporosis related to CD.

Another important mode of presentation among adults is the incidental recognition of signs of villous atrophy due to CD during endoscopy performed for any reason [41]. Upper endoscopy in adults is commonly performed for gastroesophageal reflux disease (GERD). Increasingly biopsies of the duodenum are performed at endoscopy, regardless of the appearance of the duodenal mucosa. When CD is recognized and treated in people with GERD, improvement in the reflux is frequently noted [42]. There is a reasonable argument for routine duodenal biopsies during endoscopy for adults as is the usual practice for pediatric gastroenterologists [43].

Other presentations in adults include dermatitis herpetiformis, irritable bowel syndrome, bloating, and chronic fatigue as well as a variety of neurological presentations [44]. Many of the symptoms of CD are common, frequently seen among patients attending primary care visits [45]. In a multicenter North American primary care screening study involving patients with a variety of symptoms, including bloating, fatigue, recurrent abdominal pain, and IBS, screening for CD resulted in a 40-fold increase in the rate of CD diagnosis [46].

Recurrent episodes of abdominal pain are seen prior to diagnosis in adults and children [19, 47], but seems to occur less frequently in adults. These episodes of pain may be due to small intestinal intussusceptions that appear commonly in CD [48, 49]. Intussusceptions are more prevalent among children with CD than the general population [50].

The reason that some patients present with diarrhea and others are asymptomatic is not clear, for there is no correlation of a diarrheal presentation with severity of villous atrophy [51], nor length of bowel involved as assessed by video capsule endoscopy [52]. Neurohumoral mechanisms may be important in determining the presence of symptoms. In one study, patients with CD had increased mucosal 5-hydroxy tryptamine content and enhanced release from the upper small bowel, which correlates with postprandial dyspepsia [53].

There are geographic differences in the presentation of CD. While our institutional observations of age-related differences in disease presentation have been described by other authors as well [10, 11], greater frequencies of diarrheal presentations among children have been noted in countries such as Spain [15], India [54], and Sudan [55]. Particularly in developing countries, the malnutrition associated with CD in children may be severe, and in some cases refeeding syndrome is seen upon treatment [56]. Among adults, similar differences have been cited, with Turkish adults presenting at a younger age and more frequently with classic symptoms than American adults [57].

Childhood Factors Influencing Disease Onset and Presentation

Several factors determined during the perinatal period and infancy may impact the presentation of CD. Route of delivery seems to play a role, as there is an association between cesarean delivery and development of CD [58], especially elective cesarean section [59]. Summer birth was associated with an increased risk of CD diagnosis in children [60], as well as in adults [61]. In the latter study, however, the effect was less pronounced among adults, and the association overall did not seem to be influenced by infectious exposure [60]. Breast-feeding practices additionally appear to influence the mode of presentation. Children who were exclusively breast-fed were less likely to present with failure to thrive and short stature [62]. Breast-feeding also contributes to delaying the age of presentation of the disease [63–65]. Differences in the microbiota of the infant gut caused by genetics, methods of delivery, and infant feeding, and resulting immune alterations, may explain these observations [66–69].

The timing of gluten introduction in infancy is a subject of ongoing study. Gluten introduction either too early or too late in infancy may pose a risk of CD autoimmunity in genetically predisposed infants [70, 71]. In another study, infants appeared to be at less risk of celiac autoimmunity with delayed gluten introduction, and differences in the microbiota were observed between infants with genetic risk for CD and those from a general pool of controls [72]. In addition, large quantities of gluten at the time of introduction were associated with a greater risk for developing CD [64].

At-Risk Individuals and Associated Conditions

The most frequently screened group is family members of individuals with CD, and this mode of presentation is important in both adults and children [25]. Several studies have shown that about 4–10 % of first-degree relatives have the disease [73]. The greatest risk is among siblings of affected individuals [74], but the risk extends to second-degree relatives as well [25, 74].

The list of conditions associated with CD is quite extensive, and there are specific individuals who are frequently screened for CD. The association between CD and type 1 diabetes in children is well described [75]. The coexistence of both diseases also occurs in adults [76, 77]. The presentation of diabetes generally precedes that of CD. While an increased prevalence of CD has been described in adults with autoimmune thyroid disease [78, 79], this association may not exist in children [80].

Children and adolescents with autoimmune liver disease, including biliary disease, have a high prevalence of CD [81, 82]. An increased prevalence of CD has additionally been identified in children with Down syndrome (7 %) [83], Turner syndrome (6.4 %) [84], and Williams syndrome (9.5 %) [85].

Other conditions that have been associated with CD include autoimmune myocarditis; idiopathic dilated cardiomyopathy; Sjögren's syndrome; IgA deficiency; Addison's disease; IgA nephropathy; sarcoidosis; primary hyperparathyroidism; alopecia areata; neurological abnormalities including epilepsy, ataxia, and neuropathy; atopy; inflammatory bowel disease; psoriasis; and chronic urticaria.

The association with CD and autoimmune disorders is great. About 30 % of adult patients with CD have one or more autoimmune disorders [86, 87], compared to about 3 % in the general population [88]. The mechanism of this prominent association is unclear. It has been suggested that the increase is associated with the duration of exposure to gluten [87]; however, this was not confirmed by other studies [89, 90]. In a study from France, however, after the diagnosis of CD, those that were strictly adherent to the gluten-free diet acquired fewer autoimmune disorders than those who were not compliant with the diet [91]. This suggests that the diet is protective against the development of autoimmune diseases. However, initiation of a gluten-free diet did not prevent progression of established autoimmune thyroid disease after the diagnosis of CD [92].

CD is also associated with infertility, in both women [93–95] and men [96]. Screening infertile women detects undiagnosed CD [97], and fertility improves after diagnosis of CD [98].

The Shifting Presentation of Celiac Disease

Most adults with CD diagnosed prior to 1980 presented with diarrhea [22]. With the advent of serological tests in the 1980s, the spectrum of clinical manifestations became apparent. Additionally, since the initial availability of sensitive and specific serological assays over the past two decades, the gap between initial presentation and diagnosis in symptomatic children has been gradually fading [99, 100]. This reduction in duration of symptoms has also been documented in adults [22]. Serological screening was an important mode of presentation among our patients, representing nearly one-quarter of all children recently diagnosed [19] and 17 % of adults diagnosed since 1990 [24].

Independent of the impact of improved screening tools, the presentation of CD is changing over time, and "classical" presentations are becoming less common. An overall decrease in the prevalence of diarrheal presentations over the past two decades, accompanied by an increase in atypical manifestations of the disease, has been well described in both adults and children [10, 16, 22, 24]. Children are being diagnosed at an older age [20, 101]. Overweight and obese children and adolescents with CD are now frequently identified [19, 102, 103]. The majority of North American children, in our series, had a normal body mass index, whereas the minority of children studied were underweight [19]. While more widespread use of serologic markers has facilitated diagnosis of CD in children [10], this alone does not entirely explain the decrease in diarrheal manifestations, as many long-term studies of adult and pediatric patients predating the use of these markers have documented this shift in clinical presentation [20, 22]. Awareness of the various manifestations of this disease is critical in rendering the diagnosis.

References

1. Rubio-Tapia A, Ludvigsson JF, Brantner TL, Murray JA, Everhart JE. The prevalence of celiac disease in the United States. Am J Gastroenterol. 2012;107(10):1538–44. quiz 7, 45.
2. West J, Logan RF, Hill PG, Lloyd A, Lewis S, Hubbard R, et al. Seroprevalence, correlates, and characteristics of undetected coeliac disease in England. Gut. 2003;52(7):960–5.
3. Andersen DH. Celiac syndrome. J Pediatr. 1947;30:564–82.
4. Dickie WK. Coeliac disease. Investigation of the harmful effects of certain types of cereal on patients with coeliac disease. Utrecht: Thesis, University of Utrecht; 1950.
5. Wilson R. The coeliac syndrome with adolescent rickets. Ir J Med Sci. 1951;6(301):39–42.
6. Sleisenger MH, Rynbergen HJ, Pert JH, Almy TP. Treatment of non-tropical sprue: a wheat-, rye-, and oat-free diet. J Am Diet Assoc. 1957;33(11):1137–40.
7. Benson GD, Kowlessar OD, Sleisenger MH. Adult celiac disease with emphasis upon response to the gluten-free diet. Medicine (Baltimore). 1964;43:1–40.
8. Mortimer PE, Stewart JS, Norman AP, Booth CC. Follow-up study of coeliac disease. Br Med J. 1968;3(5609):7–9.
9. Ludvigsson JF, Leffler DA, Bai JC, Biagi F, Fasano A, Green PH, et al. The Oslo definitions for coeliac disease and related terms. Gut. 2013;62(1):43–52.

10. McGowan KE, Castiglione DA, Butzner JD. The changing face of childhood celiac disease in north america: impact of serological testing. Pediatrics. 2009;124(6):1572–8.
11. Tanpowpong P, Broder-Fingert S, Katz AJ, Camargo Jr CA. Age-related patterns in clinical presentations and gluten-related issues among children and adolescents with celiac disease. Clin Transl Gastroenterol. 2012;3:e9.
12. Ravikumara M, Tuthill DP, Jenkins HR. The changing clinical presentation of coeliac disease. Arch Dis Child. 2006;91(12):969–71.
13. White LE, Bannerman E, McGrogan P, Kastner-Cole D, Carnegie E, Gillett PM. Childhood coeliac disease diagnoses in Scotland 2009-2010: the SPSU project. Arch Dis Child. 2013;98(1):52–6.
14. Llorente-Alonso MJ, Fernandez-Acenero MJ, Sebastian M. Gluten intolerance: sex and age-related features. Can J Gastroenterol. 2006;20(11):719–22.
15. Vivas S, Ruiz de Morales JM, Fernandez M, Hernando M, Herrero B, Casqueiro J, et al. Age-related clinical, serological, and histopathological features of celiac disease. Am J Gastroenterol. 2008;103(9):2360–5. quiz 2366.
16. Telega G, Bennet TR, Werlin S. Emerging new clinical patterns in the presentation of celiac disease. Arch Pediatr Adolesc Med. 2008;162(2):164–8.
17. Ludvigsson JF, Ansved P, Falth-Magnusson K, Hammersjo JA, Johansson C, Edvardsson S, et al. Symptoms and signs have changed in Swedish children with coeliac disease. J Pediatr Gastroenterol Nutr. 2004;38(2):181–6.
18. Branski D, Troncone R. Celiac disease: a reappraisal. J Pediatr. 1998;133(2):181–7.
19. Reilly NR, Aguilar K, Hassid BG, Cheng J, Defelice AR, Kazlow P, et al. Celiac disease in normal-weight and overweight children: clinical features and growth outcomes following a gluten-free diet. J Pediatr Gastroenterol Nutr. 2011;53(5):528–31.
20. Garampazzi A, Rapa A, Mura S, Capelli A, Valori A, Boldorini R, et al. Clinical pattern of celiac disease is still changing. J Pediatr Gastroenterol Nutr. 2007;45(5):611–4.
21. Rizkalla Reilly N, Dixit R, Simpson S, Green PH. Celiac disease in children: an old disease with new features. Minerva Pediatr. 2012;64(1):71–81.
22. Rampertab SD, Pooran N, Brar P, Singh P, Green PH. Trends in the presentation of celiac disease. Am J Med. 2006;119(4):355. e9–14.
23. Mukherjee R, Egbuna I, Brar P, Hernandez L, McMahon DJ, Shane EJ, et al. Celiac disease: similar presentations in the elderly and young adults. Dig Dis Sci. 2010;55(11):3147–53.
24. Lo W, Sano K, Lebwohl B, Diamond B, Green PH. Changing presentation of adult celiac disease. Dig Dis Sci. 2003;48(2):395–8.
25. Fasano A, Berti I, Gerarduzzi T, Not T, Colletti RB, Drago S, et al. Prevalence of celiac disease in at-risk and not-at-risk groups in the United States: a large multicenter study. Arch Intern Med. 2003;163(3):286–92.
26. Aggarwal S, Lebwohl B, Green PH. Screening for celiac disease in average-risk and high-risk populations. Therap Adv Gastroenterol. 2012;5(1):37–47.
27. Rodrigo-Saez L, Fuentes-Alvarez D, Perez-Martinez I, Alvarez-Mieres N, Nino-Garcia P, de-Francisco-Garcia R, et al. Differences between pediatric and adult celiac disease. Rev Esp Enferm Dig. 2011;103(5):238–44.
28. Harper JW, Holleran SF, Ramakrishnan R, Bhagat G, Green PH. Anemia in celiac disease is multifactorial in etiology. Am J Hematol. 2007;82(11):996–1000.
29. Bergamaschi G, Markopoulos K, Albertini R, Di Sabatino A, Biagi F, Ciccocioppo R, et al. Anemia of chronic disease and defective erythropoietin production in patients with celiac disease. Haematologica. 2008;93(12):1785–91.
30. Valdimarsson T, Toss G, Ross I, Lofman O, Strom M. Bone mineral density in coeliac disease. Scand J Gastroenterol. 1994;29(5):457–61.
31. Meyer D, Stavropolous S, Diamond B, Shane E, Green PH. Osteoporosis in a north american adult population with celiac disease. Am J Gastroenterol. 2001;96(1):112–9.

32. Vasquez H, Mazure R, Gonzalez D, Flores D, Pedreira S, Niveloni S, et al. Risk of fractures in celiac disease patients: a cross-sectional, case-control study. Am J Gastroenterol. 2000;95(1):183–9.
33. West J, Logan RF, Card TR, Smith C, Hubbard R. Fracture risk in people with celiac disease: a population-based cohort study. Gastroenterology. 2003;125(2):429–36.
34. Garcia-Manzanares A, Tenias JM, Lucendo AJ. Bone mineral density directly correlates with duodenal Marsh stage in newly diagnosed adult celiac patients. Scand J Gastroenterol. 2012;8–9(47):927–36.
35. Stenson WF, Newberry R, Lorenz R, Baldus C, Civitelli R. Increased prevalence of celiac disease and need for routine screening among patients with osteoporosis. Arch Intern Med. 2005;165(4):393–9.
36. Legroux-Gerot I, Leloire O, Blanckaert F, Tonnel F, Grardel B, Ducrocq JL, et al. Screening for celiac disease in patients with osteoporosis. Joint Bone Spine. 2009;76(2):162–5.
37. Kavuncu V, Dundar U, Ciftci IH, Evcik D, Yigit I. Is there any requirement for celiac disease screening routinely in postmenapausal women with osteoporosis? Rheumatol Int. 2009;29(7):841–5.
38. Kalayci AG, Kansu A, Girgin N, Kucuk O, Aras G. Bone mineral density and importance of a gluten-free diet in patients with celiac disease in childhood. Pediatrics. 2001;108(5):E89.
39. Kavak US, Yuce A, Kocak N, Demir H, Saltik IN, Gurakan F, et al. Bone mineral density in children with untreated and treated celiac disease. J Pediatr Gastroenterol Nutr. 2003;37(4):434–6.
40. Turner J, Pellerin G, Mager D. Prevalence of metabolic bone disease in children with celiac disease is independent of symptoms at diagnosis. J Pediatr Gastroenterol Nutr. 2009;49(5):589–93.
41. Green PH, Shane E, Rotterdam H, Forde KA, Grossbard L. Significance of unsuspected celiac disease detected at endoscopy. Gastrointest Endosc. 2000;51(1):60–5.
42. Nachman F, Vazquez H, Gonzalez A, Andrenacci P, Compagni L, Reyes H, et al. Gastroesophageal reflux symptoms in patients with celiac disease and the effects of a gluten-free diet. Clin Gastroenterol Hepatol. 2011;9(3):214–9.
43. Green PH, Murray JA. Routine duodenal biopsies to exclude celiac disease? Gastrointest Endosc. 2003;58(1):92–5.
44. Chin RL, Latov N, Green PH, Brannagan 3rd TH, Alaedini A, Sander HW. Neurologic complications of celiac disease. J Clin Neuromuscul Dis. 2004;5(3):129–37.
45. Hin H, Bird G, Fisher P, Mahy N, Jewell D. Coeliac disease in primary care: case finding study. BMJ. 1999;318(7177):164–7.
46. Catassi C, Kryszak D, Louis-Jacques O, Duerksen DR, Hill I, Crowe SE, et al. Detection of celiac disease in primary care: a multicenter case-finding study in North America. Am J Gastroenterol. 2007;102(7):1454–60.
47. Sanders DS, Hopper AD, Azmy IA, Rahman N, Hurlstone DP, Leeds JS, et al. Association of adult celiac disease with surgical abdominal pain: a case-control study in patients referred to secondary care. Ann Surg. 2005;242(2):201–7.
48. Gonda TA, Khan SU, Cheng J, Lewis SK, Rubin M, Green PH. Association of intussusception and celiac disease in adults. Dig Dis Sci. 2010;55(10):2899–903.
49. Sanders DS, Azmy IA, Kong SC, Lee FK. Symptomatic small bowel intussusception: a surgical opportunity to diagnose adult celiac disease? Gastrointest Endosc. 2004;59(1):161–2.
50. Reilly NR, Aguilar KM, Green PH. Should intussusception in children prompt screening for celiac disease? J Pediatr Gastroenterol Nutr. 2013;56:56–9.
51. Brar P, Kwon GY, Egbuna I, Holleran S, Ramakrishnan R, Bhagat G, et al. Lack of correlation of degree of villous atrophy with severity of clinical presentation of coeliac disease. Dig Liver Dis. 2007;39(1):26–9.
52. Murray JA, Rubio-Tapia A, Van Dyke CT, Brogan DL, Knipschield MA, Lahr B, et al. Mucosal atrophy in celiac disease: extent of involvement, correlation with clinical presentation, and response to treatment. Clin Gastroenterol Hepatol. 2008;6(2):186–93. quiz 25.

53. Coleman NS, Foley S, Dunlop SP, Wheatcroft J, Blackshaw E, Perkins AC, et al. Abnormalities of serotonin metabolism and their relation to symptoms in untreated celiac disease. Clin Gastroenterol Hepatol. 2006;4(7):874–81.
54. Kochhar R, Jain K, Thapa BR, Rawal P, Khaliq A, Bhadada S, et al. Clinical presentation of celiac disease among pediatric compared to adolescent and adult patients. Indian J Gastroenterol. 2012;31(3):116–20.
55. Ageep AK. Celiac disease in the Red Sea state of Sudan. Trop Gastroenterol. 2012;33(2): 118–22.
56. Agarwal J, Poddar U, Yachha SK, Srivastava A. Refeeding syndrome in children in developing countries who have celiac disease. J Pediatr Gastroenterol Nutr. 2012;54(4):521–4.
57. Palabykoglu M, Botoman VA, Coban S, Ormeci N, Bonner GF, Woodhouse S, et al. A tale of two cities: typical celiac sprue presenting symptoms are significantly more common in Turkish than in US Patients. J Clin Gastroenterol. 2008;42(1):62–5.
58. Decker E, Engelmann G, Findeisen A, Gerner P, Laass M, Ney D, et al. Cesarean delivery is associated with celiac disease but not inflammatory bowel disease in children. Pediatrics. 2010;125(6):e1433–40.
59. Marild K, Stephansson O, Montgomery S, Murray JA, Ludvigsson JF. Pregnancy outcome and risk of celiac disease in offspring: a nationwide case-control study. Gastroenterology. 2012;142(1):39–45. e3.
60. Lebwohl B, Green PH, Murray JA, Ludvigsson JF. Season of birth in a nationwide cohort of coeliac disease patients. Arch Dis Child. 2013;98(1):48–51.
61. Ivarsson A, Hernell O, Nystrom L, Persson LA. Children born in the summer have increased risk for coeliac disease. J Epidemiol Community Health. 2003;57(1):36–9.
62. D'Amico MA, Holmes J, Stavropoulos SN, Frederick M, Levy J, DeFelice AR, et al. Presentation of pediatric celiac disease in the United States: prominent effect of breastfeeding. Clin Pediatr (Phila). 2005;44(3):249–58.
63. Vella C, Grech V. Increasing age at diagnosis of celiac disease in Malta. Indian J Pediatr. 2004;71(7):581–2.
64. Ivarsson A, Hernell O, Stenlund H, Persson LA. Breast-feeding protects against celiac disease. Am J Clin Nutr. 2002;75(5):914–21.
65. Peters U, Schneeweiss S, Trautwein EA, Erbersdobler HF. A case-control study of the effect of infant feeding on celiac disease. Ann Nutr Metab. 2001;45(4):135–42.
66. Penders J, Thijs C, Vink C, Stelma FF, Snijders B, Kummeling I, et al. Factors influencing the composition of the intestinal microbiota in early infancy. Pediatrics. 2006;118(2):511–21.
67. Kau AL, Ahern PP, Griffin NW, Goodman AL, Gordon JI. Human nutrition, the gut microbiome and the immune system. Nature. 2011;474(7351):327–36.
68. Sjogren YM, Tomicic S, Lundberg A, Bottcher MF, Bjorksten B, Sverremark-Ekstrom E, et al. Influence of early gut microbiota on the maturation of childhood mucosal and systemic immune responses. Clin Exp Allergy. 2009;39(12):1842–51.
69. Palma GD, Capilla A, Nova E, Castillejo G, Varea V, Pozo T, et al. Influence of milk-feeding type and genetic risk of developing coeliac disease on intestinal microbiota of infants: the PROFICEL study. PLoS One. 2012;7(2):e30791.
70. Norris JM, Barriga K, Hoffenberg EJ, Taki I, Miao D, Haas JE, et al. Risk of celiac disease autoimmunity and timing of gluten introduction in the diet of infants at increased risk of disease. JAMA. 2005;293(19):2343–51.
71. Szajewska H, Chmielewska A, Piescik-Lech M, Ivarsson A, Kolacek S, Koletzko S, et al. Systematic review: early infant feeding and the prevention of coeliac disease. Aliment Pharmacol Ther. 2012;36(7):607–18.
72. Sellitto M, Bai G, Serena G, Fricke WF, Sturgeon C, Gajer P, et al. Proof of concept of microbiome-metabolome analysis and delayed gluten exposure on celiac disease autoimmunity in genetically at-risk infants. PLoS One. 2012;7(3):e33387.
73. Murray JA. Celiac disease in patients with an affected member, type 1 diabetes, iron-deficiency, or osteoporosis? Gastroenterology. 2005;128(4 Pt 2):S52–6.

74. Book L, Zone JJ, Neuhausen SL. Prevalence of celiac disease among relatives of sib pairs with celiac disease in U.S. families. Am J Gastroenterol. 2003;98(2):377–81.
75. Carlsson AK, Axelsson IE, Borulf SK, Bredberg AC, Lindberg BA, Sjoberg KG, et al. Prevalence of IgA-antiendomysium and IgA-antigliadin autoantibodies at diagnosis of insulin-dependent diabetes mellitus in Swedish children and adolescents. Pediatrics. 1999;103(6 Pt 1):1248–52.
76. Walsh CH, Cooper BT, Wright AD, Malins JM, Cooke WT. Diabetes mellitus and coeliac disease: a clinical study. Q J Med. 1978;47(185):89–100.
77. Bouguerra R, Ben Salem L, Chaabouni H, Laadhar L, Essais O, Zitouni M, et al. Celiac disease in adult patients with type 1 diabetes mellitus in Tunisia. Diabetes Metab. 2005;31(1):83–6.
78. Sategna-Guidetti C, Volta U, Ciacci C, Usai P, Carlino A, De Franceschi L, et al. Prevalence of thyroid disorders in untreated adult celiac disease patients and effect of gluten withdrawal: an Italian multicenter study. Am J Gastroenterol. 2001;96(3):751–7.
79. Sategna-Guidetti C, Bruno M, Mazza E, Carlino A, Predebon S, Tagliabue M, et al. Autoimmune thyroid diseases and coeliac disease. Eur J Gastroenterol Hepatol. 1998;10(11):927–31.
80. Sattar N, Lazare F, Kacer M, Aguayo-Figueroa L, Desikan V, Garcia M, et al. Celiac disease in children, adolescents, and young adults with autoimmune thyroid disease. J Pediatr. 2011;158(2):272–5. e1.
81. Caprai S, Vajro P, Ventura A, Sciveres M, Maggiore G. Autoimmune liver disease associated with celiac disease in childhood: a multicenter study. Clin Gastroenterol Hepatol. 2008;6(7):803–6.
82. Diamanti A, Basso MS, Pietrobattista A, Nobili V. Prevalence of celiac disease in children with autoimmune hepatitis. Dig Liver Dis. 2008;40(12):965.
83. George EK, Hertzberger-ten Cate R, van Suijlekom-Smit LW, von Blomberg BM, Stapel SO, van Elburg RM, et al. Juvenile chronic arthritis and coeliac disease in The Netherlands. Clin Exp Rheumatol. 1996;14(5):571–5.
84. Bonamico M, Pasquino AM, Mariani P, Danesi HM, Culasso F, Mazzanti L, et al. Prevalence and clinical picture of celiac disease in Turner syndrome. J Clin Endocrinol Metab. 2002;87(12):5495–8.
85. Bonamico M, Mariani P, Danesi HM, Crisogianni M, Failla P, Gemme G, et al. Prevalence and clinical picture of celiac disease in italian down syndrome patients: a multicenter study. J Pediatr Gastroenterol Nutr. 2001;33(2):139–43.
86. Bai D, Brar P, Holleran S, Ramakrishnan R, Green PH. Effect of gender on the manifestations of celiac disease: evidence for greater malabsorption in men. Scand J Gastroenterol. 2005;40(2):183–7.
87. Ventura A, Magazzu G, Greco L. Duration of exposure to gluten and risk for autoimmune disorders in patients with celiac disease. SIGEP study group for autoimmune disorders in celiac disease. Gastroenterology. 1999;117(2):297–303.
88. Jacobson DL, Gange SJ, Rose NR, Graham NM. Epidemiology and estimated population burden of selected autoimmune diseases in the United States. Clin Immunol Immunopathol. 1997;84(3):223–43.
89. Sategna Guidetti C, Solerio E, Scaglione N, Aimo G, Mengozzi G. Duration of gluten exposure in adult coeliac disease does not correlate with the risk for autoimmune disorders. Gut. 2001;49(4):502–5.
90. Viljamaa M, Kaukinen K, Huhtala H, Kyronpalo S, Rasmussen M, Collin P. Coeliac disease, autoimmune diseases and gluten exposure. Scand J Gastroenterol. 2005;40(4):437–43.
91. Cosnes J, Cellier C, Viola S, Colombel JF, Michaud L, Sarles J, et al. Incidence of autoimmune diseases in celiac disease: protective effect of the gluten-free diet. Clin Gastroenterol Hepatol. 2008;6(7):753–8.

92. Metso S, Hyytia-Ilmonen H, Kaukinen K, Huhtala H, Jaatinen P, Salmi J, et al. Gluten-free diet and autoimmune thyroiditis in patients with celiac disease. A prospective controlled study. Scand J Gastroenterol. 2012;47(1):43–8.
93. Molteni N, Bardella MT, Bianchi PA. Obstetric and gynecological problems in women with untreated celiac sprue. J Clin Gastroenterol. 1990;12(1):37–9.
94. Sher KS, Mayberry JF. Female fertility, obstetric and gynaecological history in coeliac disease. A case control study. Digestion. 1994;55(4):243–6.
95. Stazi AV, Mantovani A. A risk factor for female fertility and pregnancy: celiac disease. Gynecol Endocrinol. 2000;14(6):454–63.
96. Baker PG, Read AE. Reversible infertility in male coeliac patients. Br Med J. 1975;02(5966):316–7.
97. Choi JM, Lebwohl B, Wang J, Lee SK, Murray JA, Sauer MV, et al. Increased prevalence of celiac disease in patients with unexplained infertility in the United States. J Reprod Med. 2011;56(5–6):199–203.
98. Zugna D, Richiardi L, Akre O, Stephansson O, Ludvigsson JF. A nationwide population-based study to determine whether coeliac disease is associated with infertility. Gut. 2010;59(11):1471–5.
99. Sun S, Puttha R, Ghezaiel S, Skae M, Cooper C, Amin R. The effect of biopsy-positive silent coeliac disease and treatment with a gluten-free diet on growth and glycaemic control in children with Type 1 diabetes. Diabet Med. 2009;26(12):1250–4.
100. Savilahti E, Pelkonen P, Visakorpi JK. IgA deficiency in children. A clinical study with special reference to intestinal findings. Arch Dis Child. 1971;46(249):665–70.
101. Roma E, Panayiotou J, Karantana H, Constantinidou C, Siakavellas SI, Krini M, et al. Changing pattern in the clinical presentation of pediatric celiac disease: a 30-year study. Digestion. 2009;80(3):185–91.
102. Venkatasubramani N, Telega G, Werlin SL. Obesity in pediatric celiac disease. J Pediatr Gastroenterol Nutr. 2010;51(3):295–7.
103. Arslan N, Esen I, Demircioglu F, Yilmaz S, Unuvar T, Bober E. The changing face of celiac disease: a girl with obesity and celiac disease. J Paediatr Child Health. 2009;45(5):317–8.

Chapter 9
Diagnosis of Celiac Disease

Anna Tavakkoli and Benjamin Lebwohl

Introduction

Celiac disease (CD), often described as the "clinical chameleon," is an autoimmune disorder with a range of clinical symptoms and presentations. This chapter will review which patients should get tested for CD, the serological markers available to diagnose CD, and the role of genetic testing and small bowel endoscopy in the diagnosis of this disease.

Patients and Populations to Consider

CD is a complex and often difficult disorder to diagnose considering its wide range of clinical presentations that have been observed. While the overall diagnosis rate of CD is increasing in the United States and worldwide, the vast majority of patients in the United States remain undiagnosed [3–5]. Therefore, determining which patients to test for CD outside of those who present with classical CD symptoms has been difficult to characterize. Testing for CD should be considered in the following group of individuals.

A. Tavakkoli, M.D.
Department of Internal Medicine, Columbia University Medical Center, New York, NY, USA

B. Lebwohl, M.D., M.S. (✉)
Department of Gastroenterology, Columbia University Medical Center, 180 Fort Washington Avenue, Suite 936, New York, NY 10032, USA
e-mail: bl114@columbia.edu

S.D. Rampertab and G.E. Mullin (eds.), *Celiac Disease*, Clinical Gastroenterology,
DOI 10.1007/978-1-4614-8560-5_9, © Springer Science+Business Media New York 2014

Gastrointestinal Symptoms

The classical presentation of CD includes bulky, foul-smelling diarrhea that often occurs in parallel with malabsorptive symptoms including weight loss, vitamin deficiencies, and anemia [1, 2, 6]. Although there has been a shift in recent years from the classical presentation of CD to atypical or asymptomatic presentations [7], the diagnosis of CD should be pursued in patients with chronic or recurrent diarrhea, malabsorption, and unexplained weight loss. In addition, patients with CD can often present with symptoms that are initially misdiagnosed as irritable bowel syndrome (IBS), including abdominal pain and bloating associated with a change in bowel habit. A meta-analysis of patients with established CD discovered that IBS-like symptoms can occur in upwards of 40 % of established CD patients and occur more often in CD patients than controls [8]. Considering the overlap between symptoms among patients with IBS and CD, patients who meet ROME III criteria should additionally be evaluated for CD prior to the diagnosis of IBS. This approach is supported by a meta-analysis that found a fourfold in increase in the prevalence of CD among patients with IBS [9].

Nonclassical Presentations

Clinicians often recognize the classical presentation of CD; however, diarrhea has been the presenting symptom in fewer than 50 % of patients diagnosed with CD in recent past decades [7]. Increasingly, patients are presenting with nonclassical symptoms that have been linked to CD, including elevated transaminases, osteoporosis, neurological symptoms (ataxia, peripheral neuropathy), migraine headache, depression, and a variety of metabolic derangements (Table 9.1) [10, 11]. Since the majority of these symptoms resolve upon adoption of a gluten-free diet, there is a clear benefit in diagnosing these patients with CD [11]. While the presentations can vary extensively, it is especially important for clinicians to be familiar with these nonclassical presentations to diagnose and treat patients with CD.

Higher Prevalence Populations

While screening the general population for CD is not recommended at this time, there are several populations that have an increased prevalence of CD. First-degree relatives of patients with CD have a higher risk than the general population for developing CD, with an overall prevalence of approximately 10 % [2, 12, 13]. In addition, patients with type 1 diabetes mellitus, autoimmune thyroid disease, autoimmune liver disease, genetic disorders (Down syndrome and Turner's syndrome), and IgA deficiency have a higher prevalence of CD as well (Table 9.2) [2, 14–18].

Table 9.1 Nonclassical presentations and metabolic abnormalities associated with celiac disease[a]

Neurological–psychiatric manifestations
Cerebellar ataxia
Peripheral neuropathy
Headache (tension and migraine)
Depression/anxiety
Epilepsy
Intracranial calcifications
Hematological manifestations
Anemia
Vitamin B_{12} deficiency
Dermatological manifestations
Dermatitis herpetiformis
Metabolic derangements
Hypercalcemia
Hypophosphatemia
Hypoalbuminemia
Folate deficiency
Hyperamylasemia
Hypocholesterolemia (low HDL and LDL)
Bone disease
Osteoporosis
Osteopenia

[a]Adapted from [11]

While there has been debate for and against screening these high-risk populations, most guidelines currently recommend testing for CD only if patients in these groups develop classical or nonclassical symptoms of CD [2, 19].

Screening for Celiac Disease

CD meets the World Health Organization (WHO) criteria for diseases that warrant mass screening: early clinical detection is difficult; the condition is common; screening tests are highly sensitive and specific; effective treatment is available; and untreated disease can lead to complications [20]. In addition, initiation of a gluten-free diet reduces mortality risk, and screening for CD has been found to be cost-effective under certain circumstances [21]. However, as will be discussed below, serological testing is not 100 % sensitive or specific, and due to the CD prevalence of 0.7–1.0 % in the general population, mass screening will cause a high number of false-positive test results, leading to unnecessary procedures and complications [20]. While a case-finding approach has also been proposed, in which health-care providers would order serologic tests for patients who exhibit signs or symptoms or have a disease associated with CD, this approach may be difficult to implement in clinical

Table 9.2 Clinical and genetic conditions associated with celiac disease[a]

Endocrine
Type 1 diabetes mellitus
Autoimmune thyroid disease
Addison's disease
Secondary hyperparathyroidism
Immunological-rheumatologic
Sjögren syndrome
Arthritis
Systemic lupus erythematosus
Rheumatoid arthritis
IgA deficiency
Immune thrombocytopenic purpura
Myasthenia gravis
Dermatological
Vitiligo
Alopecia areata
Psoriasis
Malnutrition-related changes (petechiae; vitamin K, edema; hypoproteinemia, follicular hyperkeratosis; vitamin A, dermatitis; B vitamins)
Cardiopulmonary
Idiopathic dilated cardiomyopathy
Autoimmune myocarditis
Cystic fibrosis
Fibrosing alveolitis
Sarcoidosis
Idiopathic pulmonary hemosiderosis
Extrinsic allergic alveolitis (bird fancier's lung)
Recurrent pericarditis
Gastrointestinal
Crohn's disease
Microscopic colitis
Pancreatic insufficiency
Ulcerative colitis
Eosinophilic esophagitis
Hematological
Anemia
Autoimmune hemolytic anemia
Hemorrhage
Howell–Jolly bodies
Thrombocytosis
Hyposplenism
Hepatic
Elevated liver biochemical tests
Primary biliary cirrhosis
Primary sclerosing cholangitis
Autoimmune hepatitis
Autoimmune cholangitis

(continued)

Table 9.2 (continued)

Neurologic and Psychiatric
Ataxia
Behavioral abnormalities
Demyelinating central nervous system lesions
Peripheral neuropathy
Reproductive disorders
Delayed menarche
Recurrent miscarriage
Infertility
Impotence
Renal
IgA nephropathy
Musculoskeletal
Muscular atrophy and weakness
Osteoarthropathy
Polymyositis
Pathological fractures
Genetic disorders
Down syndrome
Turner syndrome
Williams syndrome
IgA deficiency

[a]Adapted from [11] and [77]

practice. At this time, there is no universally accepted threshold at which to test patients for CD, and as such, it is incumbent upon health-care providers to recognize both classical and nonclassical signs and symptoms of CD in addition to understanding the steps necessary to diagnose CD.

Serological Evaluation

Serological evaluation is the initial step in diagnosing CD and may be helpful in monitoring adherence to a gluten-free diet [2, 20]. Antibody testing is the first step in diagnosing patients with CD. Characteristics of commonly used serologies are listed below and summarized in Table 9.3.

Antigliadin Antibody

The antigliadin antibody was the first serological test developed for the diagnosis of CD in the early 1980s [22, 23]. The assay measures both IgG and circulating IgA antigliadin antibodies. While the IgA antigliadin antibodies were found to have a

Table 9.3 Sensitivity, specificity, and positive and negative predictive values of serologic tests for untreated celiac disease[a]

Test	Sensitivity (reported range) (%)	Specificity (reported range) (%)	Positive predictive value (%), pretest probability of 5 %	Negative predictive value (%), pretest probability of 5 %
IgA AGA	85 (57–100)	90 (47–94)	18	99
IgG AGA	85 (42–100)	80 (50–94)	31	99
EMA	95 (86–100)	99 (97–100)	83	99
IgA anti-TTG[b]	98 (78–100)	98 (90–100)	72	99
IgG anti-TTG[c]	70 (45–95)	95 (94–100)	42	99
IgA anti-DGP	88 (74–100)	95 (90–99)	44	99
IgG anti-DGP	80 (63–95)	98 (90–99)	68	99
IgA/IgG anti-DGP	97 (75–99)	95 (87–100)	51	99

AGA, antigliadin antibody; *DGP*, deamidated gliadin peptide; *EMA*, endomysial antibody; *TTG*, tissue transglutaminase

[a]Reprinted by permission from Macmillan Publishers Ltd: The American Journal of Gastroenterology. Leffler DA, Schuppan D. Update on serologic testing in celiac disease, 105 (12), copyright 2010

[b]Antihuman TTG-based assays only; older tests based on guinea pig antibodies have lower sensitivity and specificity

[c]Sensitivity is significantly higher, about 90–95 %, in IgA-deficient populations but lower in the overall celiac population

higher sensitivity and specificity as compared to its IgG subclass, the assay's overall sensitivity and specificity are dependent on manufactured-based arbitrary cutoff values [2, 22, 24–26]. Despite the variability seen among different commercial assays, it has generally been thought that the sensitivity and specificity of both the IgG and IgA antigliadin antibodies lie between 80 and 90 % with a positive predictive value of less than 30 % in most populations [20, 24, 25]. Considering the low positive predictive value and the development of superior antibody testing for CD, both IgG and IgA antigliadin antibody testing are no longer recommended to diagnose CD.

Deamidated Gliadin Peptide Antibody

Deamidated gliadin peptide (DGP) represents the conversion of certain gluten peptides to deamidated peptides via intestinal transglutaminase (TTG). The deamidated peptides then activate the inflammatory T-cell response by binding to antigen-presenting cells in patients with CD [27]. This results in an antibody response that has a higher specificity for CD than antibodies to native gluten [28]. The combined sensitivity and specificity for IgA and IgG anti-deamidated gliadin peptide are above 80 % and above 95 %, respectively [22]. However, studies have shown that IgA anti-TTG performs better and is less costly than the IgA-DGP [29]. Currently, DGP antibody testing is recommended for use in IgA-deficient patients to diagnose CD and in the pediatric population.

IgA Anti-endomysial Antibody

Endomysial antibody (EMA) testing was developed in the mid-1980s after the development of antigliadin antibody testing. EMA testing is based on indirect immunofluorescence, requires either monkey esophagus or human umbilical cord tissue as a substrate, and uses TTG as the target antigen [2, 22]. This test introduces interobserver and inter-site variability since one individual reads each sample under the microscope and reports the test as either positive or negative at a given titer [22]. Despite these factors, the sensitivity of IgA anti-EMA can vary, i.e., on the level of villous atrophy present, but is generally >90 % with a specificity of 97–100 % [2, 22, 30, 31].

IgA anti-EMA antibody testing is not currently recommended as the first-line therapy due to the high cost, variability, and subsequent development of IgA anti-TTG. In addition, studies have not shown a benefit to concurrently testing both anti-TTG and IgA anti-EMA simultaneously, but the test can be used as a confirmatory test in patients with borderline positive or possibly false-positive anti-TTG antibodies [31, 32].

Anti-tissue Transglutaminase Antibody

TTG was identified as a CD autoantigen in the late 1990s, [33] which allowed the development of an enzyme-linked immunosorbent assay (ELISA) test using guinea pig liver (first-generation assays), human red-cell derived, and human recombinant TTG [20, 22, 23]. Not only did the development of an ELISA-based assay avoid the time-consuming, expensive, and operator-dependent indirect immunofluorescence testing done with anti-EMA testing, but the high sensitivity and specificity found with the study are comparable to the anti-EMA testing currently available [22, 31, 34]. For these reasons, IgA anti-TTG is recommended as the initial test of choice for CD. IgG anti-TTG is also available for commercial use; however, the sensitivity and specificity of this test are wildly variable and are reserved for use in patients with IgA deficiency [31].

A new anti-TTG point-of-care test using a drop of whole blood has recently been developed. The test does bring ease to diagnosing CD but lacks the sensitivity and specificity of the ELISA-based test and lacks a titer that can be followed throughout patients' clinical illness. At this time, the test is not recommended for diagnosis due to possible false-negative results [35–37].

IgA Deficiency

Selective IgA deficiency is more prevalent among patients with CD versus non-CD control patients (2 % vs. 0.2–0.5 %) [38–41]. With an increased prevalence, IgA-based serological tests are more likely to be falsely negative in untreated CD among this patient population. Therefore, it is recommended to measure total serum IgA levels along with IgA-based serologic tests [22]. Among patients who are IgA deficient, a number of IgG-based serologic tests have been developed for CD diagnosis, including IgG antigliadin antibody, IgG anti-TTG antibody, and IgG anti-DGP [2, 22]. Traditionally, the IgG antigliadin assay has been used for these patients but frequently yields false-positive results. Therefore, using serum IgG anti-TTG assays or IgG anti-DGP tests is preferable [2, 22, 42].

There are subsets of patients who have detectable but low levels of IgA, and it is important to note that the accuracy of IgA-based tests is not thought to be significantly compromised in this group of patients [22, 43].

Genetic Testing

Approximately, 40 % of all individuals in the USA are positive for either the HLA class II heterodimer HLA-DQ2 (DQA1*05/DQB1*02) or HLA-DQ8 (DQA1*03/DQB1*0302) [2], but nearly all patients with CD are either DQ2 (95 %) or DQ8 (5 %) positive [20, 44]. Due to the fact that nearly all patients with CD will either be DQ2 or DQ8 positive, the absence of these loci provides an almost 100 % negative predictive value for the diagnosis of CD [2]. Since the routine addition of genetic testing to the standard serological evaluation described above does not increase diagnostic performance [45], genetic testing is not indicated in most initial evaluations of CD. However, due to the high negative predictive value, genetic testing is useful in excluding CD in cases where the diagnosis is unclear or among patients who are already on a gluten-free diet, as the test is not affected by gluten exclusion.

Small Intestinal Biopsy

Although serological testing has high sensitivity and specificity for the diagnosis of CD, is routinely available, and is noninvasive with minimal risks, small intestinal biopsy remains the gold standard for diagnosis of CD [2, 20]. Duodenal biopsy is routinely performed and recommended in patients after testing positive with a serological marker for CD. In addition, patients with normal serological markers but with signs and symptoms that are highly suspicious for CD should undergo endoscopic evaluation since approximately 10 % of patients with CD may be seronegative [22].

The histologic findings of CD are described using the Marsh–Oberhuber classification (Table 9.4) [46]. The hallmarks of CD include increased intraepithelial lymphocytes (IELs), crypt hyperplasia, and villous atrophy [47–50]. Endoscopic markers of villous atrophy have also been described, including a reduction in the number of duodenal folds, scalloping, mucosal grooves, and a mosaic appearance of the mucosa. However, the endoscopic appearance of small bowel has not been

Table 9.4 Marsh–Oberhuber classification of celiac disease[a]

Marsh class	Type of lesion	Villous architecture	Crypts	IELs
Marsh I	Infiltrative	Normal	Normal	>30/100 enterocytes
Marsh II	Infiltrative–hyperplastic	Normal	Hyperplasia	>30/100 enterocytes
Marsh III				
3A	Flat destructive	Mild villous atrophy	Hyperplasia	>30/100 enterocytes
3B	Flat destructive	Moderate villous atrophy	Hyperplasia	>30/100 enterocytes
3C	Flat destructive	Total villous atrophy	Hyperplasia	>30/100 enterocytes
Marsh 4	Atrophic–hypoplastic	Total villous atrophy	Hyperplasia	>30/100 enterocytes

IELs intraepithelial lymphocytes
[a]Adapted from [46]

shown to be sensitive or specific for the diagnosis of CD [2]. These findings have also been noted to occur in patients with tropical sprue, HIV enteropathy, and HIV-associated opportunistic infections, such as cytomegalovirus and *Cryptosporidium* [51]. Furthermore, studies have shown that a normal endoscopic appearance does not rule out CD. In one study of 129 patients with newly diagnosed CD, researchers found that about one-third of patients had a completely normal endoscopic appearance despite histological evidence of CD [52]. Therefore, diagnosing or excluding CD on the basis of the appearance of a patient's small bowel is not recommended.

Although progress has been made with serological markers for CD and the varying presentations of CD have been described, patients with signs and symptoms consistent with CD do not always undergo duodenal biopsy during EGD. In a study of the Clinical Outcomes Research Initiative (CORI), which is a national endoscopic database, almost 4,000 patients underwent EGD for diarrhea, iron deficiency, anemia, and weight loss from 2000 to 2003 [53]. All of the patients had normal-appearing duodenums, but a biopsy was performed in only 11 % of patients. When the CORI database was revisited recently, the rate of duodenal biopsy from 2004 to 2009 for the same symptoms increased to 43 %, which is improved but still low [54]. In the same study, they found that male patients and elderly individuals were less likely to receive a duodenal biopsy [54]. The improved but still low rate of duodenal biopsy argues that a potential cause for the underdiagnosis of CD is related to a lack of recognition of both the typical and atypical presentations of CD, the equal seroprevalence rates among men and women, the fact that CD can present at any age, and the important role that duodenal biopsies play in its diagnosis [55, 56].

The location and number of biopsies taken during EGD plays an important role in the accurate diagnosis of CD. Due to the patchy nature of villous atrophy and the predilection to affect areas of the duodenum with varying degrees of severity, multiple biopsies of both the duodenal bulb and the distal duodenum maximize the diagnostic yield [57, 58]. Traditionally, duodenal bulb biopsies had been avoided by gastroenterologists due to the acid-induced damage, gastric metaplasia, Brunner gland hyperplasia, or the presence of lymphoid follicles that may serve as a potential confounding element in the histopathological assessment of the small bowel [59]. However, a number of studies have shown that duodenal bulb biopsies can sometimes be the only evidence of villous atrophy [2, 58, 59]. When biopsying the duodenal bulb, the 9 or 12 o'clock position appears to have the highest diagnostic yield [57].

The number of distal duodenal biopsies obtained during EGD affects its sensitivity for the diagnosis of CD. The sensitivity of biopsy for the diagnosis of CD increases when four duodenal specimens are taken [60, 61]. Therefore, AGA recommendations state that four to six specimens should be submitted during duodenal biopsy for optimal detection of CD [2]. However, despite the improved sensitivity of diagnosing CD with at least four duodenal biopsies, clinical practice seems to be lagging behind. In one study analyzing a national pathology database, 132,352 patients underwent duodenal biopsy from 2006 to 2009 [62]. Among these patients, four or more specimens were submitted during duodenal biopsy in only 35 % of patients. Older patients were less likely than younger patients to have an adequate number of duodenal biopsies submitted. Even when the clinical indication was labeled as suspected CD, adherence to the recommended number of duodenal biopsies occurred in only 38.5 % of submissions. Furthermore, this study found that when fewer than four specimens were submitted for histological evaluation, the proportion of patients diagnosed with CD was only 0.7 % as compared to 1.8 % when four or more specimens were submitted. As a result of the number of studies showing that the submission of four or more duodenal biopsies and biopsies of the duodenal bulb improves the diagnosis of CD, we recommend that for adequate diagnosis of CD, at least four specimens be submitted, including a specimen from the duodenal bulb.

Duodenal biopsy may be subject to misinterpretation by pathologists, which may lead to false negatives and false positives. Review by a pathologist expert in the diagnosis of CD is advised, especially in the case of subtle findings or discrepancy between serologic and histologic results [63].

The Impact of Gluten-Free Diet on the Diagnosis of CD

The popularity of the gluten-free diet (GFD) has been increasing in the USA [64]. While previously difficult to find outside of specialty stores, gluten-free ingredients, snacks, and meals have become more available in grocery stores and restaurants. As a result, patients may present to a medical provider already on a GFD but still seeking a diagnosis for their symptoms.

Serological markers for CD normalize after 6–12 months of adherence to a GFD, though this rate is variable. Histological changes that characterize CD can persist despite normalization of serological markers. One study of 381 patients with biopsy-proven CD found that the median time to mucosal healing was 3.8 years [65]. Furthermore, many patients with confirmed mucosal healing have IELs that persisted despite normal crypt-to-villous ratio [66, 67]. While it is not recommended to begin a GFD prior to diagnostic evaluation, a patient with CD who is compliant with a GFD might still have persistent histopathology consistent with CD. Despite this, the AGA recommends that patients on a GFD at the time of biopsy undergo a gluten challenge to prevent any impact the diet might have on the pathological interpretation [2]. While an 8-week challenge had previously been recommended, a shorter challenge period may be adequate as illustrated in Appendix 8 [68]. Genetic testing for DQ2 and DQ8, as described above, is another option in patients who are on a GFD at the time of biopsy. Because of the almost 100 % negative predictive value, a negative test, even on a GFD, completely rules out CD.

Diagnosis in Children

Once thought to be a disease of infants and young children, presenting after the introduction of gluten, CD has been shown to now present at any age. Children with CD often present with gastrointestinal symptoms including diarrhea, abdominal pain, vomiting, constipation, abdominal distention, and failure to thrive [69]. Non-gastrointestinal manifestations of CD in the pediatric population are quite extensive but include idiopathic short stature, neurological and behavioral symptoms, dental enamel defects, unexplained elevation in serum transaminases, and unexplained iron deficiency. Furthermore, high-risk populations for CD among children are similar to those in the adult population, including type 1 diabetes, Turner syndrome, Williams syndrome, Down syndrome, and first-degree relatives of CD patients. Of note, patients with Down syndrome appear to have a high risk of CD, since up to 16 % of these patients are affected [70].

Recommendations on whom to test and screen for CD differ in the pediatric population as compared to adults, mostly in that screening for CD is recommended in asymptomatic patients that belong to a high-risk pediatric population. The North American Society for Pediatric Gastroenterology, Hepatology and Nutrition (NASPGHAN) recommends that testing be done in patients with gastrointestinal symptoms, non-gastrointestinal symptoms (including dermatitis herpetiformis, short stature, and delayed puberty), and asymptomatic patients who reside in a high-risk population. Testing of these asymptomatic patients is recommended to begin around 3 years of age as long as the child has been on a gluten-containing diet for at least 1 year prior to testing [69].

Serological Markers for Diagnosis of CD in Pediatric Patients

The initial test of choice for the diagnosis of CD in pediatric patients is IgA anti-TTG and total serum IgA level [69]. In those patients with IgA deficiency, IgG anti-TTG or IgG anti-DGP can be used [69]. However, even among patients with normal total IgA levels, IgA anti-TTG and EMA antibodies are often negative in children with CD who are younger than 2 years of age [20]. A series of studies have shown that anti-DGP antibodies will test positive despite normal TTG and EMA values (and correlate to histological findings confirming CD on endoscopy) and that IgA and IgG anti-DGP had a sensitivity of almost 100 % in pediatric patients less than 3 years old [71, 72]. As a result, DGP appears to be a reliable alternative to testing for CD in very young children who might present with symptoms concerning for CD.

Intestinal Biopsy

Intestinal biopsy, which includes multiple distal duodenal biopsies and sampling of the duodenal bulb, has been the gold standard for definitive diagnosis of CD in both adults and children. Several recent studies have suggested that symptomatic patients with TTG about ten times the upper limit of normal could be reliably diagnosed with CD without EGD and histological confirmation [73–75]. As a result, The European Society for Pediatric Gastroenterology, Hepatology, and Nutrition (ESPGHAN) released a new set of recommendations for the diagnosis of CD delineating two groups of patients with different diagnostic formulas. These recommendations indicate that among children with symptoms suggestive of CD, an IgA anti-TTG antibody level greater than ten times the upper limit of normal and a positive HLA haplotype can be sufficient to diagnose CD without a duodenal biopsy [76]. However, asymptomatic patients at high risk of CD still need both positive serology and histological findings on duodenal biopsy in order to diagnose CD [76]. While these are general guidelines to follow, they may reduce the amount of invasive testing pediatric patients undergo during the diagnosis of CD. It is unclear whether this practice will be widely adopted in Europe or North America.

Conclusion

The diagnosis of CD in both adults and children can be straightforward, as in the cases of those who present with classical gastrointestinal symptoms, or protracted due to the nonclassical or silent presentations that can often occur. The groundwork for diagnosing CD lies in serological markers, followed by characteristic histological changes on duodenal biopsy. Genetic testing can sometimes be useful due to its high negative predictive value.

References

1. Green PH, Cellier C. Celiac disease. N Engl J Med. 2007;357(17):1731–43. PubMed PMID: 17960014.
2. Rostom A, Murray JA, Kagnoff MF. American Gastroenterological Association (AGA) Institute technical review on the diagnosis and management of celiac disease. Gastroenterology. 2006;131(6):1981–2002. PubMed PMID: 17087937.

3. Rubio-Tapia A, Ludvigsson JF, Brantner TL, Murray JA, Everhart JE. The prevalence of celiac disease in the United States. Am J Gastroenterol. 2012;107(10):1538–44. quiz 7, 45. PubMed PMID: 22850429.
4. Murray JA, Van Dyke C, Plevak MF, Dierkhising RA, Zinsmeister AR, Melton 3rd LJ. Trends in the identification and clinical features of celiac disease in a North American community, 1950-2001. Clin Gastroenterol Hepatol. 2003;1(1):19–27. PubMed PMID: 15017513.
5. Catassi C, Kryszak D, Bhatti B, Sturgeon C, Helzlsouer K, Clipp SL, et al. Natural history of celiac disease autoimmunity in a USA cohort followed since 1974. Ann Med. 2010;42(7):530–8. PubMed PMID: 20868314.
6. Ludvigsson JF, Leffler DA, Bai JC, Biagi F, Fasano A, Green PH, et al. The Oslo definitions for coeliac disease and related terms. Gut. 2013;62(1):43–52. PubMed PMID: 22345659. Pubmed Central PMCID: 3440559.
7. Rampertab SD, Pooran N, Brar P, Singh P, Green PH. Trends in the presentation of celiac disease. Am J Med. 2006;119(4):355. e9–14. PubMed PMID: 16564784.
8. Sainsbury A, Sanders DS, Ford AC. Prevalence of irritable bowel syndrome-type symptoms in patients with celiac disease: a Meta-analysis. Clin Gastroenter Hepatol. 2013;11:359–65. PubMed PMID: 23246645.
9. Ford AC, Chey WD, Talley NJ, Malhotra A, Spiegel BM, Moayyedi P. Yield of diagnostic tests for celiac disease in individuals with symptoms suggestive of irritable bowel syndrome: systematic review and meta-analysis. Arch Intern Med. 2009;169(7):651–8. PMID 19364994.
10. Admou B, Essaadouni L, Krati K, Zaher K, Sbihi M, Chabaa L, et al. Atypical celiac disease: from recognizing to managing. Gastroenterol Res Pract. 2012;2012:637187. PubMed PMID: 22811701. Pubmed Central PMCID: 3395124.
11. Hernandez L, Green PH. Extraintestinal manifestations of celiac disease. Curr Gastroenterol Rep. 2006;8(5):383–9. PubMed PMID: 16968605.
12. Freeman HJ. Risk factors in familial forms of celiac disease. World J Gastroenterol. 2010;16(15):1828–31. PubMed PMID: 20397258. Pubmed Central PMCID: 2856821.
13. Dogan Y, Yildirmaz S, Ozercan IH. Prevalence of celiac disease among first-degree relatives of patients with celiac disease. J Pediatr Gastroenterol Nutr. 2012;55(2):205–8. PubMed PMID: 22241509.
14. Volta U, Rodrigo L, Granito A, Petrolini N, Muratori P, Muratori L, et al. Celiac disease in autoimmune cholestatic liver disorders. Am J Gastroenterol. 2002;97(10):2609–13. PubMed PMID: 12385447.
15. Aktay AN, Lee PC, Kumar V, Parton E, Wyatt DT, Werlin SL. The prevalence and clinical characteristics of celiac disease in juvenile diabetes in Wisconsin. J Pediatr Gastroenterol Nutr. 2001;33(4):462–5. PubMed PMID: 11698764.
16. Cronin CC, Feighery A, Ferriss JB, Liddy C, Shanahan F, Feighery C. High prevalence of celiac disease among patients with insulin-dependent (type 1) diabetes mellitus. Am J Gastroenterol. 1997;92(12):2210–2. PubMed PMID: 9399754.
17. Cuoco L, Certo M, Jorizzo RA, De Vitis I, Tursi A, Papa A, et al. Prevalence and early diagnosis of coeliac disease in autoimmune thyroid disorders. Ital J Gastroenterol Hepatol. 1999;31(4):283–7. PubMed PMID: 10425571.
18. Aggarwal S, Lebwohl B, Green PH. Screening for celiac disease in average-risk and high-risk populations. Therap Adv Gastroenterol. 2012;5(1):37–47. PubMed PMID: 22282707. Pubmed Central PMCID: 3263981.
19. National Institutes of Health Consensus Development Conference Statement on Celiac Disease, June 28–30, 2004. Gastroenterology. 2005;128(4 Suppl 1):S1–9. PubMed PMID: 15825115.
20. Lebwohl B, Rubio-Tapia A, Assiri A, Newland C, Guandalini S. Diagnosis of celiac disease. Gastrointest Endosc Clin N Am. 2012;22(4):661–77. PubMed PMID: 23083985.
21. Hershcovici T, Leshno M, Goldin E, Shamir R, Israeli E. Cost effectiveness of mass screening for coeliac disease is determined by time-delay to diagnosis and quality of life on a gluten-free diet. Aliment Pharmacol Ther. 2010;31(8):901–10. PubMed PMID: 20096017.

22. Leffler DA, Schuppan D. Update on serologic testing in celiac disease. Am J Gastroenterol. 2010;105(12):2520–4. PubMed PMID: 21131921.
23. O'Farrelly C, Kelly J, Hekkens W, Bradley B, Thompson A, Feighery C, et al. Alpha gliadin antibody levels: a serological test for coeliac disease. Br Med J. 1983;286(6383):2007–10. PubMed PMID: 6409205. Pubmed Central PMCID: 1548488.
24. Rostom A, Dube C, Cranney A, Saloojee N, Sy R, Garritty C, et al. The diagnostic accuracy of serologic tests for celiac disease: a systematic review. Gastroenterology. 2005;128(4 Suppl 1):S38–46. PubMed PMID: 15825125.
25. Hill ID. What are the sensitivity and specificity of serologic tests for celiac disease? Do sensitivity and specificity vary in different populations? Gastroenterology. 2005;128(4 Suppl 1):S25–32. PubMed PMID: 15825123.
26. Naiyer AJ, Hernandez L, Ciaccio EJ, Papadakis K, Manavalan JS, Bhagat G, et al. Comparison of commercially available serologic kits for the detection of celiac disease. J Clin Gastroenterol. 2009;43(3):225–32. PubMed PMID: 18724250.
27. Schuppan D, Junker Y, Barisani D. Celiac disease: from pathogenesis to novel therapies. Gastroenterology. 2009;137(6):1912–33. PubMed PMID: 19766641.
28. Prince HE. Evaluation of the INOVA diagnostics enzyme-linked immunosorbent assay kits for measuring serum immunoglobulin G (IgG) and IgA to deamidated gliadin peptides. Clin Vaccine Immunol. 2006;13(1):150–1. PubMed PMID: 16426013. Pubmed Central PMCID: 1356631.
29. Volta U, Granito A, Parisi C, Fabbri A, Fiorini E, Piscaglia M, et al. Deamidated gliadin peptide antibodies as a routine test for celiac disease: a prospective analysis. J Clin Gastroenterol. 2010;44(3):186–90. PubMed PMID: 20042872.
30. Rostami K, Kerckhaert J, Tiemessen R, von Blomberg BM, Meijer JW, Mulder CJ. Sensitivity of antiendomysium and antigliadin antibodies in untreated celiac disease: disappointing in clinical practice. Am J Gastroenterol. 1999;94(4):888–94. PubMed PMID: 10201452.
31. Fasano A, Catassi C. Clinical practice. Celiac disease. N Engl J Med. 2012;367(25):2419–26. PubMed PMID: 23252527.
32. Tesei N, Sugai E, Vazquez H, Smecuol E, Niveloni S, Mazure R, et al. Antibodies to human recombinant tissue transglutaminase may detect coeliac disease patients undiagnosed by endomysial antibodies. Aliment Pharmacol Ther. 2003;17(11):1415–23. PubMed PMID: 12786636.
33. Dieterich W, Ehnis T, Bauer M, Donner P, Volta U, Riecken EO, et al. Identification of tissue transglutaminase as the autoantigen of celiac disease. Nat Med. 1997;3(7):797–801. PubMed PMID: 9212111.
34. Zintzaras E, Germenis AE. Performance of antibodies against tissue transglutaminase for the diagnosis of celiac disease: meta-analysis. Clin Vaccine Immunol. 2006;13(2):187–92. PubMed PMID: 16467324. Pubmed Central PMCID: 1391934.
35. Raivio T, Korponay-Szabo I, Collin P, Laurila K, Huhtala H, Kaartinen T, et al. Performance of a new rapid whole blood coeliac test in adult patients with low prevalence of endomysial antibodies. Dig Liver Dis. 2007;39(12):1057–63. PubMed PMID: 17983878.
36. Alarida K, Harown J, Ahmaida A, Marinelli L, Venturini C, Kodermaz G, et al. Coeliac disease in Libyan children: a screening study based on the rapid determination of anti-transglutaminase antibodies. Dig Liver Dis. 2011;43(9):688–91. PubMed PMID: 21310672.
37. Raivio T, Kaukinen K, Nemes E, Laurila K, Collin P, Kovacs JB, et al. Self transglutaminase-based rapid coeliac disease antibody detection by a lateral flow method. Aliment Pharmacol Ther. 2006;24(1):147–54. PubMed PMID: 16803613.
38. Yel L. Selective IgA deficiency. J Clin Immunol. 2010;30(1):10–6. PubMed PMID: 20101521. Pubmed Central PMCID: 2821513.
39. Cunningham-Rundles C. Physiology of IgA and IgA deficiency. J Clin Immunol. 2001;21(5):303–9. PubMed PMID: 11720003.
40. Cataldo F, Marino V, Ventura A, Bottaro G, Corazza GR. Prevalence and clinical features of selective immunoglobulin A deficiency in coeliac disease: an Italian multicentre study. Italian Society of Paediatric Gastroenterology and Hepatology (SIGEP) and "Club del Tenue" Working Groups on Coeliac Disease. Gut. 1998;42(3):362–5. PubMed PMID: 9577342. Pubmed Central PMCID: 1727042.

41. Chow MA, Lebwohl B, Reilly NR, Green PH. Immunoglobulin a deficiency in celiac disease. J Clin Gastroenterol. 2012;46(10):850–4. PubMed PMID: 22476042.
42. Dahlbom I, Olsson M, Forooz NK, Sjoholm AG, Truedsson L, Hansson T. Immunoglobulin G (IgG) anti-tissue transglutaminase antibodies used as markers for IgA-deficient celiac disease patients. Clin Diagn Lab Immunol. 2005;12(2):254–8. PubMed PMID: 15699419. Pubmed Central PMCID: 549312.
43. Sinclair D, Saas M, Turk A, Goble M, Kerr D. Do we need to measure total serum IgA to exclude IgA deficiency in coeliac disease? J Clin Pathol. 2006;59(7):736–9. PubMed PMID: 16489174. Pubmed Central PMCID: 1860425.
44. Sollid LM. Molecular basis of celiac disease. Annu Rev Immunol. 2000;18:53–81. PubMed PMID: 10837052.
45. Hadithi M, von Blomberg BM, Crusius JB, Bloemena E, Kostense PJ, Meijer JW, et al. Accuracy of serologic tests and HLA-DQ typing for diagnosing celiac disease. Ann Intern Med. 2007;147(5):294–302. PubMed PMID: 17785484.
46. Oberhuber G, Granditsch G, Vogelsang H. The histopathology of coeliac disease: time for a standardized report scheme for pathologists. Eur J Gastroenterol Hepatol. 1999;11(10):1185–94. PubMed PMID: 10524652.
47. Rubin CE, Brandborg LL, Phelps PC, Taylor Jr HC. Studies of celiac disease. I. The apparent identical and specific nature of the duodenal and proximal jejunal lesion in celiac disease and idiopathic sprue. Gastroenterology. 1960;38:28–49. PubMed PMID: 14439871.
48. Marsh MN. Gluten, major histocompatibility complex, and the small intestine. A molecular and immunobiologic approach to the spectrum of gluten sensitivity ('celiac sprue'). Gastroenterology. 1992;102(1):330–54.
49. Marsh MN, Crowe PT. Morphology of the mucosal lesion in gluten sensitivity. Baillieres Clin Gastroenterol. 1995;9(2):273–93. PubMed PMID: 7549028.
50. Ferguson A, Arranz E, O'Mahony S. Clinical and pathological spectrum of coeliac disease–active, silent, latent, potential. Gut. 1993;34(2):150–1. PubMed PMID: 8432463. Pubmed Central PMCID: 1373959.
51. Shah VH, Rotterdam H, Kotler DP, Fasano A, Green PH. All that scallops is not celiac disease. Gastrointest Endosc. 2000;51(6):717–20. PubMed PMID: 10840307.
52. Dickey W, Hughes D. Disappointing sensitivity of endoscopic markers for villous atrophy in a high-risk population: implications for celiac disease diagnosis during routine endoscopy. Am J Gastroenterol. 2001;96(7):2126–8. PubMed PMID: 11467643.
53. Harewood GC, Holub JL, Lieberman DA. Variation in small bowel biopsy performance among diverse endoscopy settings: results from a national endoscopic database. Am J Gastroenterol. 2004;99(9):1790–4. PubMed PMID: 15330920.
54. Lebwohl B, Tennyson CA, Holub JL, Lieberman DA, Neugut AI, Green PH. Sex and racial disparities in duodenal biopsy to evaluate for celiac disease. Gastrointest Endosc. 2012;76(4):779–85. PubMed PMID: 22732871. Pubmed Central PMCID: 3445758.
55. Fasano A, Berti I, Gerarduzzi T, Not T, Colletti RB, Drago S, et al. Prevalence of celiac disease in at-risk and not-at-risk groups in the United States: a large multicenter study. Arch Intern Med. 2003;163(3):286–92. PubMed PMID: 12578508.
56. Mukherjee R, Egbuna I, Brar P, Hernandez L, McMahon DJ, Shane EJ, et al. Celiac disease: similar presentations in the elderly and young adults. Dig Dis Sci. 2010;55(11):3147–53. PubMed PMID: 20165980.
57. Kurien M, Evans KE, Hopper AD, Hale MF, Cross SS, Sanders DS. Duodenal bulb biopsies for diagnosing adult celiac disease: is there an optimal biopsy site? Gastrointest Endosc. 2012;75(6):1190–6. PubMed PMID: 22624810.
58. Evans KE, Aziz I, Cross SS, Sahota GR, Hopper AD, Hadjivassiliou M, et al. A prospective study of duodenal bulb biopsy in newly diagnosed and established adult celiac disease. Am J Gastroenterol. 2011;106(10):1837–42. PubMed PMID: 21606978.
59. Gonzalez S, Gupta A, Cheng J, Tennyson C, Lewis SK, Bhagat G, et al. Prospective study of the role of duodenal bulb biopsies in the diagnosis of celiac disease. Gastrointest Endosc. 2010;72(4):758–65. PubMed PMID: 20883853.

60. Hopper AD, Cross SS, Sanders DS. Patchy villous atrophy in adult patients with suspected gluten-sensitive enteropathy: is a multiple duodenal biopsy strategy appropriate? Endoscopy. 2008;40(3):219–24. PubMed PMID: 18058655.
61. Pais WP, Duerksen DR, Pettigrew NM, Bernstein CN. How many duodenal biopsy specimens are required to make a diagnosis of celiac disease? Gastrointest Endosc. 2008;67(7):1082–7. PubMed PMID: 18308317.
62. Lebwohl B, Kapel RC, Neugut AI, Green PH, Genta RM. Adherence to biopsy guidelines increases celiac disease diagnosis. Gastrointest Endosc. 2011;74(1):103–9. PubMed PMID: 21601201.
63. Arguelles-Grande C, Tennyson CA, Lewis SK, Green PH, Bhagat G. Variability in small bowel histopathology reporting between different pathology practice settings: impact on the diagnosis of coeliac disease. J Clin Pathol. 2012;65(3):242–7. PubMed PMID: 22081783.
64. Di Sabatino A, Corazza GR. Nonceliac gluten sensitivity: sense or sensibility? Ann Intern Med. 2012;156(4):309–11. PubMed PMID: 22351716.
65. Rubio-Tapia A, Rahim MW, See JA, Lahr BD, Wu TT, Murray JA. Mucosal recovery and mortality in adults with celiac disease after treatment with a gluten-free diet. Am J Gastroenterol. 2010;105(6):1412–20. PubMed PMID: 20145607. Pubmed Central PMCID: 2881171.
66. Iltanen S, Holm K, Partanen J, Laippala P, Maki M. Increased density of jejunal gammadelta+T cells in patients having normal mucosa – marker of operative autoimmune mechanisms? Autoimmunity. 1999;29(3):179–87. PubMed PMID: 10433098.
67. Tuire I, Marja-Leena L, Teea S, Katri H, Jukka P, Paivi S, et al. Persistent duodenal intraepithelial lymphocytosis despite a long-term strict gluten-free diet in celiac disease. Am J Gastroenterol. 2012;107(10):1563–9. PubMed PMID: 22825364.
68. Leffler D, Schuppan D, Pallav K, Najarian R, Goldsmith JD, Hansen J, et al. Kinetics of the histological, serological and symptomatic responses to gluten challenge in adults with coeliac disease. Gut. 2013;62:996–1004. PubMed PMID: 22619366. Pubmed Central PMCID: 3525791.
69. Hill ID, Dirks MH, Liptak GS, Colletti RB, Fasano A, Guandalini S, et al. Guideline for the diagnosis and treatment of celiac disease in children: recommendations of the North American Society for Pediatric Gastroenterology, Hepatology and Nutrition. J Pediatr Gastroenterol Nutr. 2005;40(1):1–19. PubMed PMID: 15625418.
70. Carlsson A, Axelsson I, Borulf S, Bredberg A, Forslund M, Lindberg B, et al. Prevalence of IgA-antigliadin antibodies and IgA-antiendomysium antibodies related to celiac disease in children with Down syndrome. Pediatrics. 1998;101(2):272–5. PubMed PMID: 9445503.
71. Barbato M, Maiella G, Di Camillo C, Guida S, Valitutti F, Lastrucci G, et al. The anti-deamidated gliadin peptide antibodies unmask celiac disease in small children with chronic diarrhoea. Dig Liver Dis. 2011;43(6):465–9. PubMed PMID: 21257356.
72. Monzani A, Rapa A, Fonio P, Tognato E, Panigati L, Oderda G. Use of deamidated gliadin peptide antibodies to monitor diet compliance in childhood celiac disease. J Pediatr Gastroenterol Nutr. 2011;53(1):55–60. PubMed PMID: 21694536.
73. Mubarak A, Wolters VM, Gerritsen SA, Gmelig-Meyling FH, Ten Kate FJ, Houwen RH. A biopsy is not always necessary to diagnose celiac disease. J Pediatr Gastroenterol Nutr. 2011;52(5):554–7. PubMed PMID: 21240025.
74. Barker CC, Mitton C, Jevon G, Mock T. Can tissue transglutaminase antibody titers replace small-bowel biopsy to diagnose celiac disease in select pediatric populations? Pediatrics. 2005;115(5):1341–6. PubMed PMID: 15867045.
75. Alessio MG, Tonutti E, Brusca I, Radice A, Licini L, Sonzogni A, et al. Correlation between IgA tissue transglutaminase antibody ratio and histological finding in celiac disease. J Pediatr Gastroenterol Nutr. 2012;55(1):44–9. PubMed PMID: 22197946.
76. Husby S, Koletzko S, Korponay-Szabo IR, Mearin ML, Phillips A, Shamir R, et al. European society for pediatric gastroenterology, hepatology, and nutrition guidelines for the diagnosis of coeliac disease. J Pediatr Gastroenterol Nutr. 2012;54(1):136–60. PubMed PMID: 22197856.
77. Farrell RJ, Kelly CP. Celiac disease and refractory celiac disease. In: Feldman M, Friedman LS, Brandt LJ, editors. Sleisenger and Fordtrans gastrointestinal and liver disease – pathophysiology diagnosis management. 9th ed. Philadelphia, PA: Elsevier; 2010.

Chapter 10
Nutrition in Celiac Disease

Suzanne Simpson and Tricia Thompson

According to the Academy of Nutrition and Dietetics (formerly the American Dietetic Association) evidence analysis library, "medical nutrition therapy provided by a registered dietitian is strongly recommended for individuals with celiac disease" [1]. Therefore, consultation with a dietitian/nutritionist that has expertise in CD should be mandatory for all patients with CD at diagnosis as well as in follow-up (Table 10.1). The gluten-free diet is currently the only treatment for CD, a genetically based autoimmune disease with chronic inflammation of the small intestinal mucosa. Individuals with CD have an immunologic reaction to the proteins in wheat, rye, and barley. Patients with CD must be monitored closely by the dietitian to assess the healthfulness of the gluten-free diet as well as to discuss motivation, quality of life, symptom improvement, and barriers to compliance.

Nutrition assessment is the first step in the nutrition care process. During the assessment, pertinent data are gathered and compared to normative values. A nutrition diagnosis is determined and a nutrition care plan is developed and prescribed. The nutrition intervention should include goals that are quantifiable, achievable, time defined, and negotiated with the patient so as to improve dietary intake and reduce risk factors. The assessment continues at each patient visit. A complete nutrition assessment includes a review of dietary intake, anthropometric measures, biochemical data, medical tests, and procedures (Table 10.2). Communication with the referring physician/gastroenterologist is advisable for optimal patient care. During the assessment, the dietitian may determine that a diagnosed patient with gastrointestinal symptoms, not related to gluten intake, could be related to another food intolerance or a medical issue that the physician must investigate. Similarly, the dietitian may determine that a micronutrient deficiency or weight

S. Simpson, Ba.Sc., B.A.H., R.D. (✉)
Columbia University, Celiac Disease Center, 180 Fort Washington Avenue,
Suite 936, New York, NY 10034, USA
e-mail: sms2246@columbia.eu

T. Thompson, M.S., R.D.
Gluten Free Watchdog, LLC, Manchester, MA, USA

S.D. Rampertab and G.E. Mullin (eds.), *Celiac Disease*, Clinical Gastroenterology, 123
DOI 10.1007/978-1-4614-8560-5_10, © Springer Science+Business Media New York 2014

Table 10.1 When to refer patients with celiac disease to a dietitian

Initial assessment at diagnosis as well as two to three more visits within the first year of diagnosis as well as annual visits thereafter
Suspicion of gluten ingestion (positive serologies after 1 year or more of being on a gluten-free diet)
Food intolerances (lactose, fructose), food allergies
Constipation/diarrhea/reflux
Fluctuations in body mass index—weight gain or loss
Micronutrient deficiencies or toxicities
Gastroparesis
Hypercholesterolemia
Type 1 diabetes
Refractory celiac disease

Table 10.2 Nutrition assessment checklist

Obtain a complete dietary history—foods and beverages consumed at all meals and snacks, including name brands
Ensure adequate calories, protein, micronutrient intake (the typical gluten-free diet can increase the risk of calcium, iron, fiber, vitamin D, folate, niacin, zinc, vitamin B_{12} deficiencies due to lack of fortification of gluten-free packaged foods including breads, pastas)
Review intake of foods away from the home—restaurant frequency, fast food, take out, order in, cafeteria, other people's homes, social and work events
Travel—foods consumed, frequency of travel
Supplements—herbal remedies, over-the-counter diet aids
Vitamins and minerals—review name brands and check if gluten-free; compare and correct micronutrients compared to recommended intake
Prescription medications—must be gluten-free
Cross-contamination prevention measures
Review past medical history, family history, symptoms, laboratory measures; review of all tests and procedures
Anthropometrics—height, weight, BMI
Social support—family, work, peers
Quality of life—work, family, exercise, risk of depression
Activity level
Assess knowledge of gluten-free diet food labels—make sure client knows how to identify gluten in an ingredient list, understands the meaning of nutrition food claims such as no gluten, gluten-free, wheat-free, made in the same factory that processes wheat, low gluten
Readiness for change—assess patient willingness to change diet and patient's goals for learning and meeting with the dietitian
Family history—other family members with celiac disease; family members tested for celiac disease
Potential nutrition diagnoses—follows a strict gluten-free diet, ingesting gluten inadvertently in restaurants, ingesting gluten on purpose monthly, inadequate calcium/vitamin D intake, inadequate fiber intake, risk of iron deficiency, constipation due to inadequate fiber intake, excessive caloric intake resulting in weight gain, at risk of overweight

loss is not caused by inadequate intake. Dietitians can also recommend the physician to screen for CD in patients that do not have a diagnosis but exhibit symptoms or in those who have significant medical history or family history or unexplained nutrient deficiencies.

Dietary Intake Assessment

Assessment of typical dietary intake in CD must be thorough. All food and beverages consumed on weekdays and weekends should be reviewed including name brands of products and frequency of food eaten away from the home (restaurants, social events, other people's homes, travel). It is helpful for the patient to complete a food diary for the dietitian to review. Dietary restrictions such as food intolerances, food allergies, religious observances, and self-imposed restrictions are considered.

Patients should be queried about their compliance to a strict gluten-free diet and the frequency of gluten ingestion (purposely or inadvertently). It is important to assess patients' knowledge and understanding of the diet by reviewing their label reading principles, how they order foods in restaurants, and what cross-contamination procedures are utilized in shared kitchens.

Patients may have obtained information about the gluten-free diet elsewhere, and it is important to assess the source for its accuracy (internet, other nutritionists, books, peers, magazines). Medications, vitamins, and dietary supplements must be reviewed for their gluten status, their purpose, and whether they meet or exceed the Dietary Reference Intake (brands are required). It is important to assess quality of life, social history/social support, sufficiency of income, and ability to access gluten-free food. Inquiry should be made as to who prepares food at home, particularly in a shared kitchen. A review of gastrointestinal symptoms (such as type, frequency, and volume of bowel movements, abdominal pain, bloating, nausea or vomiting, delayed gastric emptying, reflux, flatulence) is required. Compliance with a strict gluten-free diet usually reduces gastrointestinal symptoms in CD [2–13] and should always be encouraged.

Anthropometric Assessment

Assess age, height, weight, body mass index, growth parameters in children, weight history, physical activity, disordered eating, and/or diets (currently or in the past).

Table 10.3 Laboratory measures recommended

Laboratory tests	Include	Frequency
Celiac disease antibodies	Anti-endomysial antibody Anti-tissue transglutaminase antibody Deamidated gliadin protein Serum IgA level	One to two times a year post diagnosis
Anemia profile	Hemoglobin Hematocrit MCV Folate Ferritin Transferrin saturation Vitamin B_{12}	One to two times a year
Vitamin profile	Vitamin B_6 Thiamin Riboflavin 25-Hydroxy vitamin D Vitamins A, E	Annually—if abnormal must be repeated 3 months after treatment
Mineral profile	Copper Zinc Magnesium Calcium	Annually
Lipid profile	LDL HDL Triglycerides Total cholesterol	Annually—more frequently if abnormal
Electrolytes	Sodium Potassium	Annually
Other	PTH Albumin ESR	Annually
Renal profile	BUN Creatinine GFR	Annually

Biochemical Data, Medical Tests, and Procedure Assessment

Review all laboratory tests. If these are not accessible, a request should be made to access such information. See Table 10.3 for a list of tests that should be accessed and/or recommended.

Medical Procedures

All medical procedures must be reviewed including endoscopy report (classification of Marsh scores, number, and location of segments biopsied), bone mineral density,

Table 10.4 Nutrition education for the gluten-free diet

Label reading 101—review the list of ingredients that must be avoided, labeling laws, surprising sources of gluten, cross-contamination procedures, nutrition claims (e.g., gluten-free, wheat-free, low gluten, made in the same facility as wheat, no gluten ingredients), sources of important nutrients such as calcium, vitamin D, iron, fiber
Provide recommendations for portions and variety of foods from all food groups
Heart-healthy recommendations to prevent high cholesterol
Recommend high fiber, as tolerated, to prevent weight gain and constipation
Review of gluten-free grains—50 % of grains consumed should be gluten-free whole grains
Discuss risk of vitamin deficiencies
Encourage healthful gluten-free food choices
Discuss risks associated with ingesting gluten
Discuss vitamin supplementation as needed
Discuss use of supplements such as probiotics, over-the-counter remedies
Discuss family testing
Discuss restaurant eating, social situations, menu planning, recipes, grocery shopping
Coordinate care with other healthcare providers
Discuss other dietary restrictions within the confines of the gluten-free diet: lactose-free diet, low-fructose diet, diabetes meal plan/carbohydrate counting, kosher diet, low-fat diet, weight-control diet
Implement weight-centered guidelines as needed

breath tests (bacterial overgrowth, fructose intolerance, lactose intolerance), gastric emptying study, surgeries, medical treatments, and colonoscopy. Review past medical history (e.g., gastrointestinal, immune, neurological, and psychological), other health conditions, autoimmune diseases, family history of CD, allergies, body-muscle stores, and fat stores. Inquire about appetite, current gastrointestinal symptoms, and symptoms prior to diagnosis of CD.

Physical

Assess appearance of hair, skin, nails, and body shape.

Nutrition Intervention and Education

The gluten-free diet is the medical and nutritional treatment for CD. A gluten-free diet is discussed in a later section of this chapter. Gluten must be removed from the diet completely and permanently. Table 10.4 includes a list of items that must be included in the nutrition education for patients with CD. It is important to answer questions the patient may have, establish a trustful rapport, and set goals with the patient that can be addressed in follow-up.

Table 10.5 Nutrition items to monitor in follow-up visits

Implementation of nutrition goals
Adherence to gluten-free living
Factors affecting quality of life
Medical status (e.g., gastrointestinal, immune, neurological, and psychological)
Social supports
Body mass index
Label reading principles
Restaurant habits and frequency
Diet history and gluten-free dietary pattern—specific focus on intake of nutrients at risk of deficiency (iron, calcium, vitamin D, B vitamins, fiber, folate, niacin, zinc), intake compared to recommendations (food pyramid), recommend not ingesting excessive sugar and fat from prepared gluten-free foods, overall caloric intake
Vitamin intake
Medications and supplements
Antibody levels, potential exposure to cross-contamination, surprising sources of gluten in foods
Answer patient questions

Follow-up

CD is a lifelong systemic disease with a burdensome treatment that requires regular follow-up visits with the expert dietitian and gastroenterologist; patients must be monitored for compliance, symptoms, well-being, and medical issues. See Table 10.5 for items that need to be monitored during follow-up visits.

If someone with CD is not treated with the gluten-free diet, there can be serious consequences. The intake of gluten may result in gastrointestinal symptoms, malabsorption and micronutrient deficiencies, villous atrophy and the development of neurological complications, fertility problems, reduced quality of life, intestinal lymphoma, and reduced bone mineral density. The dietitian must assess compliance in follow-up, particularly in patients with symptoms. If gluten exposure is determined not to be the cause of symptoms, other potential causes could be lactose, fructose, and carbohydrate intolerances, bacterial overgrowth, refractory sprue, related cancers, and other gastrointestinal diseases and conditions. These would require investigation by a gastroenterologist.

Individuals with CD have been found to show improved quality of life after compliance with a gluten-free dietary pattern for at least 1 year particularly if they had symptoms prior to diagnosis [12, 14]. However, they may not attain the same level of quality of life as the general population; this has been reported more frequently by women than men and particularly in those that continue to have gastrointestinal symptoms despite adherence to a gluten-free diet [15, 16].

The Gluten-Free Diet

Currently, the only treatment for CD is a strict, lifelong gluten-free diet. A gluten-free diet is defined as being free of all but miniscule amounts of protein from wheat, barley, rye, and crossbred varieties of these grains, such as triticale. In the USA, labeled gluten-free foods must contain less than 20 ppm of gluten from ingredients and/or cross-contact with gluten. In place of gluten-containing cereal foods (breads, pastas, breakfast cereals), foods containing corn, rice, millet teff, sorghum, wild rice, oats, amaranth, buckwheat, and quinoa are used.

Labeled Gluten-Free Foods

There are an ever-increasing number of labeled gluten-free cereal foods available in both natural foods stores and mainstream grocery stores. At the time of this writing, the Food and Drug Administration (FDA) had not yet released the final rule for labeling foods gluten-free. Under the FDA's proposed rule, a food may not be labeled gluten-free if any of the following applies [17]:

- The food contains an ingredient that is a prohibited grain. Prohibited grains include wheat, barley, rye, and triticale (a cross between wheat and rye).
- The food contains an ingredient derived from a prohibited grain that has not been processed to remove gluten. Examples of these types of ingredients include wheat flour, hydrolyzed wheat protein, wheat germ, malt, and barley malt flavoring.
- The food contains an ingredient derived from a prohibited grain that has been processed to remove gluten but use of the ingredient results in the final food product containing 20 ppm or more gluten. Examples of these types of ingredients are wheat starch and modified food starch made from wheat.
- The food contains 20 ppm or more of gluten.

The definition of gluten-free in the USA differs slightly from the codex standard for foods for special dietary use for persons intolerant to gluten [18]. Under this standard, gluten-free foods are dietary foods that fit one of the two definitions below.

- Foods that are made only from ingredients that do not contain wheat, barley, rye, oats,[1] or their crossbred varieties and with a gluten content not greater than 20 ppm.
- Foods made using one or more ingredients from wheat, barley, rye, oats, or their crossbred varieties which have been specially processed to remove gluten and with a gluten content not greater than 20 ppm.

---

[1] Under Codex, the use of oats uncontaminated with wheat, barley, and rye may be determined at a national level. In the United States, oats are not considered a prohibited grain and may be included in labeled gluten-free foods as long as the final food product contains less than 20 ppm of gluten and the food meets the other criteria for gluten-free labeling.

Reading Labels of Foods Not Labeled Gluten-Free

In the USA, gluten-free consumers are advised to trust the food label. If a food is labeled gluten-free, the manufacturer has determined that the product meets the criteria for labeling established by the FDA. For food not labeled gluten-free, the consumer has to read the ingredients list and contains statement for six words. If any of the following words are included on the food label, the food should be avoided:

1. "Wheat." Under the FDA's Food Allergen Labeling and Consumer Protection Act (FALCPA), if an ingredient in a packaged food product regulated by the FDA includes protein from wheat, the word "wheat" must be included on the food label either in the ingredients list or Contains statement [19]. If the word "wheat" is not included on the food label, none of the ingredients in the product contain protein from wheat.
2. "Barley."
3. "Rye."
4. "Oats." Only oats and products containing oats labeled gluten-free should be eaten by individuals with CD [20]. While oats are considered inherently gluten-free, they also are highly likely to be contaminated with wheat, barley, or rye [21, 22].
5. "Malt." The single word "malt" in an ingredients list means "barley malt" [23]. If another source of malt is used, such as corn, the ingredients list will read "corn malt."
6. "Brewer's yeast." This type of yeast may be a product of the beer brewing process (i.e., spent brewer's yeast) [24]. As a result, it may be contaminated with malt and grain.

Foods Regulated by the USDA

While the labeling of most food in the USA is under the jurisdiction of the FDA, some foods are regulated by the United States Department of Agriculture (USDA). These products are meat products, poultry products, egg products (defined as liquid, dried, and frozen whole eggs, egg yolks, and egg whites with or without added ingredients), and mixed food products containing in general more than 3 % raw meat or 2 % or more cooked meat or poultry meat [25–27]. While the FDA has mandatory allergen labeling under FALCPA, the USDA does not. Manufacturers under the jurisdiction of the USDA are encouraged to voluntarily follow FALCPA-like allergen labeling, and the USDA believes 80–90 % of product labels are in voluntary compliance [25].

There are a few additional ingredients consumers must look for in the ingredients lists of foods regulated by the USDA if the manufacturer is not voluntarily following FALCPA-like allergen labeling. These ingredients (in addition to the ingredients already listed above) should be avoided until the manufacturer is contacted and it is confirmed that the source of the ingredient is not wheat.

1. "Modified food starch." Modified food starch in a food regulated by the USDA may contain protein from wheat and "wheat" may not be included on the food label if the manufacturer is not voluntarily complying with FALCPA-like allergen labeling [28].
2. "Dextrin." Dextrin in a food regulated by the USDA may contain protein from wheat, and "wheat" may not be included on the food label if the manufacturer is not voluntarily complying with FALCPA-like allergen labeling [28].
3. "Starch." The single word "starch" in the ingredients list of a food product regulated by the USDA may mean either "corn starch" or "wheat starch" [29]. If the starch is derived from wheat and contains wheat protein, the word wheat may not be included on the food label if the manufacturer is not voluntarily complying with FALCPA-like allergen labeling [28]. Note: In foods regulated by the FDA, the single word "starch" in the ingredients list means "cornstarch."

For all of these ingredients—modified food starch, dextrin, and starch—the source is most likely cornstarch if the ingredient is manufactured in the USA. If the ingredient is manufactured outside the USA, there is a greater likelihood that the source is wheat starch.

Beverages Regulated by the TTB

The Alcohol and Tobacco Tax and Trade Bureau (TTB) recently released an interim policy on gluten content statements in the labeling and advertising of wines, distilled spirits, and malt beverages [30]. The TTB regulates almost all alcohol sold in the USA. Exceptions include beer made without malted barley and hops and wines containing less than 7 % alcohol by volume. These beverages are regulated by the FDA and must comply with FDA labeling laws.

Under the TTB's interim policy, a gluten-free claim cannot be included on product labels if the alcohol is made with any amount of wheat, barley, rye, or crossbred varieties of these grains. Manufacturers can include a gluten-free claim on product labels if the beverage is made without gluten-containing grains, but manufacturers must ensure that the raw materials, ingredients, production facilities, storage materials, and finished products are not cross-contaminated with gluten. Alcoholic beverages that may qualify for a gluten-free claim include wine, rum, and vodka distilled from potatoes.

The TTB is allowing the statement "Processed (or treated or crafted) to remove gluten" on product labels if the grains used or ingredients used in the beverage have been processed to remove all or some of the gluten, but an explanatory statement must also be included. For fermented products, the statement must read, "Product fermented from grains containing gluten and processed (or treated or crafted) to remove gluten. The gluten content of this product cannot be verified, and this product may contain gluten." For distilled products the statement must read, "This product was distilled from grains containing gluten which removed some or all of the gluten. The gluten content of this product cannot be verified, and this product may contain gluten."

Cross-Contamination with Wheat, Barley, or Rye

Naturally gluten-free grains may become contaminated with gluten-containing grain anywhere along the line from the field where they are grown (due to crop rotation with wheat, barley, or rye or one of these grains being grown in a adjacent field) to the plant where they are processed (due to shared harvesting, transporting, and/or processing equipment). A study by Thompson et al. found that of 22 samples of naturally gluten-free grains and flours sold in the USA, nine contained mean levels of gluten ranging from 8.5 to 2,925.0 ppm of gluten [31]. Seven of these samples contained mean levels of gluten at or above 20 ppm and would not be considered gluten-free under the FDA's proposed gluten-free labeling rule. To help decrease the risk of cross-contamination, the Academy of Nutrition and Dietetics Celiac Disease Toolkit recommends that individuals with CD buy naturally gluten-free grains and flours that are labeled gluten-free [32]. It is also recommended that products that are predominantly grain-based be labeled gluten-free [32]. A comparison of the gluten content of labeled versus not labeled gluten-free millet, rice, soy, and sorghum flours is provided in Table 10.6. The labeled gluten-free brands tested contained lower amounts of gluten than the brands not labeled gluten-free [31, 33].

Inadvertent gluten intake through contamination must be considered if it is believed that an individual is consuming gluten despite the appearance of a strict gluten-free diet based on symptoms and/or follow-up serological testing. A registered dietitian well versed in CD must be consulted to help determine the source of contamination. Food may be contaminated at point of purchase or become contaminated in the home. If a lot of eating is done outside the home (e.g., restaurant), then this will have to be investigated too.

Nutritional Quality of the Gluten-Free Diet

The nutritional quality of the gluten-free diet depends upon the food choices of consumers. According to the Academy of Nutrition and Dietetics Evidence Analysis Library, "adherence to the gluten-free dietary pattern may result in a diet that is high in fat and low in carbohydrates and fiber, as well as low in iron, folate, niacin, vitamin B_{12}, calcium, phosphorus and zinc" [34]. There is also evidence that gluten-free diets may contain inadequate amounts of thiamin [35]. As a result, the Academy's Evidence-Based Nutrition Practice Guideline for Celiac Disease recommends the consumption of whole and enriched gluten-free grains and products [20]. The addition of a gluten-free age and gender-specific multivitamin and mineral supplement is advised if "usual food intake shows nutritional inadequacies that cannot be alleviated through improved eating habits" [20].

There are several possible reasons for this macro- and micronutrient profile of the gluten-free diet. Individuals with CD may not consume the recommended number of servings of grain foods. A study conducted by Thompson et al. found that only 21 % of US adult female participants consumed the minimum recommended

Table 10.6 Gluten content of labeled versus not labeled gluten-free flours[a]

Flour	Mean gluten content ppm[b]
Labeled gluten-free	
Millet	15.5
Rice	<5
Sorghum	<5[c]
Soy	<5[d]
Not labeled gluten-free	
Millet	305.0
Millet	327.0
Rice	8.5
Sorghum	234.0
Soy	2,925.0
Soy	92.0

[a]Data from [31, 33]
[b]Flours not labeled gluten-free: one sample tested in duplicate (mean of two extractions); flours labeled gluten-free: three samples of same brand tested in duplicate (six extractions)
[c]Five extractions tested <5 ppm gluten; one extraction tested at 7 ppm gluten
[d]Five extractions tested <5 ppm gluten; one extraction tested at 6 ppm gluten

number of grain food servings [36]. A retrospective review of diet histories of patients with CD at a US celiac disease center conducted by Lee et al. found that 38 % of meals and snacks eaten by study participants did not contain a grain or starch component [37]. Low overall grain consumption can result in diets that are low in carbohydrates and fiber and proportionally higher in fat [38]. It also can result in diets that are low in iron, folate, niacin, and zinc [38].

Many of the grain-based foods that individuals with CD eat may be higher in fat than their gluten-containing counterparts. This is due to manufacturers adding ingredients, including fat, to mimic the mouthfeel and texture of gluten. Increased fat content of foods not generally thought to contain fat can result in diets that are inadvertently high in fat.

Individuals with CD may consume grain foods made primarily from refined gluten-free grains and starch, such as white rice, milled corn, rice starch, cornstarch, and tapioca starch. A study conducted by Thompson found that of 268 gluten-free breads, pastas, and breakfast cereals for sale in the USA and reviewed for ingredients, 73 % listed a refined grain or starch as the first ingredient [39]. Of these refined grain foods, only 16 % were enriched or fortified with B vitamins and iron. Since this study was conducted, there has been an increase in availability and use of alternative gluten-free whole grains and flours, including millet, teff, sorghum, wild rice, amaranth, buckwheat, and quinoa. Regardless, too many gluten-free cereal products are made that still list maize, starch, or white rice flour as the first ingredient. Additionally, there has not been much of an increase in the numbers of manufacturers enriching or fortifying refined gluten-free products. An overreliance on refined grain-based foods (versus whole grains) that are not enriched or fortified can result in diets that are low in fiber, iron, folate, niacin, vitamin B_{12}, and zinc [38].

In addition, many individuals newly diagnosed with CD also are diagnosed with secondary lactose intolerance. While this type of lactose intolerance generally resolves as the small intestine heals, individuals may limit their intake of milk-based products. This may result in decreased intakes of calcium, vitamin B_{12}, and phosphorous [38].

To help ensure a healthy gluten-free diet, individuals with CD should be:

- Referred to a dietitian well versed in CD as soon as possible after diagnosis. Dietitians can be found at http://www.eatright.org and http://www.glutenfreedietitian.com/newsletter/dietitians-specializing-in-celiac-disease/.
- Encouraged to consume foods made from gluten-free whole grains (e.g., quinoa, gluten-free oats, teff), especially those products that list a whole grain as the first ingredient, and to choose whole grain products over those made with refined gluten-free grains (e.g., white rice, milled corn, tapioca starch).
- Counseled to choose enriched or fortified refined grain foods over refined grain foods that are not enriched. Consumers should be advised that they can determine whether a product is enriched or fortified by reading the ingredients list. Added vitamins and minerals will be included in the list or immediately following the list.
- Advised to use the Nutrition Facts panel to compare the fat and fiber content of gluten-free grain foods and to choose products with more fiber and less fat whenever possible.
- Encouraged to eat or drink calcium-rich foods even if they are lactose intolerant, such as calcium-fortified soy milk, calcium-fortified orange juice, and calcium-processed plain tofu, as well as foods naturally containing calcium, such as leafy greens and beans.

Weight Gain and the Gluten-Free Diet

Contrary to what is often reported in the media, a gluten-free diet is not a weight loss plan. In fact, many individuals complain of weight gain after being diagnosed with CD and starting a gluten-free diet. According to the Academy of Nutrition and Dietetics Evidence Analysis Library, "A small number of studies in adults show a trend toward weight gain after diagnosis; further research is needed in this area" [34]. One reason why individuals with CD might gain weight after diagnosis is that caloric intake requirements may decrease once the gluten-free diet is begun [36]. Prior to diagnosis, individuals may have experienced varying degrees of malabsorption. In order to maintain their weight or decrease the rate of weight loss, they may have become used to eating a certain number of calories. Once a diagnosis is made, a gluten-free diet is started, and the intestine heals. Therefore, fewer calories may be needed to maintain weight. Individuals may have to adjust their caloric intake and relearn appropriate portion control to prevent unwanted weight gain.

References

1. Academy of Nutrition and Dietetics. Evidence analysis library. Celiac disease. Evidence-based nutrition practice guideline. http://www.adaevidencelibrary.com/topic.cfm?cat=3726.
2. Cucchiara S, Bassotti G, Castellucci G, Minella R, Betti C, Fusaro C, et al. Upper gastrointestinal motor abnormalities in children with active celiac disease. J Pediatr Gastroenterol Nutr. 1995;21:435–42.
3. Usai P, Bassotti G, Usai Satta P, Cherchi M, Plesa A, Boy F, et al. Oesophageal motility in adult coeliac disease. Neurogastroenterol Motil. 1995;7:239–44.
4. Chiarioni G, Bassotti G, Germani U, Battaglia E, Brentegani MT, Morelli A, et al. Gluten-free diet normalizes mouth-to-cecum transit of a caloric meal in adult patients with celiac disease. Dig Dis Sci. 1997;42:2100–5.
5. Fine KD, Meyer RL, Lee EL. The prevalence and causes of chronic diarrhea in patients with celiac sprue treated with a gluten-free diet. Gastroenterology. 1997;112:1830–8.
6. Benini L, Sembenini C, Salandini L, Dall OE, Bonfante F, Vantini I. Gastric emptying of realistic meals with and without gluten in patients with coeliac disease. Effect of jejunal mucosal recovery. Scand J Gastroenterol. 2001;36:1044–8.
7. Cuomo A, Romano M, Rocco A, Budillon G, Del Vecchio Blanco C, Nardone G. Reflux oesophagitis in adult coeliac disease: beneficial effect of a gluten free diet. Gut. 2003;52:514–7.
8. Midhagen G, Hallert C. High rate of gastrointestinal symptoms in celiac patients living on a gluten-free diet: controlled study. Am J Gastroenterol. 2003;98:2023–6.
9. Tursi A, Brandimarte G, Giorgetti G. High prevalence of small intestinal bacterial overgrowth in celiac patients with persistence of gastrointestinal symptoms after gluten withdrawal. Am J Gastroenterol. 2003;98:839–43.
10. Murray JA, Watson T, Clearman B, Mitros F. Effect of a gluten-free diet on gastrointestinal symptoms in celiac disease. Am J Clin Nutr. 2004;79:669–73.
11. Hopper AD, Leeds JS, Hurlstone DP, Hadjivassiliou M, Drew K, Sanders DS. Are lower gastrointestinal investigations necessary in patients with coeliac disease? Eur J Gastroenterol Hepatol. 2005;17:617–21.
12. Viljamaa M, Collin P, Huhtala H, Sievanen H, Maki M, Kaukinen K. Is coeliac disease screening in risk groups justified? A fourteen-year follow-up with special focus on compliance and quality of life. Aliment Pharmacol Ther. 2005;22:317–24.
13. Casellas F, Lopez Vivancos J, Malagelada JR. Current epidemiology and accessibility to diet compliance in adult celiac disease. Rev Esp Enferm Dig. 2006;98:408–19.
14. Green PHR, Stavropoulos SN, Panagi SG, Goldstein SL, Mcmahon DJ, Absan H, et al. Characteristics of adult celiac disease in the USA: results of a national survey. Am J Gastroenterol. 2001;96:126–31.
15. Lee SK, Lo W, Memeo L, Rotterdam H, Green PH. Duodenal histology in patients with celiac disease after treatment with a gluten-free diet. Gastrointest Endosc. 2003;57:187–91.
16. Rashid M, Cranney A, Zarkadas M, Graham ID, Switzer C, Case S, et al. Celiac disease: evaluation of the diagnosis and dietary compliance in Canadian children. Pediatrics. 2005;116:e754–9.
17. US Food and Drug Administration. Federal register proposed rule-72 FR 2795 January 23 2007: food labeling; gluten-free labeling of foods. http://www.fda.gov/Food/LabelingNutrition/FoodAllergensLabeling/GuidanceComplianceRegulatoryInformation/ucm077926.htm.
18. Codex Alimentarius Commission. Standard for gluten-free foods (Stan 118) Revised 2008. http://www.codexalimentarius.net/web/more_info.jsp?id_sta=291.
19. US Food and Drug Administration. Center for Food Safety and Applied Nutrition. Food Allergen Labeling and Consumer Protection Act of 2004 (Title II of Public Law 108-282). August 2004. http://www.fda.gov/food/labelingnutrition/FoodAllergensLabeling/GuidanceComplianceRegulatoryInformation/ucm106187.htm.

20. Academy of Nutrition and Dietetics. Evidence analysis library. Celiac disease. Evidence-based nutrition practice guideline. http://www.adaevidencelibrary.com/topic.cfm?cat=3677.
21. Thompson T. Gluten contamination of commercial oat products in the United States. N Engl J Med. 2004;351:2021–2.
22. Koerner TB, Cleroux C, Poirier C, Cantin I, Alimkulov A, Elamparo H. Gluten contamination in the Canadian commercial oat supply. Food Addit Contam Part A Chem Anal Control Expo Risk Assess. 2011;28:705–10.
23. US Food and Drug Administration. Code of Federal Regulations. Malt. 21CFR184.1443a. Revised April 2009. http://www.accessdata.fda.gov/scripts/cdrh/cfdocs/cfcfr/CFRSearch.cfm?fr=184.1443a&SearchTerm=malt.
24. Thompson T. Is marmite gluten-free? Diet.com website. http://www.diet.com/dietblogs/read_blog.php?title=Is+Marmite+Gluten+Free%3F&blid=1853 (2010).
25. Thompson T. Labeling of USDA-regulated foods. Diet.com website. http://www.diet.com/dietblogs/read_blog.php?title=&blid=17330 (2009).
26. US Department of Agriculture. A guide to federal food labeling requirements for meat and poultry products. http://www.fsis.usda.gov/pdf/labeling_requirements_guide.pdf (2007).
27. US Department of Agriculture. Food safety and inspection service. Definition egg product. 9 CFR 590.5. http://edocket.access.gpo.gov/cfr_2008/janqtr/pdf/9cfr590.5.pdf.
28. US Department of Agriculture. Food safety and inspection service. Questions and answers related to ingredients of public health concern.
29. US Department of Agriculture. Food Safety and Inspection Service. Food safety. Food Standards and Labeling Policy Book. http://www.fsis.usda.gov/OPPDE/larc/Policies/Labeling_Policy_Book_082005.pdf (August 2005).
30. Department of Treasury. Alcohol and Tobacco Tex and Trade Bureau. Interim Policy on Gluten Content Statements in the Labeling and Advertising of Wines DSaMBTR. May 24, 2012 Number 2012-2.
31. Thompson T, Lee AR, Grace T. Gluten contamination of grains, seeds, and flours in the United States: a pilot study. J Am Diet Assoc. 2010;110:937–40.
32. Academy of Nutrition and Dietetics. Celiac disease toolkit. Chicago, IL: American Dietetic Association; 2011.
33. Gluten-free Watchdog, LLC. http://www.glutenfreewatchdog.org.
34. Academy of Nutrition and Dietetics. Evidence analysis library. Celiac disease. Evidence analysis library project. http://www.adaevidencelibrary.com/topic.cfm?cat=1403.
35. Shepherd SJ, Gibson PR. Nutritional inadequacies of the gluten-free diet in both recently-diagnosed and long-term patients with coeliac disease. J Hum Nutr Diet. 2012.
36. Thompson T, Dennis M, Higgins LA, Lee AR, Sharrett MK. Gluten-free diet survey: are Americans with coeliac disease consuming recommended amounts of fibre, iron, calcium and grain foods? J Hum Nutr Diet. 2005;18:163–9.
37. Lee AR, Ng DL, Dave E, Ciaccio EJ, Green PH. The effect of substituting alternative grains in the diet on the nutritional profile of the gluten-free diet. J Hum Nutr Diet. 2009;22:359–63.
38. Thompson T. ADA pocket guide to gluten-free strategies for clients with multiple dietary restrictions. Chicago, IL: American Dietetic Association; 2011.
39. Thompson T. Thiamin, riboflavin, and niacin contents of the gluten-free diet: is there cause for concern? J Am Diet Assoc. 1999;99:858–62.

Chapter 11
Dietary Supplements in Celiac Disease

Michelle Maria Pietzak

Why Are There Nutritional Deficiencies in Patients with Celiac Disease?

Celiac disease (CD) is more than just an "allergy" or "sensitivity" to wheat and gluten. It is a lifelong, permanent intolerance to the gliadin fraction of wheat protein and its related alcohol-soluble proteins (prolamins) found in rye and barley. In patients with the genetic susceptibility to CD, ingesting these proteins leads to an autoimmune enteropathy that will self-perpetuate as long as these foods remain in the diet. The good news is that, unlike most autoimmune conditions, removal of the environmental trigger (gluten) from the diet of a biopsy-proven celiac results in complete symptomatic and histologic resolution of the disease in the majority of patients [1, 2].

Differentiating CD from wheat allergy, gluten sensitivity, and other autoimmune gastrointestinal (GI) diseases (such as Crohn's disease) can be challenging. Likewise, CD can present at any age with "classic" GI features, such as diarrhea and weight loss, or outside the GI tract with anemia, rashes, infertility, osteoporosis, joint pain, short stature, delayed puberty, and even malignancy. It is common that patients experience chronic ill health and nutritional deficiencies prior to the correct diagnosis being made. These patients commonly incur high healthcare costs because of the multiple subspecialists and tests performed on them prior to the confirmation of CD [3].

The duodenum and proximal small bowel play an important role in the digestion and absorption of many key nutrients, such as carbohydrates, protein, lipids, and iron. The bulk flow of water occurs primarily through the porous junctions of the proximal

M.M. Pietzak, M.D. (✉)
Department of Pediatric Gastroenterology, University of Southern California Keck School of Medicine, Intern's and Resident's Building Room 124, 2020 Zonal Avenue, Los Angeles, CA, USA
e-mail: Pietzak@usc.edu

S.D. Rampertab and G.E. Mullin (eds.), *Celiac Disease*, Clinical Gastroenterology, DOI 10.1007/978-1-4614-8560-5_11,

small intestinal epithelial cells. The distal part of the small bowel, the terminal ileum, is preferentially responsible for the absorption of B_{12} and bile acids. In a patient with CD, depending upon the severity of intestinal damage, there may be varying amounts of edema, atrophy, and loss of disaccharidases (in particular, lactase) within the villous structures. This can lead to malabsorption of the above nutrients, as well as excessive osmotic load by undigested sugars, causing watery diarrhea.

The colon is an important salvage organ and is mainly responsible for the reabsorption of water. Also, indigestible fibers are broken down by enzymes in the colonic bacteria, producing short-chain fatty acids (acetate, proprionate, and butyrate), which are then efficiently absorbed by the colon. Some patients with CD will also have a lymphocytic colitis if biopsies are taken during a colonoscopy. Patients with CD-associated lymphocytic colitis may experience urgency and tenesmus in addition to watery diarrhea.

Lifelong compliance with the gluten-free diet (GFD) is challenging, with frequent temptations towards dietary transgressions, which will lead to further enteropathy and malabsorption. Adherence to the GFD is improved by patient education, close supervision by an interested physician, and regular nutritional counseling by a registered dietician with expertise in CD [4]. Compliance can be improved, even in adolescents, who are seen by a physician on a regular basis [5, 6]. One of the best and least expensive markers for dietary compliance is assessment by a trained interviewer (either a physician or dietician) due to the low cost, noninvasiveness, and a strong correlation to intestinal damage [6]. Healthcare providers should encourage the patient to join local chapters of national support organizations (see Appendix 1), which can aid in finding local resources such as supermarkets, food manufacturers, literature, and restaurants that are familiar with the GFD [4]. It is important to be familiar with the recommended dietary allowances of micronutrients of CD patients who are at risk for deficiencies. Likewise, the practitioner caring for the patient with CD should be able to recognize the signs of micronutrients deficiency, be able to provide guidelines for corrective supplementation, and monitor safety of therapy. We have provided the Food and Nutrition Board and the Institute of Medicine's Dietary Reference Intakes (DRI) for vitamins and elements in Appendix 10 and the DRI for Tolerable Upper Intake for vitamins and elements in Appendix 11 (http://www.iom.edu/About-IOM/Leadership-Staff/Boards/Food-and-Nutrition-Board.aspx).

Anemia in CD: Iron, B_{12}, and Folic Acid Deficiencies

Background

A routine complete blood cell count may reveal many hematologic abnormalities in an untreated patient with CD. Anemia, leukopenia, and thrombocytopenia have all been reported. The anemia is usually microcytic and hypochromic, due to iron deficiency [7]. Iron is absorbed by villus enterocytes in the proximal duodenum [8]. A macrocytic anemia should warrant an investigation into deficiencies of B12 (cobalamin) and/or folic acid. A large study in a cohort of patients with newly diagnosed CD found anemia in 20 %, with iron deficiency in 33 % of men and 19 % of women, folate deficiency in 12 % of the total, and B_{12} deficiency in 5 % of the total [9]. In addition to malabsorption, inflammation and poor dietary intake may explain these deficiencies since the GFD in and of itself may be deficient in nutrients such as folate. Since elevated ferritin and sedimentation rates were seen in some, these authors hypothesized that inflammation may be responsible for this anemia of chronic disease. In a 3-day GFD survey, only 44 % of the female respondents consumed the daily recommended amounts of iron [10]. In addition, research done on gluten-free cereals indicates that these products contain lower amounts of iron and folic acid than their gluten-containing counterparts [11].

Symptoms

Common symptoms of anemia include pallor, fatigue, frontal headache, decreased appetite, and shortness of breath on exertion. Iron deficiency, in particular, is associated with abdominal pain, disturbed sleep, sore red tongue, and brittle hair and nails. Patients may demonstrate pica, which is a strong desire to eat nonfoods such as ice, paint, dirt, and hair. Iron-deficiency anemia may also lead to problems with fertility and maintenance of pregnancy. Profound B_{12} deficiency may also manifest as mania, impaired balance, depression, and peripheral neuropathy.

Diagnosis

A complete blood cell count with peripheral smear, mean corpuscular volume, and other red cell indices is a routine screen for these anemias. The degree of iron deficiency can be further delineated by serum iron, ferritin, percent saturation, and total iron binding capacity. Since serum B_{12} levels are not very sensitive for B_{12} function, a serum methylmalonic acid (MMA) level is recommended. Serum folic acid is easily measured in red blood cells.

Treatment

Dietary sources rich in iron include meats (beef, shrimp, turkey, and liver), seafood (oysters, clams, and scallops), beans (lentils, chick peas, soybeans), dark green leafy vegetables, and iron-fortified cereals. Iron supplements come in liquids, tablets, and slow-release capsules. Dosages range from 1 to 5 mg/kg/day of iron for 3–6 months, depending upon the severity of the anemia. Foods rich in folic acid include green leafy vegetables (spinach, lettuce, broccoli, asparagus), soybeans, salmon, bananas, fortified cereals, and orange and tomato juice. Since folate is heat sensitive, it may be inactivated in overcooked foods. Medications that may lower folic acid levels include metformin, anti-inflammatory drugs (aspirin), and acid blockers (Pepcid, Tagamet, Zantac). The typical dose of folate for megaloblastic anemia and malabsorption ranges from 250 to 1,000 μg per day. B_{12} is found in high concentrations in eggs, liver, beef, lamb, cheese, and seafood (clams, oysters, mussels, caviar, octopus, crab, lobster, and bony fish). Supplementation of B_{12} can be done via oral, sublingual, intramuscular, intravenous, or nasal routes, depending upon the degree of malabsorption. Doses range from 10 μg per day for prevention of anemia to upwards of 1,000–2,000 μg in scheduled doses to treat severe anemia. Fortification of folate to gluten-free dietary products should be strongly considered [12].

Deficiencies of the Fat-Soluble Vitamins (A, E, D, K) in CD

Background

The fat-soluble vitamins are solubilized into micelles in the intestinal lumen by bile acids, which are then absorbed through the duodenal epithelium into the bloodstream [13, 14]. Fat malabsorption may occur in CD due to intestinal damage, liver disease, underlying pancreatic insufficiency, or drugs that bind to bile acids such as cholestyramine [15]. The inability to properly digest and absorb fat can lead to deficiencies in vitamins A, E, D, and K, some of which have profound lifelong morbidities. Requirements and recommended daily allowances for these and all vitamins and minerals are dependent upon age, reproductive status, and underlying health conditions and are provided in Appendix 10 and Appendix 11. The reader is also encouraged to refer to the intake recommendations for nutrients developed by the Food and Nutrition Board at the Institute of Medicine of the National Academies (http://www.iom.edu/About-IOM/Leadership-Staff/Boards/Food-and-Nutrition-Board.aspx) as well as the NIH Office of Dietary Supplements (http://ods.od.nih.gov/).

Vitamin A (Retinol and Provitamin A Carotenoids)

Symptoms

Vitamin A is important for epithelial cell development in the eyes, heart, lungs, and kidneys [16]. It also plays a role in the maintenance of the skin and mucous membranes of the mouth, nose and sinuses, bone formation, reproduction, and collagen synthesis and wound healing [17–19]. Deficiency often presents during periods of high nutritional demand, such as during pregnancy, lactation, infancy, and childhood. Vitamin A deficiency increases the risk of diarrhea; while chronic diarrhea can also lead to excessive losses [13]. The most common symptoms are xerophthalmia and night blindness [20]. In fact, vitamin A deficiency is one of the leading causes of blindness in children worldwide [21]. Vitamin A deficiency also increases the severity and mortality risk of infections, especially with measles [13, 21]. Higher intakes of carotenoids may be associated with lower risks of lung cancer, prostate cancer, cataracts, and macular degeneration [22–24].

Diagnosis

Retinol and carotenoid levels can be measured in plasma; however, their value for assessing marginal vitamin A status is limited, as they do not decline until hepatic stores are almost depleted [25].

Treatment

Preformed vitamin A is found in animal sources, such as meat (especially liver), dairy, and fish, as well as fruits, leafy green vegetables, orange and yellow vegetables, and tomato products [25]. In the USA, the top food sources of vitamin A are dairy products, liver, fish, and fortified cereals, while the top sources of provitamin A are carrots, broccoli, cantaloupe, and squash [22]. Dietary supplements are available as retinyl acetate or retinyl palmitate (preformed vitamin A), beta-carotene (provitamin A), or a combination of the two. Caution must be used with preformed vitamin A supplementation to avoid hypervitaminosis A, which has been associated with pseudotumor cerebri, skin irritation, joint pain, fractures, coma, and even death [13, 16, 26]. Fortification of GF foods with vitamin A should be considered [12].

Vitamin E (Alpha-Tocopherol)

Symptoms

Vitamin E is an antioxidant that protects cells from the damaging effects of free radicals. It also plays a role in immune function and the inhibition of platelet aggregation [22, 27]. Deficiency symptoms include peripheral neuropathy, ataxia, skeletal myopathy, retinopathy, and impairment of the immune response [22, 28]. Vitamin E is being studied for the prevention of coronary heart disease, cataracts, age-related macular degeneration, Alzheimer's disease, and prostate, bladder, and colon cancers [22, 24, 29–33].

Diagnosis

Alpha-tocopherol and beta-gamma-tocopherol are easily measured in serum. Early manifestations of vitamin E deficiency include hyporeflexia, ataxia, limitations in upward/outward gaze, and deficits in proprioception and vibratory sense. Late symptoms of continued deficiency include severe ataxia, diffuse muscle weakness, nystagmus, dysphagia, dysarthria, blindness, and dementia [34].

Treatment

The vitamin may be administered via oral, intramuscular, or parenteral routes. Overdose, though rare, is associated with decreased platelet aggregation and possible increased risk for hemorrhagic stroke [35]. In the USA, most vitamin E in the diet is in the form of gamma-tocopherol from vegetable oils (soybean, canola, corn), although small amounts of alpha-tocopherol are found in nuts, tomato, kiwi, mango, spinach, and broccoli [36].

Vitamin D

Symptoms

There is a long list of potential benefits with vitamin D, including improved bone health and resistance to infections, cancer, and cardiovascular diseases. In children, the classic diseases associated with deficiency are rickets and osteomalacia. Adults may also manifest with bone pain, muscle weakness, dental disease, limited joint mobility, osteopenia, and osteoporosis [37, 38]. Ongoing research is exploring the impact of vitamin D on diabetes, multiple sclerosis, hypertension, and rheumatoid arthritis [39–44].

Diagnosis

The best test to determine vitamin D status is serum 25-hydroxy vitamin D. Levels less than <20 ng/mL (<50 mmol/L) are consistent with vitamin D deficiency, while levels of 21–29 ng/mL (52.5–72.5 mmol/L) are considered consistent with vitamin D insufficiency [45]. Serum parathyroid hormone levels are often elevated, indicating secondary hyperparathyroidism. Skeletal radiographs and bone density measurements may reveal rickets, osteopenia, or osteoporosis (see subsequent section "Issues in Bone Health in CD").

Treatment

There are a limited number of foods that naturally contain vitamin D. Some of the best sources are fish liver oil and bony fish (salmon, tuna, mackerel, herring, sardines) [37]. Small amounts are found in cheese, egg yolk, mushrooms, and beef liver. Thc majority of vitamin D in the U.S. diet comes from fortified foods. These include milk as well as some breakfast cereals, orange juice, yogurt, and margarine. Of note, products made from milk, such as cheese and ice cream, are not generally fortified in the United States [46]. Vitamin D supplements, which are readily available over the counter, can vary widely in their potencies [47], and thus caution should be used to avoid overdose. Excessive vitamin D intake can be associated with anorexia, arrhythmias and calcifications in the renal and cardiovascular systems [37]. Vitamin D is also made by the body as a result of exposure to the sun.

Vitamin K

Symptoms

This vitamin is absorbed mainly in the terminal ileum and is important for the synthesis of vitamin K–dependent clotting factors, which are made in the liver [48]. It is also important for the formation of the bone matrix. There are three types: phylloquinone from plants, menaquinone from bacteria in the GI tract, and menadione, which is synthetic and water soluble. Deficient patients have increased risk for spontaneous bruising and bleeding as well as osteoporosis [49, 50].

Diagnosis

A significant amount of this vitamin in the human body is synthesized by bacteria in the colon; therefore, overuse of broad-spectrum antibiotics can lead to deficiency. Prothrombin time (PT) and prothrombin antigen assay readily detect deficiencies of factor VII, a vitamin K-dependent factor with a very short half-life of only 30 min. Although plasma vitamin K can be measured, checking a PT is less expensive and more readily available.

Treatment

The vitamin K deficiency found in malabsortive GI disorders such as CD is easily treated and monitored by the correction of the PT [51]. Oral VK-3, a menadione, is a synthetic, water-soluble form used to treat deficiency associated with GI malabsorption. IV or IM preparations can be administered for more severe cases. However, the IV form must be given very slowly as it can be associated with hypersensitivity, anaphylaxis, shock, and cardiopulmonary arrest. This nutrient can be found in green leafy vegetables and vegetable oils (soybean, cottonseed, olive, canola) [52].

Malabsorption of Minerals and Trace Metals in CD: Zinc, Selenium, Copper, Calcium, and Magnesium

High percentages of magnesium, calcium, and phosphorous deficiencies have been reported in both adolescents and adults with CD [10, 53].

Zinc

Background

This trace element is absorbed throughout the small intestine by a number of transporters and binding proteins located in the villus epithelial cells [54]. As zinc is important for DNA synthesis, it plays a role in wound healing and maintenance of the intestinal mucosa. It is a coenzyme for over 100 enzymes, some of which are involved with the immune system, linear growth, hemoglobin synthesis, male fertility, and taste and smell. Deficiency of zinc has been reported in newly diagnosed and severely malnourished adults and children with CD [55, 56]. GF breads may not be routinely fortified with zinc.

Symptoms

Patients may complain of anorexia, fatigue, depression, diarrhea, and compromised taste and smell discrimination. Physical exam may reveal hypothyroidism, short stature, white spots in the nail beds, and various skin rashes (psoriasis and eczema). As zinc is stored intracellularly, including in enterocytes, excessive amounts can be lost through diarrhea.

Diagnosis

Serum levels of zinc, red blood cells, and alkaline phosphatase can all be used as indices for zinc status [57]. Fractional absorption of oral or IV zinc isotopes can be used as a research tool for measuring gut integrity [58].

Treatment

Food products containing zinc include meats, fish, shellfish (especially oysters), and nuts, beans, and seeds. The supplement is readily available over the counter as either separate pills or in multivitamins. Zinc absorption is increased by red wine and decreased by copper, iron, calcium, folic acid, and phytates from plants (corn, rice) [59]. Toxicity with zinc has been associated with nausea, and emesis is rare if more than 100 mg a day are ingested. Given the competition of cooper and zinc for binding sites in the gut lining, zinc excess can cause copper deficiency.

Selenium

Background

Selenium is absorbed in the proximal small bowel. Severe GI malabsorptive disorders, such as CD, may result in its depletion or deficiency [60]. This nutrient is important for the function of muscle, the immune system, and thyroid hormone.

Symptoms

Although rare in the USA, three specific conditions have been reported with severe selenium deficiency: Keshan disease (enlarged heart with poor function in children), Kashin–Beck disease (osteoarthropathy), and myxedematous endemic cretinism (hypothyroidism with mental retardation) [61].

Diagnosis

CD patients deficient in selenium may complain of generalized fatigue and muscle weakness. Physical exam and labwork may reveal low serum selenium levels, hypertension, cardiomyopathy, elevated transaminases, autoimmune thyroid disease, and perhaps even psychiatric manifestations (schizophrenia) [62, 63].

Treatment

Selenium is found in high amounts in nuts (Brazil nuts), beans, organ meats (kidney, liver), fish, shellfish, and mushrooms. GFD sources include products made from corn and rice flour where the grains were grown in selenium-rich soil [64]. As opposed to zinc, selenium toxicity (selenosis) is relatively easy to develop, with symptoms including diarrhea, fatigue, nerve damage, and brittle hair and nails [65, 66].

Copper

Background

Copper deficiency can be seen in severe malabsorption states, but it is uncommonly screened for in CD. One report describes five CD patients with neurologic complaints, three of which also had hematological abnormalities due to copper deficiency [67].

Symptoms

The most common complaints of copper deficiency are neurologic and include ataxia and sensory loss in the limbs which could be confusing in the CD patient who may present with diverse neurological sequale [68]. Hypochromic anemia (despite iron sufficiency), neutropenia, and thrombocytopenia may present as fatigue, increased infections, and easy bruising and bleeding. Other findings include bone and joint issues, osteoporosis, and changes in skin color [67].

Diagnosis

Serum copper and ceruloplasmin (the major copper carrying protein) can be used to measure levels. A CBC with differential may show the above hematologic abnormalities.

Treatment

Dietary copper comes from liver, shellfish, legumes, chocolate, nuts, and sun-dried tomatoes. Oral copper sulfate is usually adequate to correct mild deficiencies seen in malabsorption. Parenteral copper histidine can be given subcutaneously for severe deficiency. Most copper in the blood is bound to proteins. Free copper is toxic, and overdose results in nausea, vomiting, diarrhea, and even fatal kidney and liver disease. Absorption is decreased by taking zinc and calcium. A hidden source of zinc is denture creams which are frequently ingested by consumers in significant and toxic quantities enough to cause serious sequale [69].

Calcium

Background

Calcium deficiency is common in untreated CD, as its ionized form is actively transported through the duodenum. Comorbid vitamin D deficiency, as described prior, also decreases calcium absorption. A 3-day diet history showed that less than one-third of females with CD consumed the daily-recommended amounts of calcium [10].

Symptoms

Oral paresthesias are often the earliest symptom of hypocalcemia. Acutely low levels of serum calcium are associated with muscle cramps and mental status changes (anxiety and insomnia). Severe hypocalcemia can be life threatening, and is associated with bone pain, convulsions, arrhythmias, tetany, and numbness of the extremities.

Diagnosis

Measurements of total serum calcium, ionized calcium, albumin, magnesium, phosphorus, PTH, and vitamin D can be revealing for the etiology of hypocalcemia. On physical exam, hyperactive tendon reflexes, Trousseau sign (carpal spasm with inflation of the blood pressure cuff), and Chvostek's sign (facial spasms with tapping the cheek) may be elicited. Other physical findings can include petechiae, purpura, and hand tetany. EKG may reveal intermittent prolongation of the QTc, which puts the patient at risk for torsades de pointes, a specific type of ventricular fibrillation. Skeletal radiographs and bone density measurements may reveal rickets, osteopenia, or osteoporosis (see subsequent section "Issues in Bone Health in CD").

Treatment

Calcium-rich foods include dairy products (milk, yogurt, cheese, ice cream), dark-green leafy vegetables (broccoli, spinach, bok choy), boney fish (salmon, sardines), firm tofu, and those which are fortified (orange juice, soymilk, some juices). Vitamin D helps with the absorption of calcium. Intestinal absorption of calcium is interfered by the ingestion of soda, proton pump inhibitors, and diets high in fiber, phytic acid (whole grains), and oxalic acid (green vegetables, berries, nuts, grains, and seeds) [70–73]. Oral calcium citrate and calcium carbonate are available and are dosed by sex, age, and severity of deficiency, along with vitamin D supplementation. For severe, life-threatening, acute hypocalcemia, IV calcium gluconate and calcium chloride can be used. Excessive calcium ingestion can interfere with the absorption of iron, magnesium, and manganese. Hypercalcemia leads to nausea, vomiting, constipation, delirium, kidney stones, and excessive calcification of the soft tissues [74].

Magnesium

Background

Hypomagnesima occurs commonly in CD due to both malabsorption and inadequate dietary intake from the GFD, which is naturally low in this mineral. Most magnesium is absorbed, along with fat, in the jejunum. Multiple studies have shown inadequate dietary intake of magnesium in both newly diagnosed CD patients and those who have been on the GFD for years [12, 75, 76].

Symptoms

Magnesium is important in all nerve conduction and muscle contraction, including those in the heart and GI tract. Patients may complain of vague symptoms, including anorexia, fatigue, vomiting, constipation, insomnia, anxiety, and depression. Chronic deficiency contributes to hypertension, osteoporosis, impaired PTH secretion (leading to hypocalcemia), hypertension, and myocardial ischemia and dysrhythmias [77, 78].

Diagnosis

Serum magnesium, calcium, PTH, and fat-soluble vitamins may be measured concomitantly. In research studies, magnesium status has been examined by intravenous Mg loading test, serum and erythrocyte magnesium concentrations, and urinary excretion [75]. Bone density measurements may reveal osteoporosis (see subsequent section "Issues in Bone Health in CD").

Treatment

Foods that naturally contain magnesium include seafood, nuts, and beans. Patients with CD should embrace GF dietary sources such as buckwheat, quinoa, amaranth, and flours made from soy, corn, and brown rice. Oral supplements are available as liquid, powder, and capsules and are dosed based upon sex and age. A parenteral form can be used for severe deficiency. Hypermagnesemia can occur with supplements, with symptoms such as diarrhea and lethargy. Drugs that inhibit magnesium absorption include proton pump inhibitors, some antibiotics, diuretics, warfarin, steroids, cyclosporin, and oral contraceptives. Fortification of GF foods with magnesium should be considered [12, 79, 80].

Fiber

Background

Patients on the GFD often go "fiber-free" when they eat "gluten-free." One study reported that less than half of the females surveyed during a 3-day GFD history consumed the daily-recommended amounts of fiber [10]. In addition, the dietary fiber content of GF cereals do not compare favorably to gluten-containing flours, breads, and pastas made from whole wheat sources [11].

Symptoms

CD patients who do not get enough fiber in their diet will often complain of constipation, nausea, fatigue, and irritable bowel syndrome-like symptoms. Since fiber contributes to satiety, and non-fiber carbohydrates are more easily absorbed and digested, weight gain may also be an issue. Studies show that a diet high in whole grains is preventative for diabetes, hypertension, cancer, and hypercholesterolemia.

Diagnosis

Patients may appear bloated and distended, as well as have hemorrhoids, due to constipation. A flat plate X-ray of the abdomen may reveal obstipation.

Treatment

It is recommended that adults consume at least 25 g of fiber per day. The two most commonly prescribed fiber supplements include psyllium and inulin/fructo-oligosaccharide containing compounds (prebiotics). Other sources include cellulose, dextrins, guar gum, and acacia fibers. Gluten-free dietary sources of fiber should be strongly encouraged as part of the GFD. Fruits, vegetables, and legumes are excellent sources of fiber. Gluten-free sources include enriched, fortified, whole grain gluten-free cereals and breads and pastas made from brown rice, bean flour, corn, millet, nuts, quinoa, buckwheat, teff, tapioca, amaranth, flax, soybean, and sorghum [11]. Unfortunately, products made from these inherently gluten-free grains, seeds, and flours can become contaminated with wheat, barley, or rye anywhere from the field to the packaging plant, making them unsafe for those on a GFD [81]. Improvements in gluten-free labeling, as per the "Food Allergen Labeling and Consumer Protection Act of 2004 (Title II of Public Law 108–282)" will hopefully address these issues with contamination [82].

It remains controversial whether or not oats should be eliminated from the GFD. The prolamin of oats, avenin, only accounts for 5–15 % of the total seed protein. This is in marked contrast to gliadin, which comprises about 50 % of the wheat protein [83]. Since avenin does not elicit the same immune response as gliadin, it is thought by some to be safe for patients with CD to ingest. Children with newly diagnosed CD in a U.S. study were provided oats as part of the GFD and demonstrated symptomatic and histologic resolution of the disease comparable to those who were denied oats [84]. However, since oats are often crop rotated, harvested, and milled with wheat, the risk for contamination with wheat gluten is potentially somewhat greater than with other grains such as quinoa.

Are Probiotics Useful in CD?

Background

The intestinal barrier plays an important role in various inflammatory diseases of the GI tract, including CD. Alterations in the intestinal microbiota that are normally involved in gut-associated lymphoid tissue (GALT) homeostasis may also play a role in CD [85]. Probiotics have shown benefit in a number of disorders such as ulcerative colitis, antibiotic-associated diarrhea, *Clostridium difficle* colitis, infectious diarrheas, and the irritable bowel syndrome (IBS), but not specifically in CD in humans to date. Basic science studies show that specific probiotics may have preservative effects on the intestinal epithelial barrier in regard to increasing mucus, defensins, and tight junction protein expression, and an inhibition of epithelial apoptosis, proinflammatory cytokines, and pathogenic bacterial adhesion [86].

A combination of bacterial probiotic supplement, VSL#3, has shown ability to decrease the toxicity of wheat flour by completely hydrolyzing the alpha2-gliadin-derived epitopes 62–75 and 33-mer *in vitro* [87]. The probiotic *yeast Saccharomyces boulardii* has been shown to hydrolyze the 28-kDa-gliadin fraction and improve enteropathy and inflammation in gluten sensitive mice [88].Oral administration of probiotic bacteria *Lactobacillus casei* induced a complete recovery of villus blunting and improved GALT homeostasis in a mouse model of gliadin-induced enteropathy [85]. As reviewed in Chap. 7, dysbiosis may be a key etiologic factor in the pathobiology of CD.

Symptoms

Symptoms of IBS and dysbiosis such as small intestine bacterial overgrowth (SIBO) commonly include gassiness, bloating, diarrhea, and abdominal distension.

Diagnosis

SIBO can be measured by breath hydrogen testing or via culture of jejunal aspirates obtained during endoscopy.

Treatment

Probiotics can be ingested via foods and supplements. Fermented products containing live active cultures, such as yogurts with Bifidobacteria and *Lactobacillus* strains, can alleviate IBS symptoms. Oral probiotic bacterial and yeast supplements in sachets, liquids, and capsule form are commonly available that promote "GI health."

Issues for Bone Health in CD

Background

Low bone density is a common morbidity in CD, and it can lead to vertebral fractures, kyphosis, hip fractures, and Colles fracture of the lower radius. One review summarized the published literature to state that, at diagnosis, approximately one-third of adult CD patients have osteoporosis, one-third have osteopenia, and one-third have normal bone mineral density [89]. Although osteopenia can begin in early childhood, prompt initiation of the GFD can halt progression, and may even reverse bone loss and low height velocity in pediatric patients [90–92]. Severe osteoporosis, however, from CD diagnosed late in life will not improve on the GFD and puts the patient at increased risk of fracture over the general population [93]. The prevalence of CD among osteoporotic individuals has been reported as high as 17-fold higher than among nonosteoporotic individuals, justifying a recommendation to screen all those with low bone density for CD [94].

Diagnosis

Bone density should be measured in newly diagnosed CD, as numerous studies have documented low bone density in both children and adults at the time of initial diagnosis. Plain bone radiographs may reveal osteopenia, but this is not a sensitive measure of bone density. Bone mineral density can be measured via dual-energy X-ray absorptiometry (DXA, previously DEXA) or quantitative CT (QCT) of the spine and femur. Abnormal scans should be repeated 1–2 years after initiation of the GFD. Serum measurements of calcium, phosphorus, albumin, copper, and vitamins A, D, and K (as outlined prior) and 24 h urine calcium can reveal specific nutrient deficiencies [89]. Parathyroid hormone (PTH) may be high due to hypocalcemia (secondary hyperparathyroidism) [95]. Serum alkaline phosphatase may be elevated due to a high bone fraction.

Treatment

The most important treatment for CD-associated bone disease in both pediatrics and adults is the GFD [96]. The GFD can improve bone mineral health even in postmenopausal women and those with incomplete mucosal recovery [97]. Oral calcium, magnesium, and vitamin D supplements may be prescribed. Impact sports and weight-bearing exercises can also improve bone density. Moderation of alcohol and caffeine, and cessation of smoking, also improves bone health. Supplemental antiresorptives, which prevent excessive bone remodeling (bisphosphonates, estrogen replacement, selective estrogen receptor modulators [raloxifene], and denosumab (a human antibody that inactivates RANKL)), may be required in those at high fracture risk despite the GFD such as postmenopausal women and older men [89, 98].

Special Issues for Women: Pregnancy and Fertility

CD is diagnosed at a higher rate in women than in men [99]; however, a large serologic screening in the USA showed that the prevalence rates in both sexes are the same [100].

Background

Women with CD have been reported older at menarche, younger at menopause, having a lower mean number of children, and having more spontaneous miscarriages [101]. GFD in CD women reduced the relative risk of abortion ninefold, reduced the number of low birth weight babies from 29 % to zero ($p<0.05$), and increased duration of breast-feeding twofold [102].

Symptoms

Failure to follow a GFD during pregnancy can have effects on the fetus, including increased risk for spina bifida and other neural tube defects due to poor folic acid absorption [103]. The fatigue associated with iron-deficiency anemia can make pregnancy and newborn care more difficult. Depression in CD can interfere with maternal-child bonding. Duration of breast-feeding has been reported to be three times shorter in untreated mothers with CD [102]. Low levels of maternal plasma zinc are associated with toxemia, vaginitis, prolonged labor, and a history of previous stillbirth [57].

Diagnosis

Serology for CD should be performed in idiopathic infertility cases, as initiation of a GFD during pregnancy can decrease the risk of spontaneous abortions and low birth weight infants [102, 104]. Levels of the above vitamins and nutrients, especially iron, folate and zinc, should be measured in the pregnant women with CD [99, 102].

Treatment

Women with known CD should follow a strict GFD during pregnancy and ensure that iron, folic acid, zinc, calcium, B and D vitamins, and gluten-free sources of fiber are included in the diet (or supplemented) in addition to routine prenatal vitamins. Supplementing magnesium and calcium may decrease the risk of preeclampsia (high blood pressure, proteinuria, edema) [105]. In the GFD, the major source of dietary folic acid is lost because fortified commercial cereals, breads, and pasta products are excluded. Without supplementation during the child-bearing years, women with CD might not receive enough dietary folate to maintain protective levels against neural tube defects [106]. Fortification of gluten-free foods with folate should be considered.

Nutritional Issues in Refractory Celiac Disease

Background

A minority of CD patients will continue to have GI symptoms and biopsy-proven enteropathy, despite vigorous adherence to the GFD.

Symptoms

Patients with refractory celiac disease (RCD) have profound diarrhea and malabsorption, exhibiting many of the nutritional deficiencies described prior in this chapter.

Diagnosis

Non-adherence to the GFD accounts for the majority of patients who are not better on the GFD. In those unresponsive to the GFD, a thorough dietary history should exclude inadvertent gluten ingestion; compliance should be assessed with serum antibodies; workup including endoscopic evaluation should be performed to exclude other causes of continued symptoms despite strict compliance with a GFD [2, 107].

Treatment

In addition to the GFD, these patients often require immunosuppression with steroids, azathioprine, cyclosporine, and methotrexate [107–112]. Oral or parenteral supplementation with iron, copper, magnesium, folic acid, zinc, and albumin has been used with some benefit. With proven osteopenia (and steroid use), vitamin D, calcium, and biphosphonates have been utilized [113, 114]. A 4-week elemental (amino acid-based) diet has been shown in one study to reduce inflammatory cytokines and improve clinical symptoms, histology, and serum albumin in RCD [115]. If malabsorption and weight loss are severe, total parenteral nutrition may be required [107].

References

1. Rubin CE, Brandborg LL, Flick AL. Biopsy studies on the pathogenesis of celiac sprue. In: Wolstenholme GEW, Cameron CM, editors. Intestinal biopsy. Boston: Little, Brown & Co; 1962. p. 67.
2. Lee SK, Lo W, Memeo L, Rotterdam H, Green PH. Duodenal histology in patients with celiac disease after treatment with a gluten-free diet. Gastrointest Endosc. 2003;57:187–91.
3. Hankey GL, Holmes GK. Coeliac disease in the elderly. Gut. 1994;35:65–7.
4. Pietzak M. The follow-up of patients with celiac disease – achieving compliance with treatment. Gastroenterology. 2005;128:S135–41.
5. Ljungman G, Myrdal U. Compliance in teenagers with coeliac disease—a Swedish follow-up study. Acta Paediatr. 1993;82:235–8.
6. Mäki M, Lähdehaho ML, Hällström O, Viander M, Visakorpi JK. Postpubertal gluten challenge in coeliac disease. Arch Dis Child. 1989;64:1604–7.
7. Carroccio A, Iannitto E, Cavataio F, Montalto G, Tumminelo M, Campagna P, et al. Sideropenic anemia and celiac disease: one study, two points of view. Dig Dis Sci. 1998;43:673–8.
8. Wessling-Resnick M. Iron transport. Annu Rev Nutr. 2000;20:129–51.
9. Harper JW, Holleran SF, Ramakrishnan R, Bhagat G, Green PHR. Anemia in celiac disease is multifactorial in etiology. Am J Hematol. 2007;11:996–1000.
10. Thompson T, Dennis M, Higgins LA, Lees AR, Sharrett MK. Gluten-free diet survey: are Americans with celiac disease consuming recommended amounts of fibre, iron, calcium and grain foods? J Hum Nutr Dietet. 2005;18:163–9.
11. Thompson T. Folate, iron, and dietary fiber contents of the gluten-free diet. J Am Diet Assoc. 2000;100:1389–96.
12. Shepherd SJ, Gibson PR. Nutritional inadequacies of the gluten-free diet in both recently-diagnosed and long-term patients with coeliac disease. J Hum Nutr Diet. 2012. doi:10.1111/jhn.12018.
13. Institute of Medicine, Food and Nutrition Board. Dietary reference intakes for vitamin A, vitamin K, arsenic, boron, chromium, copper, iodine, iron, manganese, molybdenum, nickel, silicon, vanadium, and zinc. Washington, DC: National Academy Press; 2001.
14. Hofmann AF, Borgström B. The intraluminal phase of fat digestion in man: the lipid content of the micellar and oil phases of intestinal content obtained during fat digestion and absorption. J Clin Invest. 1964;43(2):247.
15. Carroccio A, Iacono G, Lerro P, Cavataio F, Malorgio E, Soresi M, et al. Role of pancreatic impairment in growth recovery during gluten-free diet in childhood celiac disease. Gastroenterology. 1997;112:1839–44.

16. Ross CA. Vitamin A. In: Coates PM, Betz JM, Blackman MR, editors. Encyclopedia of dietary supplements. 2nd ed. London: Informa Healthcare; 2010. p. 778–91.
17. Alberts D, Ranger-Moore J, Einspahr J. Safety and efficacy of dose-intensive oral vitamin A in subjects with sun-damaged skin. Clin Cancer Res. 2004;10:1875–80.
18. National Institutes of Health, Office of Dietary Supplements. Facts about dietary supplements: vitamin A and carotenoids. Bethesda: National Institutes of Health; December 2001.
19. Ribaya-Mercado JD, Blumber JB. Vitamin A: is it a risk factor for osteoporosis and bone fracture? Nutr Rev. 2007;65(10):425–38.
20. Sommer A. Vitamin A, deficiency and clinical disease: an historical overview. J Nutr. 2008;138:1835–9.
21. World Health Organization. Global prevalence of vitamin A deficiency in populations at risk 1995–2005: WHO global database on vitamin A deficiency. Geneva: World Health Organization; 2009.
22. Institute of Medicine, Food and Nutrition Board. Dietary reference intakes for vitamin C, vitamin E, selenium, and carotenoids. Washington, DC: National Academy Press; 2000.
23. Neuhouser ML, Barnett MJ, Kristal AR, Ambrosone CB, King IB, Thornquist M, et al. Dietary supplement use and prostate cancer risk in the carotene and retinol efficacy trial. Cancer Epidemiol Biomarkers Prev. 2009;18:2202–6.
24. Age-Related Eye Disease Study Research Group. A randomized, placebo-controlled, clinical trial of high-dose supplementation with vitamins C and E, beta carotene, and zinc for age-related macular degeneration and vision loss: AREDS report no. 8. Arch Ophthalmol. 2001;119:1417–36.
25. Ross A. Vitamin A and carotenoids. In: Shils M, Shike M, Ross A, Caballero B, Cousins R, editors. Modern nutrition in health and disease. 10th ed. Baltimore: Lippincott Williams & Wilkins; 2006. p. 351–75.
26. Villamor E, Fawzi WW. Vitamin A supplementation: implications for morbidity and mortality in children. J Infect Dis. 2000;182 Suppl 1:S122–33.
27. Traber MG. Vitamin E. In: Shils ME, Shike M, Ross AC, Caballero B, Cousins R, editors. Modern nutrition in health and disease. 10th ed. Baltimore: Lippincott Williams & Wilkins; 2006. p. 396–411.
28. Kowdley KV, Mason JB, Meydani SN, Cornwall S, Grand RJ. Vitamin E deficiency and impaired cellular immunity related to intestinal fat malabsorption. Gastroenterology. 1992;102:2139–42.
29. Knekt P, Reunanen A, Jarvinen R, Seppanen R, Heliovaara M, Aromaa A. Antioxidant vitamin intake and coronary mortality in a longitudinal population study. Am J Epidemiol. 1994;139:1180–9.
30. Kirsh VA, Hayes RB, Mayne ST, Chatterjee N, Subar AF, Dixon LB, et al. Supplemental and dietary vitamin E, β-carotene, and vitamin C intakes and prostate cancer risk. J Natl Cancer Inst. 2006;98:245–54.
31. Bostick RM, Potter JD, McKenzie DR, Sellers TA, Kushi LH, Steinmetz KA, et al. Reduced risk of colon cancer with high intakes of vitamin E: the Iowa women's health study. Cancer Res. 1993;15:4230–17.
32. Jacobs EJ, Henion AK, Briggs PJ, Connell CJ, McCullough ML, Jonas CR, et al. Vitamin C and vitamin E supplement use and bladder cancer mortality in a large cohort of US men and women. Am J Epidemiol. 2002;156:1002–10.
33. Age-Related Eye Disease Study Research Group. A randomized, placebo-controlled, clinical trial of high-dose supplementation with vitamins C and E and beta carotene for age-related cataract and vision loss: AREDS report no. 9. Arch Opthalmol. 2011;119:1439–52.
34. Sokol RJ, Guggenheim MA, Heubi JE. Frequency and clinical progression of the vitamin E deficiency neurologic disorder in children with prolonged neonatal cholestasis. Am J Dis Child. 1985;139(12):1211–5.
35. Bjelakovic G, Nikolova D, Gluud LL, Simonetti RG, Gluud C. Mortality in randomized trials of antioxidant supplements for primary and secondary prevention: systematic review and meta-analysis. JAMA. 2007;297:842–57.

36. Dietrich M, Traber MG, Jacques PF, Cross CE, Hu Y, Block G. Does γ-tocopherol play a role in the primary prevention of heart disease and cancer? A review. Am J Coll Nutr. 2006;25:292–9.
37. Institute of Medicine, Food and Nutrition Board. Dietary reference intakes for calcium and vitamin D. Washington, DC: National Academy Press; 2010.
38. Wharton B, Bishop N. Rickets. Lancet. 2003;362:1389–400.
39. Hyppönen E, Läärä E, Reunanen A, Järvelin MR, Virtanen SM. Intake of vitamin D and risk of type 1 diabetes: a birth-cohort study. Lancet. 2001;358:1500–3.
40. Pittas AG, Dawson-Hughes B, Li T, Van Dam RM, Willett WC, Manson JE, et al. Vitamin D and calcium intake in relation to type 2 diabetes in women. Diabetes Care. 2006;29:650–6.
41. Krause R, Bühring M, Hopfenmüller W, Holick MF, Sharma AM. Ultraviolet B and blood pressure. Lancet. 1998;352:709–10.
42. Chiu KC, Chu A, Go VL, Saad MF. Hypovitaminosis D is associated with insulin resistance and beta cell dysfunction. Am J Clin Nutr. 2004;79:820–5.
43. Munger KL, Levin LI, Hollis BW, Howard NS, Ascherio A. Serum 25-hydroxyvitamin D levels and risk of multiple sclerosis. JAMA. 2006;296:2832–8.
44. Merlino LA, Curtis J, Mikuls TR, Cerhan JR, Criswell LA, Saag K. Vitamin D intake is inversely associated with rheumatoid arthritis: results from the Iowa women's health study. Arthritis Rheum. 2004;50:72–7.
45. Hollis BW, Wagner CL. Normal serum vitamin D levels. N Engl J Med. 2005;352(5):515–6.
46. Calvo MS, Whiting SJ, Barton CN. Vitamin D fortification in the United States and Canada: current status and data needs. Am J Clin Nutr. 2004;80:1710S–6S.
47. LeBlanc ES, Perrin N, Johnson JD, Ballatore A, Hillier T. Over-the-counter and compounded vitamin D: is potency what we expect? JAMA Intern Med. 2013;173(7):585–6.
48. Udall JA. Human sources and absorption of vitamin K in relation to anticoagulation stability. JAMA. 1965;194(2):127–9.
49. Ozdemir MA, Karakukcu M, Per H, Unal E, Gumus H, Patiroglu T. Late-type vitamin K deficiency bleeding: experience from 120 patients. Childs Nerv Syst. 2012;28(2):247–51.
50. Vermeer C, Theuwissen E. Vitamin K, osteoporosis and degenerative diseases of ageing. Menopause Int. 2011;17(1):19–23.
51. Krasinski SD, Russell RM, Furie BC. The prevalence of vitamin K deficiency in chronic gastrointestinal disorders. Am J Clin Nutr. 1985;41(3):639–43.
52. Suttie JW. Vitamin K. In: Machlin L, editor. Handbook of vitamins. New York: Marcel Dekker; 1984. p. 147.
53. Sdepanian VL, de Miranda Carvalho CN, de Morais MB, Colugnati FA, Fagundes-Neto U. Bone mineral density of the lumbar spine in children and adolescents with celiac disease on a gluten-free diet in São Paulo, Brazil. J Pediatr Gastroenterol Nutr. 2003;37(5):571–6.
54. Krebs NF. Overview of zinc absorption and excretion in the human gastrointestinal tract. J Nutr. 2000;130:1374S–7S.
55. Singhal N, Alam S, Sherwani R, Musarrat J. Serum zinc levels in celiac disease. Indian Pediatr. 2008;45(4):319–21.
56. Solomons NW, Rosenberg IH, Sandstead HH. Zinc nutrition in celiac sprue. Am J Clin Nutr. 1976;29(4):371–5.
57. Lazebnik N, Kuhnert BR, Kuhnert PM, Thompson KL. Zinc status, pregnancy complications, and labor abnormalities. Am J Obstet Gynecol. 1988;158(1):161–6.
58. Tran CD, Katsikeros R, Manton N, Krebs NF, Hambidge KM, Butler RN, et al. Zinc homeostasis and gut function in children with celiac disease. Am J Clin Nutr. 2011;94(4):1026–32.
59. Lonnerdal B. Dietary factors influencing zinc absorption. J Nutr. 2000;130:1378S–85S.
60. Rannem T, Ladefoged K, Hylander E, Hegnhoj J, Staun M. Selenium depletion in patients with gastrointestinal diseases: are there any predictive factors? Scand J Gastroenterol. 1998;33:1057–61.
61. National Institutes of Health Office of Dietary Supplements. Dietary Supplement Fact Sheet: Selenium. http://ods.od.nih.gov/factsheets/Selenium-HealthProfessional/#en20.

62. Stazi AV, Trinti B. Selenium deficiency in celiac disease: risk of autoimmune thyroid diseases [Article in Italian]. Minerva Med. 2008;99(6):643–53.
63. Brown JS, Foster HD. Schizophrenia: an update of the selenium deficiency hypothesis. J Orthomol Med. 1996;11(400):211–2.
64. Longnecker MP, Taylor PR, Levander OA, Howe M, Veillon C, McAdam PA, et al. Selenium in diet, blood, and toenails in relation to human health in a seleniferous area. Am J Clin Nutr. 1991;53:1288–94.
65. Koller LD, Exon JH. The two faces of selenium-deficiency and toxicity are similar in animals and man. Can J Vet Res. 1986;50:297–306.
66. Goldhaber SB. Trace element risk assessment: essentiality vs. toxicity. Regul Toxicol Pharmacol. 2003;38:232–42.
67. Halfdanarson TR, Kumar N, Hogan WJ, Murray JA. Copper deficiency in celiac disease. J Clin Gastroenterol. 2009;43(2):162–4.
68. Goodman PB, Mistry MD. Copper deficiency myeloneuropathy due to occult celiac disease. Neurologist. 2009;15(6):355–6.
69. Hedera P, Peltier A, Fink JK, Wilcock S, London Z, Brewer GJ. Myelopolyneuropathy and pancytopenia due to copper deficiency and high zinc levels of unknown origin II. The denture cream is a primary source of excessive zinc. Neurotoxicology. 2009 Nov;30(6):996–9.
70. Kopic S, Geibel JP. Gastric acid, calcium absorption, and their impact on bone health. Physiol Rev. 2013;93(1):189–268.
71. Yang YX, Lewis JD, Epstein S, Metz DC. Long-term proton pump inhibitor therapy and risk of hip fracture. JAMA. 2006;296(24):2947–53.
72. Krittaphol W, Bailey KB, Pongcharoen T, Winichagoon P, Gibson RS. Low zinc, iron, and calcium intakes of Northeast Thai school children consuming glutinous rice-based diets are not exacerbated by high phytate. Int J Food Sci Nutr. 2006;57(7–8):520–8.
73. Thomas E, von Unruh GE, Hesse A. Influence of a low- and a high-oxalate vegetarian diet on intestinal oxalate absorption and urinary excretion. Eur J Clin Nutr. 2008;62(9):1090–7.
74. Legrand SB. Modern management of malignant hypercalcemia. Am J Hosp Palliat Care. 2011;28(7):515–7.
75. Rujner J, Socha J, Syczewska M, Wojtasik A, Kunachowicz H, Stolarczyk A. Magnesium status in children and adolescents with coeliac disease without malabsorption symptoms. Clin Nutr. 2004;5:1074–9.
76. Wild D, Robins GG, Burley VJ, Howdle PD. Evidence of high sugar intake, and low fibre and mineral intake, in the gluten-free diet. Aliment Pharmacol Ther. 2010;32(4):573–81.
77. al-Ghamdi SM, Cameron EC, Sutton RA. Magnesium deficiency: pathophysiologic and clinical overview. Am J Kidney Dis. 1994;24(5):737–52.
78. Ramsay JG. Cardiac management in the ICU. Chest. 1999;115(5):138S–44S.
79. Horn EJ. A case series of proton pump inhibitor-induced hypomagnesemia. Am J Kidney Dis. 2010;56(1):112–6.
80. Sheen E, Triadafilopoulos G. Adverse effects of long-term proton pump inhibitor therapy. Dig Dis Sci. 2011;56(4):931–50.
81. Thompson T, Lee AR, Grace T. Gluten contamination of grains, seeds, and flours in the United States: a pilot study. J Am Diet Assoc. 2010;110(6):937–40.
82. Pietzak M. Gluten-free food labeling in the United States. J Pediatr Gastroenterol Nutr. 2005;41(5):567–8.
83. Holmes G, Catassi C, editors. Coeliac disease. Oxford: Health Press; 2000.
84. Hoffenberg EJ, Haas J, Drescher A, Barnhurst R, Osberg I, Bao F, et al. A trial of oats in children with newly diagnosed celiac disease. J Pediatr. 2000;137:361–6.
85. D'Arienzo R, Stefanile R, Maurano F, Mazzarella G, Ricca E, Troncone R, et al. Immunomodulatory effects of Lactobacillus casei administration in a mouse model of gliadin-sensitive enteropathy. Scand J Immunol. 2011;74(4):335–41.
86. Mennigen R, Bruewer M. Effect of probiotics on intestinal barrier function molecular structure and function of the tight junction. Ann NY Acad Sci. 2009;1165:183–9.

87. De Angelis M, Rizzello CG, Fasano A, Clemente MG, De Simone C, Silano M, et al. VSL#3 probiotic preparation has the capacity to hydrolyze gliadin polypeptides responsible for celiac sprue. Bioenergetics. 2006;1762(1):80–93.
88. Papista C, Gerakopoulos V, Kourelis A, Sounidaki M, Kontana A, Berthelot L, et al. Gluten induces coeliac-like disease in sensitised mice involving IgA, CD71 and transglutaminase 2 interactions that are prevented by probiotics. Lab Invest. 2012;92(4):625–35.
89. Fouda MA, Khan AA, Sultan MS, Rios LP, McAssey K, Armstrong D. Evaluation and management of skeletal health in celiac disease: position statement. [Review]. Can J Gastroenterol. 2012;26(11):819–29.
90. Valdimarsson T, Lofmano O, Toss G, Strom M. Reversal of osteopenia with diet in adult coeliac disease. Gut. 1996;38:322–7.
91. Mora S, Barera G, Beccio S, Proverbio MC, Weber G, Bianchi C, et al. Bone density and bone metabolism are normal after long-term gluten-free diet in young celiac patients. Am J Gastroenterol. 1999;94:398–403.
92. Prader A, Tanner JM, von Harnack GA. Catch-up growth in coeliac disease. Acta Paediatr Scand. 1969;58:311.
93. Meyer D, Stavropolous S, Diamond B, Shane E, Green PH. Osteoporosis in a North American adult population with celiac disease. Am J Gastroenterol. 2001;96:112–9.
94. Stenson WF, Newberry R, Lorenz R, Baldus C, Civitelli R. Increased prevalence of celiac disease and need for routine screening among patients with osteoporosis. Arch Intern Med. 2005;165:393–9.
95. Valdimarsson T, Toss G, Löfman O, Ström M. Three years' follow-up of bone density in adult coeliac disease: significance of secondary hyperparathyroidism. Scand J Gastroenterol. 2000;35:274–80.
96. Mora S, Barera G, Beccio S, Menni L, Proverbio MC, Bianchi C, et al. A prospective, longitudinal study of the long-term effect of treatment on bone density in children with celiac disease. J Pediatr. 2001;139:516–21.
97. Sategna-Guidetti C, Grosso SB, Grosso S, Mengozzi G, Aimo G, Zaccaria T, et al. The effects of 1-year gluten withdrawal on bone mass, bone metabolism and nutritional status in newly-diagnosed adult coeliac disease patients. Aliment Pharmacol Ther. 2000;14:35–43.
98. Recker RR, Armas L. The effect of antiresorptives on bone quality. Clin Orthop Relat Res. 2011;469(8):2207–14.
99. Danowski L, Brand LG, Connolly J. Selections from current literature: gluten-free diets, coeliac disease and associated disorders. Fam Pract. 2003;20:607–11.
100. Fasano A, Berti I, Gerarduzzi T, Not T, Colletti RB, Drago S. Prevalence of celiac disease in at-risk and not at-risk groups in the United States: a large multicenter study. Arch Intern Med. 2003;163:286–92.
101. Sher KS, Mayberry JF. Female fertility, obstetric and gynaecological history in coeliac disease: a case control study. Acta Paediatr Suppl. 1996;412:76–7.
102. Ciacci C, Cirillo M, Auriemma G, Di Dato G, Sabbatini F, Mazzacca G. Celiac disease and pregnancy outcome. Am J Gastroenterol. 1996;91:718–22.
103. Wald NJ, Hackshaw AD, Stone R. Blood folic acid and vitamin B12 in relation to neural tube defects. Br J Obstet Gynaecol. 1996;103(4):319–24.
104. Kumar A, Meena M, Begum N, Kumar N, Gupta RK, Aggarwal S, et al. Latent celiac disease in reproductive performance of women. Fertil Steril. 2011;95(3):922–7.
105. Zerfu TA, Ayele KT. Micronutrients and pregnancy; effect of supplementation on pregnancy and pregnancy outcomes: a systematic review. Nutr J. 2013;12:20.
106. Hancock R, Koren G. Celiac disease during pregnancy. Can Fam Physician. 2004;50:1361–3.
107. Daum S, Cellier C, Mulder CJJ. Refractory coeliac disease. Best Pract Res Clin Gastroenterol. 2005;19:413–24.
108. Stuart BM, Gent AE. Atrophy of the coeliac mucosa. Eur J Gastroenterol Hepatol. 1998;10: 523–5.

109. Mitchison HC, al Mardini H, Gillespie S. A pilot study of fluticasone propionate in untreated coeliac disease. Gut. 1991;32:260–5.
110. Vaidya A, Bolanos J, Berkelhammer C. Azathioprine in refractory sprue. Am J Gastroenterol. 1999;94:1967–9.
111. Rolny P, Sigurjonsdottir HA, Remotti H. Role of immunosuppressive therapy in refractory sprue-like disease. Am J Gastroenterol. 1999;94:219–25.
112. O'Mahony S, Howdle PD, Losowsky SM. Management of patients with non-responsive coeliac disease. Aliment Pharmacol Ther. 1996;10:671–80.
113. Mulder CJ, Wahab PJ, Moshaver B, Meijer JW. Refractory coeliac disease: a window between coeliac disease and enteropathy associated T cell lymphoma. Scand J Gastroenterol Suppl. 2000;232:32–7.
114. Love A, Elmes M, Golden M, McMaster D. Zinc deficiency and coeliac disease. In: McNicholl B, McCarthy C, Fottrell P, editors. Perspectives in coeliac disease. Lancaster: MTP; 1978. p. 335–42.
115. Olaussen RW, Løvik A, Tollefsen S, Andresen PA, Vatn MH, De Lange T, et al. Effect of elemental diet on mucosal immunopathology and clinical symptoms in type 1 refractory celiac disease. Clin Gastroenterol Hepatol. 2005;3(9):875–85.

Chapter 12
Monitoring and Follow-Up of Patients with Celiac Disease

Margot L. Herman, Imad Absah, Amy S. Oxentenko, and Alberto Rubio-Tapia

Introduction

The only available treatment for celiac disease (CD) is a strict, lifelong gluten-free diet, which requires avoidance of gluten-containing grains such as wheat, barley, and rye. Although oats are generally safe in those with CD, cross-contamination can lead to inadvertent gluten ingestion, so oats are often avoided for the first year after the diagnosis of CD is made, with introduction thereafter if symptoms are controlled. Patients need to be advised that many other products may contain gluten, such as medications (including vitamin and mineral supplements), cosmetics, dental products, adhesive glues (envelopes), communion wafers, and more. Research has found in some patients as little as one-thirtieth of a loaf of bread can have enough gluten to cause intestinal damage if consumed regularly [1, 2].

Given the lack of currently available pharmacologic treatments, some may perceive the management of CD to be "out of the hands of the physician." However, this is far from the truth, as physicians play a pivotal role in the counseling of patients with CD. Without such support, patients may have poor compliance with treatment, which can lead to delayed intestinal healing, ongoing symptoms, and an increased risk for associated diseases, including malignancy [3, 4]. The mortality risk for undiagnosed or noncompliant CD patients appears to be increased compared to the general population; however, when a gluten-free diet is followed, this

M.L. Herman, M.D. • A.S. Oxentenko, M.D., F.A.C.P., F.A.C.G.
A. Rubio-Tapia, M.D. (✉)
Division of Gastroenterology and Hepatology, Department of Internal Medicine, Mayo Clinic, Rochester, MN, USA
e-mail: rubiotapia.alberto@mayo.edu

I. Absah, M.D.
Division of Gastroenterology and Hepatology, Department of Pediatrics, Mayo Clinic, Rochester, MN, USA

S.D. Rampertab and G.E. Mullin (eds.), *Celiac Disease*, Clinical Gastroenterology,
DOI 10.1007/978-1-4614-8560-5_12, © Springer Science+Business Media New York 2014

risk may decrease, which can be an additional motivating factor for patients beyond control of symptoms [5–7]. In the following chapter, we will discuss the management of CD via a concerted multidisciplinary approach with attention given to the medical, dietary, and psychosocial aspects of this complex disease in order to avoid celiac-related complications.

Rationale for Follow-Up

CD is a chronic disease that is felt to be lifelong and as such requires long-term follow-up. Although there are rare reports of patients who develop latency of their CD and have resumed a gluten-containing diet, this is certainly the exception and may put these individuals at risk of developing recurrent small bowel inflammation and associated complications [8].

CD has protean manifestations. While the classic features of CD include malabsorption, diarrhea, weight loss, malnutrition, and delayed growth, there is a broad spectrum of disease manifestations including iron-deficiency anemia, metabolic bone disease, infertility, fatigue, dermatitis herpetiformis, and many more. Symptomatically, the vast majority of patients with celiac disease who start a gluten-free diet can see improvement in diarrhea within days after initiation, and most will have complete resolution of diarrhea by 6 months into treatment, with a mean improvement time of 4 weeks [7, 9]. Additionally, other gastrointestinal features of CD (bloating, abdominal pain, fecal incontinence, weight loss) tend to improve at a similar rate for most patients [9].

The gluten-free diet, albeit a challenge to ascribe to, is safe and effective in treating CD [10]. The situations where compliance with a gluten-free diet can be most challenging include a change in social situation (going to college, moving in with others, etc.), eating out at restaurants, grocery shopping, traveling, or when patients are asymptomatic or detected through family screening. The availability of regular follow-up with a multidisciplinary team that has specialized knowledge of a gluten-free diet and is familiar with overcoming barriers to adherence is absolutely necessary.

Despite an increasing awareness of CD in the community, it is concerning that patients have such a variable rate of adherence to a gluten-free diet. In a 2009 systematic review, compliance with a gluten-free diet was found to be anywhere from 42 % to 91 % among CD patients, but typically lower rates of compliance were seen when a gluten-free diet was defined more rigorously [1, 4]. Even more concerning is recent literature that highlights that physicians are failing to assess CD patients regarding compliance to a gluten-free diet, further impacting patients' perception of its importance. A 2012 retrospective assessment of medical care in a CD population living in Olmsted County revealed that nearly one-third of patients followed longitudinally had "celiac disease assessments" that did not document nor discuss compliance to a gluten-free diet [11].

A lack of appropriate dietary counseling can lead to adverse consequences, given a large portion of CD has been shown to have inadequate mucosal healing long after the disease has been diagnosed and despite ascribing to what they believe is an appropriate diet, highlighting that inadequate education can lead to inadvertent ingestion [7, 12]. Although mucosal healing may take several years to occur (especially in adults), it is a possible and desirable outcome. Noting the likelihood for ongoing disease activity in a majority of the CD population, it is not entirely surprising that patients with CD appear to have a modestly increased risk of mortality conferred by poor compliance to a gluten-free diet and ongoing intestinal inflammation [5–7].

There are diseases and conditions associated with CD such as autoimmune thyroid disease, type 1 diabetes, microscopic colitis, IgA deficiency, infertility, autoimmune liver disease, neurologic conditions, and genetic syndromes (Down, Turner, and Williams) [13–17]. It important for the clinician and patient to be aware of these associations and to also realize that untreated CD with ongoing gluten exposure and intestinal mucosal inflammation is likely to increase the severity of many extraintestinal manifestations (such as iron deficiency anemia, metabolic bone disease, and many others). Adherence to a gluten-free diet is correlated with not only improved health but also improved scores on standardized quality of life assessments [14, 18, 19].

The need for regular follow-up to promote compliance and avoid complications in CD has been well established, and it is becoming increasingly clear that many medical providers and patients may not be aware of current recommendations [11, 20].

Current Expert Opinion and Medical Society Recommendations

Despite multiple expert opinion papers and practice guidelines published on the optimal long-term monitoring of patients with CD, it remains a controversial topic due to disparate guidelines, scarce good-quality research (evidence-based recommendations), and highly variable practices among clinicians [10, 11, 14, 21–28]. A systematic review synthesizing the multiple practice guidelines also exists, which highlights the highly variable cost of care among guidelines [28]. Many guidelines focus largely on the diagnosis of CD, where more objective data have been presented. Table 12.1 reviews the currently published recommendations for longitudinal follow-up of patients with CD.

Essential Aspects of Follow-Up

The following recommendations reflect a synthesis of available guidelines and expert opinions, and in instances where there was a paucity of evidence, the authors' expert opinion and institutional practice were included. For a graphic representation of these recommendations, please see Fig. 12.1.

Table 12.1 The currently available practice guidelines for long-term monitoring and management of celiac disease

Source	Visit frequency and objective	Dietician	Serology	Other blood tests	Repeat biopsy	Bone-density	Support
AGA 2006	"Regular intervals" • Compliance assessment • History and physical • "Education, motivation and support"	Yes Diagnosis and then, "regular intervals"	Optional "regular intervals" (will not identify minor gluten exposure)				Yes
NIH 2004	"Periodic visits" • Compliance assessment • Symptom check • Monitor for complications	Diagnosis	Optional "regular intervals" (will not identify minor gluten exposure)				
BSG 2010	Cites lack of evidence, however generally supports active follow-up to assess for symptoms which would require further work-up	Diagnosis and at 3–6 months following first visit	May be of interest to assess adherence	CBC, calcium, ferritin, folate, B_{12} annually	If persistently positive serology, symptoms or diagnostic ambiguity	Once at diagnosis, then repeat at interval based on findings[a]	Yes
WGO 2012	Every 3–6 months in first year. Then, annually. • Symptom check	Diagnosis and every 3–6 months in first year. Compliance assessment	"Periodic testing" Frequency of testing depending on compliance, and time on GFD				Relatives should be "well informed"
NASPGHAN 2005	"Periodic visits" • History and physical • Compliance assessment • Growth check	Diagnosis Thereafter if/when compliance concerns	tTG at 6 months following diagnosis, then annually unless symptoms persist or recur				Yes

PCG-UK 2006	3–6 months after diagnosis, then annually and if pregnancy • Symptom check • Compliance assessment • Growth check	"Important role in follow-up care" (frequency not specified)[b]	Annually	Hemoglobin, folate, ferritin, albumin, alkaline phosphatase, nutritional deficiencies (calcium, vitamin D, B_{12})	4–6 months after initiating a GFD	Once at diagnosis, then repeat at interval based on findings[a]	
Pietzak 2005	3–6 months and 1 year after diagnosis, then annually by primary care or gastroenterologist if doing well. • History and physical • Compliance assessment • Screen for nutritional deficiencies/other autoimmune diseases/complications	Diagnosis, 3–6 months, then if persistently positive serology, symptoms or nutritional deficiencies return visit	Annually, unless elevated	CBC, iron studies, folate, vitamins A, E, D, electrolytes, albumin, total protein, liver enzymes, PT, PTH if impaired bone density at first visit, then as needed	"Gold standard" for assessing compliance, suggested at 6–12 months following diagnosis	Diagnosis	Yes
Haines 2008	6 weeks, 6 months, 12 months, then annually by either physician or dietician • Compliance assessment/reinforcement • Assess for symptoms/complications	6 weeks, 6 months, 12 months, then annually by either physician or dietician	6 and 12 months following diagnosis, then annually unless clinical concerns	CBC, electrolytes, liver function tests, TSH, iron studies, calcium, phosphate, vitamin D, folate, B_{12}, fasting glucose, ± zinc, magnesium	"At 1–2 years following diagnosis, then as indicated on clinical grounds"	Diagnosis, then every 3–5 years in high risk groups (non-compliance, refractory, female ≥50 years, fractures, men ≥55 years); annually if on treatment	Yes

Abbreviations: *CBC* complete blood count, *tTG* tissue transglutaminase, *PT* prothrombin time, *PTH* parathyroid hormone, *TSH* thyroid stimulating hormone, *AGA* American Gastroenterological Association, *NIH* National Institutes of Health, *WGO* World Gastroenterology Organization, *BSG* British Society of Gastroenterology, *NASPGHAN* North American Society for Pediatric Gastroenterology, Hepatology and Nutrition, *PCG-UK* Primary Care Gastroenterology Society-United Kingdom

[a] Repeat at 3 years if osteopenia, at age 55 in males, menopause in females

[b] Implies that nutritionist could carry out compliance assessment, growth assessment, and evaluate nutritional status and refer to physician or nurse if needed

[c] "Doing well" defined as normal antibodies and no clinical symptoms

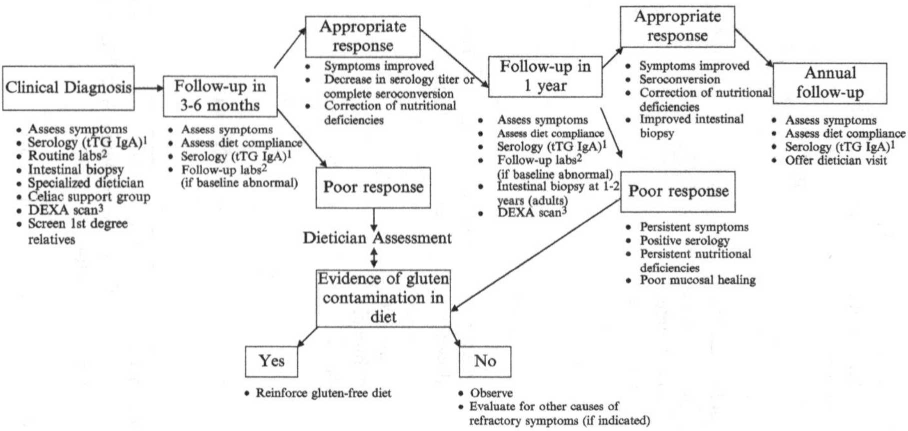

Fig. 12.1 Proposed CD management plan. [1]*TTG* tissue transglutaminase, [3]*DEXA* dual-energy X-ray absorptiometry, [2]*DGP* deaminated gliadin peptide, *EMA* endomysial antibody, *CBC* complete blood count, *TSH* thyroid-stimulating hormone. Adapted from [61]

Overall Objectives

1. Encourage dietary compliance through increased education and accountability
2. Monitor for ongoing or recurrent symptoms
3. Prevention and early detection of celiac-associated diseases and conditions

Frequency of Follow-Up

Follow-up is important in encouraging dietary compliance; however, there is no solid evidence to guide the optimal schedule for follow-up of patients with CD. A reasonable approach to follow-up is a visit in 3–6 months, then annually from date of diagnosis. In one study, annual follow-up with serology (tissue transglutaminase antibody) improved adherence to a gluten-free diet and led to seroconversion in 95 % of patients over a period of 5 years [20]. Ideally, the patient's primary care provider should be knowledgeable about CD in order to evaluate their status at routine annual visits, which are often used for other immunizations, growth assessments, screening, and medication refills. The follow-up interval can be lengthened to every 2 years, but only if patients are doing well on a gluten-free diet, have no ongoing symptoms, negative celiac serologies, and no nutritional deficiencies.

Provider Type

The concept of a multidisciplinary approach to follow-up has been of interest in a time when specialization and non-physician provider use has increased. Additionally, it has become clear that many physicians, regardless of specialty, have limited knowledge of CD and do not adequately assess compliance to the gluten-free diet or screen for disease-specific complications [11, 29]. Patient preference for follow-up is also important in aiding in compliance, given a British survey of patients with CD found that patients preferred that their annual follow-up was with a dietitian, with a doctor available if necessary [30]. It is important to note that most of these patients also felt that the annual review, associated with reassurance and blood testing, was "very useful," highlighting that the annual visit would require a physician to order and review serologic assessments in most medical systems.

In another study, 698 Finnish patients who were newly diagnosed with CD were surveyed to assess their experiences regarding the management of their disease. Patients were more pleased when they obtained dietary counseling from dieticians, and felt that the dietary counseling provided from physicians was not adequate or felt rushed [31]. Thus, the most important factor in choosing a long-term provider is selecting one with a knowledge and interest in caring for those with CD and finding a dietician well versed in the disease. In our practice, follow-up is guided by a physician. Assessment of the diet by an expert dietician is highly encouraged.

Serology

Serology can be useful in confirming response and compliance to the gluten-free diet. Adherence to a gluten-free diet is associated with a decrease in the absolute value of baseline celiac serology levels [32, 33]. The most accepted serologic studies for following CD activity include IgA tissue trans-glutaminase (TTG), IgA or IgG deaminated gliadin peptide (DGP), or IgA endomysial antibody (EMA). In patients who are known to be IgA deficient, an IgG-based serologic study (TTG or DGP) would be needed for diagnosis and monitoring. In this role, the sensitivity of TTG and EMA appear to be similar, with DGP being shown more recently to have some superiority [34]. It is important to note that the sensitivity of these markers decreases for small to moderate dietary transgressions, and so a normal value does not ensure full compliance [34, 35]. Increasingly, data have indicated that patients with normalized serology may continue to have ongoing intestinal inflammation and gluten contamination in their diets [36]. While it is expected that a patient who follows a gluten-free diet will have serologic normalization as early as 3 months after diagnosis, the converse is not always true, in that a patient who continues to consume gluten may have falsely normal serology, and therefore serology should not be the solitary means to monitor for treatment compliance [32]. There is no evidence to guide optimal frequency of serologic monitoring in CD patients; however, most guidelines suggest a reasonable approach would be annual serology, with consideration given to extending the interval only after a patient has proven to be very stable and successful on the gluten-free diet.

Assessing Mucosal Recovery: Repeat Duodenal Biopsy

Mucosal recovery generally requires several years of strict gluten avoidance in adults and is often patchy or incomplete [7, 12, 37, 38]. Duodenal biopsy is the gold standard for assessing mucosal healing. While it has been proposed that repeating duodenal biopsy to confirm healing should be a regular measure in all CD patients after 12 months on a gluten-free diet, the cost and invasive nature of endoscopic biopsy must be considered, as well as the lack of solid evidence supporting this practice. It is notable that adult celiac specialists often favor repeat intestinal biopsy over pediatric celiac specialists, which may be due to a variety of factors; adults often have delayed healing and are at increased risk for refractory CD and lymphoproliferative disease if inflammation is persistent [39].

In patients with persistent or recurrent symptoms, detailed dietary review is indicated, and if necessary, small bowel biopsy or other investigations should be employed. If a patient has persistent symptoms, despite strictly following a gluten-free diet, it is essential to repeat biopsy to look for evidence of refractory CD [40].

Capsule endoscopy is a new technique that can detect mucosal lesions that suggest villous atrophy (fissures, loss of folds, cobblestone pattern, scalloping), but this method has not been widely used or systematically evaluated as a method of clinical follow-up and may be reserved for those presenting with refractory symptoms, assuming there are no obstructing processes within the small bowel such as intussusception or malignancy [41]. Additionally, capsule endoscopy may be useful for patients unwilling or unable to undergo upper endoscopy.

Use of Routine Laboratory Studies

The use of routine laboratory studies in following CD has also not been systematically studied, but should be used to confirm resolution of nutritional deficiencies or abnormalities that were present at diagnosis. At diagnosis, it is recommended that patients be assessed for anemia, malnutrition, vitamin or mineral deficiencies, liver test abnormalities, and thyroid dysfunction [14, 42]. This can be done by checking a complete blood count (with serum ferritin if anemia is present), vitamin B_{12}, folate, albumin, calcium, 25-hydroxyvitamin D_3, alkaline phosphatase, alanine aminotransferase, and thyroid stimulating hormone levels. If indicated based on clinical symptoms or features of fat malabsorption, vitamin A and E levels could be checked, and similarly, trace minerals as indicated by the clinical presentation (may include zinc or copper). These should be followed until corrected and then periodically thereafter if there are ongoing concerns. If there is delayed or no recovery from baseline laboratory abnormalities, this may suggest gluten contamination in the diet, refractory CD, or another underlying disorder.

Hyposplenism and Immunization

CD is commonly correlated with functional hyposplenia (33–76 % prevalence) and increased risk of sepsis [43, 44]. Thus, immunization for encapsulated organisms in celiac patients including *Streptococcus pneumonia*, *Haemophilus influenza* type B, and *Neisseria meningitides* is recommended if not already immunized at time of diagnosis.

Screening for Associated Diseases

Decreased Bone Density

Patients with CD have an increased risk of low bone mineral density and an increased risk of fracture [45]. There is evidence that bone demineralization will improve and possibly reverse upon institution of a gluten-free diet after adequate time for recovery [46, 47]. Thus, the most important preventive measure is gluten avoidance. The 2012 British Society for Gastroenterology recommends that only those patients with CD who have additional risk factors (age, smoking, low BMI, persistent malabsorptive symptoms, etc.) undergo dual X-ray absorptiometry (DEXA) scan at diagnosis. Others have recommended DEXA in all adult patients diagnosed with CD, with repeat testing in subsequent years only if the baseline study was abnormal or if other risk factors for metabolic bone disease are present (i.e., menopause) [2]. All patients with CD should have periodic assessment of risk and repeat DEXA scanning if appropriate. Patients should have adequate dietary calcium and vitamin D supplementation for their age, or based on laboratory or DEXA testing. Baseline assessment of calcium, alkaline phosphatase, and 25-hydroxyvitamin D_3 levels should be considered [45]. Antiresorptive agents should be considered in patients with persistent or progressive bone loss in addition to continuing a gluten-free diet, calcium, and vitamin D supplementation [48, 49].

Screening for Malignancy

The increased risk of malignancy in CD is attributable to non-Hodgkin lymphoma, particularly enteropathy associated T-cell lymphoma (EATL). For patients who follow a strict gluten-free diet and achieve mucosal healing, the risk of EATL is felt to be on par with that of the general population [50]. Thus, regular follow-up to encourage compliance of a gluten-free diet is the best method for reducing risk of malignancy. Aside from this, there is no evidence to support routine screening for malignancy in celiac patients beyond what would be recommended for the general population. However, if a patient has refractory symptoms, they must undergo further evaluation to assess for lymphoproliferative changes of the small bowel [39]. Patients with CD have a higher risk of small bowel adenocarcinoma, nasopharyngeal carcinoma, and carcinoma of the esophagus, but these reports have not always been fully validated in multiple geographic locations [51]. The presence of symptoms or signs suggestive of these malignancies should prompt immediate clinical evaluation [2, 39].

Other Autoimmune Diseases

Many autoimmune diseases do appear to have increased prevalence among patients with CD, which include type 1 diabetes melitus (DM), autoimmune thyroid disease, autoimmune liver disease, alopecia areata, and microscopic colitis [14].

While no routine screening is required for these conditions, patients should have thyroid testing and baseline liver biochemistries at time of diagnosis, and only repeated later if a baseline study was abnormal or there are new clinical symptoms or concerns.

Alarm Features

The following symptoms and signs should prompt further work-up to investigate the potential complications and associated diseases involved in CD including enteropathy associated T-cell lymphoma, ulcerative jejunitis, or refractory CD (types I and II.)

- "B symptoms" (night sweats, fevers, weight loss)
- Increasing titers or persistently positive celiac serology
- New or persistent nutritional abnormalities
- New or persistent symptoms

Special Considerations for Children

Like in adults, the majority of children with CD are asymptomatic [52]. Clinical features of CD in children differ by age. Intestinal symptoms are common in children diagnosed within the first 2 years of life; failure to thrive, chronic diarrhea, vomiting, and abdominal distention are present in most cases. Extraintestinal manifestations, without any accompanying digestive symptoms, are more common in older children and adolescents. Short stature and iron deficiency anemia are the most recognized non-digestive manifestation of CD in children [53, 54].

Rapid resolution of the clinical symptoms is usually noted within a few weeks after starting the gluten-free diet. Most children are compliant with a gluten-free diet, especially when diagnosed early in life. Asymptomatic older children and adolescents may experience difficulties in modifying their lifestyles and being compliant with a gluten-free diet [55].

When a child is diagnosed with CD, all immediate family members should be screened with serologic testing. There are no clear guidelines on when to screen younger siblings (infants). The current practice is to screen them between 2 and 3 years of age, sooner if symptomatic, and consider repeating at 3- to 5-year intervals if asymptomatic until adulthood.

Children with positive serology and normal intestinal mucosa are referred to as "potential celiac" patients, and unlike adults patients with latent CD, they have never experienced intestinal villous atrophy [56]. There is no agreement on the management of these patients, but they will be given the option of normal diet with close observation and follow-up.

Psycho-Social Support

Patients often struggle with attending social gatherings, which are frequently oriented around food, much of which they will be unable to consume. This can leave patients feeling frustrated, isolated, and depressed, not to mention perhaps under more financial stress given the increased cost associated with a gluten-free diet prescription. Patients with CD benefit from involvement in local celiac support groups and societies; when involved, they are more likely to be compliant on a gluten-free diet and cope better with the burden of disease [57].

Improvements on the Forefront for Celiac Disease Management

Improving Compliance and Risk Stratification

More CD research has allowed for a better understanding of patient preferences and unique risks. Certain patients with CD appear to be less likely to follow the gluten-free diet, such as those diagnosed as adolescents, those without classic symptoms and those asymptomatic individuals diagnosed through family screening programs [58]. These groups should be targeted for future research and intervention. More exploration is needed to identify genetically high-risk subgroups of CD populations and tailor our management approach as well. This could allow for closer surveillance in groups with higher risk of developing refractory CD or other complications. Drug development is an area of active research that may become a reality in the near future.

Quality Improvement

A unique approach to assess compliance with validated questionnaires has been explored and could have increased utilization and applicability within new electronic medical record systems [59, 60]. Use of medical care process models could guide physicians to a standardized approach to the diagnosis and follow-up of patients with CD and would provide a quick reference during an office visit to improve the quality and cost-effectiveness of care.

Conclusion

An active livelong follow-up strategy is necessary in patients with CD to improve clinical outcomes and patient satisfaction. Further research and refinement of guidelines are likely to occur in the next few years and will help to further guide practitioners.

Acknowledgments Supported by American College of Gastroenterology Junior Faculty Development Award (to A.R.T).

References

1. Catassi C, Fabiani E, Iacono G, D'Agate C, Francavilla R, Biagi F, et al. A prospective, double-blind, placebo-controlled trial to establish a safe gluten threshold for patients with celiac disease [Multicenter Study Randomized Controlled Trial Research Support, Non-U.S. Gov't]. Am J Clin Nutr. 2007;85(1):160–6.
2. Leffler D. Celiac disease diagnosis and management: a 46-year-old woman with anemia [Case Reports Clinical Conference]. JAMA. 2011;306(14):1582–92.
3. Godfrey JD, Brantner TL, Brinjikji W, Christensen KN, Brogan DL, Van Dyke CT, et al. Morbidity and mortality among older individuals with undiagnosed celiac disease [Research Support, N.I.H., Extramural]. Gastroenterology. 2010;139(3):763–9.
4. Hall NJ, Rubin G, Charnock A. Systematic review: adherence to a gluten-free diet in adult patients with coeliac disease [Research Support, Non-U.S. Gov't Review]. Aliment Pharmacol Ther. 2009;30(4):315–30.
5. Rubio-Tapia A, Kyle RA, Kaplan EL, Johnson DR, Page W, Erdtmann F, et al. Increased prevalence and mortality in undiagnosed celiac disease [Research Support, N.I.H., Extramural]. Gastroenterology. 2009;137(1):88–93.
6. Ludvigsson JF, Montgomery SM, Ekbom A, Brandt L, Granath F. Small-intestinal histopathology and mortality risk in celiac disease [Research Support, Non-U.S. Gov't]. JAMA. 2009;302(11):1171–8.
7. Rubio-Tapia A, Rahim MW, See JA, Lahr BD, Wu TT, Murray JA. Mucosal recovery and mortality in adults with celiac disease after treatment with a gluten-free diet [Research Support, N.I.H., Extramural]. Am J Gastroenterol. 2010;105(6):1412–20.
8. Matysiak-Budnik T, Malamut G, de Serre NPM, Grosdidier E, Seguier S, Brousse N, et al. Long-term follow-up of 61 coeliac patients diagnosed in childhood: evolution toward latency is possible on a normal diet. Gut. 2007;56(10):1379–86.
9. Murray JA, Watson T, Clearman B, Mitros F. Effect of a gluten-free diet on gastrointestinal symptoms in celiac disease [Research Support, U.S. Gov't, P.H.S.]. Am J Clin Nutr. 2004;79(4):669–73.
10. Pietzak MM. Follow-up of patients with celiac disease: achieving compliance with treatment. Gastroenterology. 2005;128(4 Suppl 1):S135–41.
11. Herman ML, Rubio-Tapia A, Lahr BD, Larson JJ, Van Dyke CT, Murray JA. Patients with celiac disease are not followed up adequately [Research Support, N.I.H., Extramural Research Support, Non-U.S. Gov't]. Clin Gastroenterol Hepatol. 2012;10(8):893–9.e1.
12. Lanzini A, Lanzarotto F, Villanacci V, Mora A, Bertolazzi S, Turini D, et al. Complete recovery of intestinal mucosa occurs very rarely in adult coeliac patients despite adherence to gluten-free diet. Aliment Pharmacol Ther. 2009;29(12):1299–308.
13. Hernandez L, Green PH. Extraintestinal manifestations of celiac disease [Review]. Curr Gastroenterol Rep. 2006;8(5):383–9.
14. Haines ML, Anderson RP, Gibson PR. Systematic review: the evidence base for long-term management of coeliac disease [Review]. Aliment Pharmacol Ther. 2008;28(9):1042–66.
15. Dias JA, Walker-Smith J. Down's syndrome and coeliac disease [Case Reports]. J Pediatr Gastroenterol Nutr. 1990;10(1):41–3.
16. Bonamico M, Pasquino AM, Mariani P, Danesi HM, Culasso F, Mazzanti L, et al. Prevalence and clinical picture of celiac disease in Turner syndrome [Multicenter Study Research Support, Non-U.S. Gov't]. J Clin Endocrinol Metab. 2002;87(12):5495–8.
17. Giannotti A, Tiberio G, Castro M, Virgilii F, Colistro F, Ferretti F, et al. Coeliac disease in Williams syndrome. J Med Genet. 2001;38(11):767–8.

18. Nachman F, del Campo MP, Gonzalez A, Corzo L, Vazquez H, Sfoggia C, et al. Long-term deterioration of quality of life in adult patients with celiac disease is associated with treatment noncompliance [Comparative Study Research Support, Non-U.S. Gov't]. Dig Liver Dis. 2010;42(10):685–91.
19. Nachman F, Maurino E, Vazquez H, Sfoggia C, Gonzalez A, Gonzalez V, et al. Quality of life in celiac disease patients: prospective analysis on the importance of clinical severity at diagnosis and the impact of treatment [Comparative Study Research Support, Non-U.S. Gov't]. Dig Liver Dis. 2009;41(1):15–25.
20. Zanini B, Lanzarotto F, Mora A, Bertolazzi S, Turini D, Cesana B, et al. Five year time course of celiac disease serology during gluten-free diet: results of a community based "CD-Watch" program. Dig Liver Dis. 2010;42(12):865–70.
21. AGA Institute Medical Position Statement on the Diagnosis and management of celiac disease [Practice Guideline]. Gastroenterology. 2006;131(6):1977–80.
22. National Institutes of Health Consensus Development Conference Statement on Celiac Disease, June 28–30, 2004 [Consensus Development Conference Consensus Development Conference, NIH Review]. Gastroenterology. 2005;128(4 Suppl 1):S1–9.
23. Hill ID, Dirks MH, Liptak GS, Colletti RB, Fasano A, Guandalini S, et al. Guideline for the diagnosis and treatment of celiac disease in children: recommendations of the North American Society for Pediatric Gastroenterology, Hepatology and Nutrition [Practice Guideline]. J Pediatr Gastroenterol Nutr. 2005;40(1):1–19.
24. Bai JF, Corazza GR, Schuppan DL, Farthing M, Catassi C, Greco L, Cohen H, Ciacci C, Fasano A, González A, Krabshuis JH, LeMair A. World Gastroenterology Organisation Global Guidelines–Celiac disease. Milwaukee, WI: World Gastroenterology Organisation; 2012.
25. Guidelines for the management of patients with coeliac disease. Glasgow: British Society for Gastroenterology; 2010.
26. The management of adults with coeliac disease in primary care. London: Primary Care Society for Gastroenterology; 2006.
27. Fasano A, Catassi C. Celiac disease. N Engl J Med. 2012;367(25):2419–26.
28. Silvester JA, Rashid M. Long-term follow-up of individuals with celiac disease: an evaluation of current practice guidelines [Review]. Can J Gastroenterol. 2007;21(9):557–64.
29. Leffler DA, Edwards George JB, Dennis M, Cook EF, Schuppan D, Kelly CP. A prospective comparative study of five measures of gluten-free diet adherence in adults with coeliac disease [Comparative Study Research Support, N.I.H., Extramural Research Support, Non-U.S. Gov't]. Aliment Pharmacol Ther. 2007;26(9):1227–35.
30. Bebb JR, Lawson A, Knight T, Long RG. Long-term follow-up of coeliac disease–what do coeliac patients want? Aliment Pharmacol Ther. 2006;23(6):827–31.
31. Ukkola A, Maki M, Kurppa K, Collin P, Huhtala H, Kekkonen L, et al. Patients' experiences and perceptions of living with coeliac disease – implications for optimizing care [Clinical Trial Research Support, Non-U.S. Gov't]. J Gastrointest Liver Dis. 2012;21(1):17–22.
32. Nachman F, Sugai E, Vazquez H, Gonzalez A, Andrenacci P, Niveloni S, et al. Serological tests for celiac disease as indicators of long-term compliance with the gluten-free diet [Research Support, Non-U.S. Gov't]. Eur J Gastroenterol Hepatol. 2011;23(6):473–80.
33. Sugai E, Nachman F, Vaquez H, Gonzalez A, Andrenacci P, Czech A, et al. Dynamics of celiac disease-specific serology after initiation of a gluten-free diet and use in the assessment of compliance with treatment [Research Support, Non-U.S. Gov't]. Dig Liver Dis. 2010;42(5):352–8.
34. Monzani A, Rapa A, Fonio P, Tognato E, Panigati L, Oderda G. Use of deamidated gliadin peptide antibodies to monitor diet compliance in childhood celiac disease [Comparative Study Research Support, Non-U.S. Gov't]. J Pediatr Gastroenterol Nutr. 2011;53(1):55–60.
35. Vahedi K, Mascart F, Mary JY, Laberenne JE, Bouhnik Y, Morin MC, et al. Reliability of antitransglutaminase antibodies as predictors of gluten-free diet compliance in adult celiac disease [Comparative Study]. Am J Gastroenterol. 2003;98(5):1079–87.
36. Tursi A, Brandimarte G, Giorgetti GM. Lack of usefulness of anti-transglutaminase antibodies in assessing histologic recovery after gluten-free diet in celiac disease. J Clin Gastroenterol. 2003;37(5):387–91.

37. Wahab PJ, Meijer JW, Mulder CJ. Histologic follow-up of people with celiac disease on a gluten-free diet: slow and incomplete recovery. Am J Clin Pathol. 2002;118(3):459–63.
38. Macdonald WC, Brandborg LL, Flick AL, Trier JS, Rubin CE. Studies of celiac sprue. IV. The response of the whole length of the small bowel to a gluten-free diet. Gastroenterology. 1964;47:573–89.
39. Rubio-Tapia A, Murray JA. Classification and management of refractory coeliac disease [Research Support, N.I.H., Extramural Review]. Gut. 2010;59(4):547–57.
40. Daum S, Ipczynski R, Schumann M, Wahnschaffe U, Zeitz M, Ullrich R. High rates of complications and substantial mortality in both types of refractory sprue. Eur J Gastroenterol Hepatol. 2009;21(1):66–70.
41. Atlas DS, Rubio-Tapia A, Van Dyke CT, Lahr BD, Murray JA. Capsule endoscopy in nonresponsive celiac disease [Comparative Study Research Support, N.I.H., Extramural Research Support, Non-U.S. Gov't]. Gastrointest Endosc. 2011;74(6):1315–22.
42. Sategna-Guidetti C, Volta U, Ciacci C, Usai P, Carlino A, De Franceschi L, et al. Prevalence of thyroid disorders in untreated adult celiac disease patients and effect of gluten withdrawal: an Italian multicenter study [Multicenter Study]. Am J Gastroenterol. 2001;96(3):751–7.
43. Di Sabatino A, Carsetti R, Corazza GR. Post-splenectomy and hyposplenic states [Review]. Lancet. 2011;378(9785):86–97.
44. Ludvigsson JF, Olen O, Bell M, Ekbom A, Montgomery SM. Coeliac disease and risk of sepsis [Multicenter Study Research Support, Non-U.S. Gov't]. Gut. 2008;57(8):1074–80.
45. Fouda MA, Khan AA, Sultan MS, Rios LP, McAssey K, Armstrong D. Evaluation and management of skeletal health in celiac disease: position statement. Can J Gastroenterol. 2012;26(11):819–29.
46. Mora S, Barera G, Beccio S, Menni L, Proverbio MC, Bianchi C, et al. A prospective, longitudinal study of the long-term effect of treatment on bone density in children with celiac disease [Clinical Trial]. J Pediatr. 2001;139(4):516–21.
47. Sategna-Guidetti C, Grosso SB, Grosso S, Mengozzi G, Aimo G, Zaccaria T, et al. The effects of 1-year gluten withdrawal on bone mass, bone metabolism and nutritional status in newly-diagnosed adult coeliac disease patients [Clinical Trial Research Support, Non-U.S. Gov't]. Aliment Pharmacol Ther. 2000;14(1):35–43.
48. Osteoporosis prevention, diagnosis, and therapy [Consensus Development Conference Consensus Development Conference, NIH Review]. JAMA. 2001;285(6):785–95.
49. Pinkerton JV, Dalkin AC, Crowe SE, Wilson BB, Stelow EB. Treatment of postmenopausal osteoporosis in a patient with celiac disease [Case Reports]. Nat Rev Endocrinol. 2010;6(3):167–71.
50. Elfstrom P, Granath F, Ekstrom Smedby K, Montgomery SM, Askling J, Ekbom A, et al. Risk of lymphoproliferative malignancy in relation to small intestinal histopathology among patients with celiac disease [Multicenter StudyResearch Support, Non-U.S. Gov't]. J Natl Cancer Inst. 2011;103(5):436–44.
51. Ludvigsson JF. Mortality and malignancy in celiac disease [Research Support, Non-U.S. Gov't]. Gastrointest Endosc Clin N Am. 2012;22(4):705–22.
52. Catassi C, Fabiani E, Ratsch IM, Coppa GV, Giorgi PL, Pierdomenico R, et al. The coeliac iceberg in Italy. A multicentre antigliadin antibodies screening for coeliac disease in school-age subjects [Clinical Trial Multicenter Study]. Acta Paediatr Suppl. 1996;412:29–35.
53. Cacciari E, Salardi S, Volta U, Biasco G, Lazzari R, Corazza GR, et al. Can antigliadin antibody detect symptomless coeliac disease in children with short stature? [Comparative Study Research Support, Non-U.S. Gov't]. Lancet. 1985;1(8444):1469–71.
54. Bottaro G, Cataldo F, Rotolo N, Spina M, Corazza GR. The clinical pattern of subclinical/silent celiac disease: an analysis on 1026 consecutive cases [Multicenter Study]. Am J Gastroenterol. 1999;94(3):691–6.
55. Rashid M, Cranney A, Zarkadas M, Graham ID, Switzer C, Case S, et al. Celiac disease: evaluation of the diagnosis and dietary compliance in Canadian children [Research Support, Non--U.S. Gov't]. Pediatrics. 2005;116(6):e754–9.

56. Paparo F, Petrone E, Tosco A, Maglio M, Borrelli M, Salvati VM, et al. Clinical, HLA, and small bowel immunohistochemical features of children with positive serum antiendomysium antibodies and architecturally normal small intestinal mucosa [Research Support, Non-U.S. Gov't]. Am J Gastroenterol. 2005;100(10):2294–8.
57. Leffler DA, Edwards-George J, Dennis M, Schuppan D, Cook F, Franko DL, et al. Factors that influence adherence to a gluten-free diet in adults with celiac disease [Research Support, N.I.H., Extramural Research Support, Non-U.S. Gov't]. Dig Dis Sci. 2008;53(6):1573–81.
58. Fabiani E, Catassi C, Villari A, Gismondi P, Pierdomenico R, Ratsch IM, et al. Dietary compliance in screening-detected coeliac disease adolescents. Acta Paediatr Suppl. 1996;412:65–7.
59. Biagi F, Bianchi PI, Marchese A, Trotta L, Vattiato C, Balduzzi D, Brusco G, Andrealli A, Cisarò F, Astegiano M, Pellegrino S, Magazzù G, Klersy C, Corazza GR. A score that verifies adherence to a gluten-free diet: a cross-sectional, multicentre validation in real clinical life. Br J Nutr. 2012;108(10):1884–8.
60. Leffler DA, Dennis M, Edwards George JB, Jamma S, Magge S, Cook EF, et al. A simple validated gluten-free diet adherence survey for adults with celiac disease [Evaluation Studies Research Support, N.I.H., Extramural]. Clin Gastroenterol Hepatol. 2009;7(5):530–6, 6 e1–2.
61. Rubio-Tapia A. Seguimiento Médico del Paciente Celiaco. In: Rodrigo L, Pena A, editors. Enfermedad Celiaca. Barcelona: OmniaScience; 2012.

Chapter 13
Special Considerations in Children and Young Adults with Celiac Disease

Stefano Guandalini and Sona Young

Although celiac disease (CD) appears to have the same pattern of pathogenesis across all ages, there are indeed special aspects of it that must be accounted for when working with children and adolescents as compared to adults

Epidemiology

Studies have demonstrated that the prevalence of CD in children is similar to adult populations at approximately 1 %, although it appears to be more prone to be influenced by factors such as infant feeding practices, as demonstrated by the persistently elevated prevalence of CD in 12-year-old children born in Sweden during the "epidemics" of the early 1990s [1].

Pathogenesis

The pathogenesis is similar between adults and children. However, one difference is in the degree of T-cell activation that occurs in response to gliadin and glutenin epitopes. In adults, there is a single region of alpha-gliadin that requires deamidation and has been described as the dominant epitope to cause an immunologic response; however, in children, T cells were reactive to multiple epitopes found in both gliadin and glutenin. In addition, both deamidation-dependent and deamidation-independent responses were seen in the pediatric population [2].

S. Guandalini, M.D. (✉) • S. Young, M.D.
Department of Pediatric Gastroenterology, University of Chicago Comer Children's Hospital, 5841 S. Maryland Ave., MC 4065, Chicago, IL, 60637, USA
e-mail: sguandalini@peds.bsd.uchicago.edu

S.D. Rampertab and G.E. Mullin (eds.), *Celiac Disease*, Clinical Gastroenterology, DOI 10.1007/978-1-4614-8560-5_13,

CD is multifactorial and requires a combination of genetic and environmental factors. A genetic component to CD is supported by its tendency to run in families. Monozygotic twins show a high concordance rate as high as 86 %, while dizygotic twins are around 20 % [3]. However, although genetic predisposition is present, the fact that only about 4 % of genetically predisposed individuals develop celiac disease shows that there are also environmental risk factors to consider in the pediatric population.

In fact, in addition to gluten as a necessary trigger, several other factors come into play. These include the presence and duration of breast-feeding, timing and amount of gluten at introduction, and infectious exposures. Breast-feeding is thought to be protective against the development of CD, but it is not clear whether this provides a permanent benefit or whether it simply delays and/or changes the presentation [4]. A meta-analysis performed by Akobeng et al. included a total of 714 cases of CD and 1,255 controls, and found that children who were breast-fed at the time of gluten introduction had a 52 % risk reduction for the development of CD [5]. Other studies have also demonstrated that a longer duration of breast-feeding does coincide with a decrease in the risk for CD [6–8]. The mechanism behind this is unclear, but may be due to the protective nature of breast-feeding against gastrointestinal infections or to the fact that the complex immune milieu created in the gut by breast milk at the time of gluten introduction favors the development of oral tolerance against antigens such as gluten [9]. The transfer of small amounts of gluten with gluten-specific IgA antibodies has been suggested as a possibility to affect the immune system response in infants [10]. Furthermore, it was shown that infants who were breast-fed had a higher percentage of peripheral CD4+CD25+ and lower CD4+CD38+ T cells when compared to formula-fed infants, again suggesting that breast milk may lead to the development of a more mature immune system.

The effect of timing of gluten introduction in CD was demonstrated for the first time in the 1970s, when it was observed that the incidence of CD decreased from 1:2228 to 1:4168 after recommendations were changed to delay introducing gluten until after 4 months of age. The amount of gluten that is introduced at the time of weaning also plays a role, and evidence suggests that introducing gluten in small amounts while breast-feeding may help to decrease risk of CD [1, 9, 11].

Infectious exposure has recently been shown to be an additional, important risk factor: children who had three or more infectious episodes prior to the age of 6 months had an increased risk of developing CD before the age of 2 years [12]. Furthermore, rotavirus infection is thought to be an independent risk factor, as it has been found to precipitate the induction of inflammatory anti-gluten responses and the generation of TG2-specific antibodies [13, 14]. In general, gastrointestinal infections cause tissue damage and inflammation, thus increasing the permeability of the intestine and allowing for enhanced penetration and presentation of the gluten peptides [15, 16]. Infections can also induce polyclonal lymphocyte activation, increase the immunogenicity of organ autoantigens secondary to inflammation, and lead to antigen mimicry molecular mechanisms. In antigen mimicry, the cross-reactivity between host epitopes and immunologically similar epitopes in the infectious organism lead to an autoimmune response [17]. This antigen mimicry and increased immune activation and expression of IFN-alpha and IL-15 secondary to infection-mediated inflammation has been hypothesized as a possible link between CD in patients with multiple infectious exposures [18].

Another question that may arise is whether vaccinations are associated with the development of CD. A study done in Sweden found no association between early vaccination and a patient's risk for developing CD [19].

Clinical Presentation

The spectrum of symptoms with CD is quite heterogeneous and can manifest at any age after gluten exposure. Compared to children, adults and adolescent are more likely to have a longer duration of symptoms prior to the diagnosis of CD, whereas younger children may be more likely to present with typical features of CD, such as diarrhea, emesis, abdominal distension, and failure to thrive. In addition, more pronounced histological features may be found in the younger children [20].

As the age of diagnosis increases, a greater proportion of children present with atypical symptoms such as anemia and short stature [21, 22]. Up to 25 % may be diagnosed based solely on targeted screening rather than symptoms [23]. Due to this increased awareness and screening, many children are discovered before having active CD and are found to have what is being termed potential CD. In this case, the child has positive serology for CD and has the predisposing HLA genotype; however, the small intestine displays normal histology. Children may or may not have symptoms and not all will go on to develop a gluten-sensitive enteropathy [15]. One study found that over a 3-year period, 33 % developed villous atrophy, while the majority did not [24]. Clearly, it is not known if those who were asymptomatic and had a normal histology after 3 years will later manifest full-blown CD. In fact, the issue of potential CD in children must still be considered an unsolved one.

A recent prospective investigation [25] in 96 children with a family risk of CD and positive serology followed up for 2 years showed that 72 had overt CD, while 24 of them had potential CD. The stronger predictors of potential CD were lack of symptoms, anti-TTG level lower than 11-fold the upper normal limit, age lower than 24 months, and breast-feeding longer than 8 months. Eighty-six percent of them, continuing a gluten-containing diet, became, however, antibody negative; 5 % eventually developed overt CD, and 9 % had fluctuating antibody levels after 2 years. Thus, the prevalence of potential CD and the percentage of short-term loss of CD-related-antibodies are high in infants at-family-risk for CD, suggesting a cautious strategy in asymptomatic children with a positive celiac serology. Table 13.1 reports a schematic classification of the various presentations of CD.

Table 13.1 Classification of celiac disease[a]

Type	Serology (TTG and/or EMA)	Age most often affected	Symptoms	Pathology
"Typical"	Positive	Toddler, young child	Abdominal pain, distention Diarrhea Vomiting Anorexia Constipation	Marsh 2–3
"Atypical"	Positive	Older child, adult	Mostly extra-intestinal (see Table 13.2)	Marsh 1–3
Silent	Positive	Adult	None	Marsh 1–3
Latent	Positive or negative	Adult	None Gastrointestinal Extra-intestinal	Marsh 0–1 (previous or future gluten enteropathy)
Potential	Positive	Any age	None Gastrointestinal Extra-intestinal	Marsh 0–1

[a]In all cases, genetic asset is HLA-DQ2 and/or DQ8

Extra-Intestinal Manifestations

Short Stature

A special consideration in the pediatric population as compared to adults is the importance in achieving full growth potential. Short stature has been described as the only presenting sign of CD in otherwise asymptomatic patients. Catch-up growth may be observed within 6 months after initiation of a gluten-free diet but can take up to 2 years [26]. There is also the possibility of an associated growth-hormone deficiency, which should be considered in children who show no catch-up growth on a gluten free diet despite conversion to negative serology [27].

Hematologic Abnormalities

Like in adults, the most common hematologic abnormality in children with CD is iron-deficiency anemia (IDA), which can be seen in up to 35 % of patients at time of diagnosis [28]. In fact, IDA refractory to oral iron supplements may be the sole presenting symptom of CD. Other hematologic abnormalities may include thrombocytosis, thrombocytopenia, megaloblastic anemia from folate/vitamin B_{12} deficiency, leucopenia, functional hyposplenism, and selective IgA deficiency [29]. In most cases, IDA regresses quite promptly after a strict gluten-free diet is instituted, and iron supplements may be required only for a short time after diagnosis.

Bone Mineral Density

Many studies have shown differences in bone health between children with CD and healthy children. These differences are corrected after following a strict gluten-free diet, often within 1 year [30–32]. Long term, the efficacy of a gluten-free diet in maintaining bone mass is supported by two studies that followed patients with CD after being on a gluten-free diet for approximately 4 and 10 years, respectively. In these patients, there was no significant difference in bone mineral density between the two populations after treatment with a gluten-free diet. In addition, those patients with good compliance demonstrated higher bone mineral content, bone density, and bone content compared to those with poor compliance [33, 34].

Hepatitis

It has been known for many years that children with CD have a high prevalence of liver disorders. Among them, an otherwise unexplained mild increase of serum transaminases is the most common. Farre et al. observed that out of 114 children diagnosed with CD, 37 patients (32 %) had elevated transaminases at the time of diagnosis, and that this was the only manifestation of CD in 5 (4.3 %) of the patients. Of note, 35 patients had follow-up, and all of them showed normalization of their liver function tests (LFTs) on a gluten-free diet either before or by the time their celiac serology also normalized [35]. A recent meta-analysis [36] on liver disease and CD encompassing more than 2,000 children concluded that CD is associated with elevated transaminases in about one-third of newly diagnosed children. Cryptogenic persistent hypertransaminasemia may signal gluten-dependent non-specific mild hepatitis (12.0 % of cases) or more rarely (6.3 %) severe CD-related autoimmune hepatitis.

Oral Manifestations

A number of oral issues can be encountered more frequently in children and teenagers with CD than in their adult counterpart. In fact, problems such as dental enamel hypoplasia, aphthous ulcers, and delayed teeth eruption are common. Dental enamel hypoplasia has been reported with prevalence ranging from 10 % to 97 % [37–40], and appears to be more prevalent in children compared with adults with CD. This defect, more common in patients with celiac disease compared to the general population [41], is thought to be secondary to nutritional deficiencies and immune disturbances during this period of enamel formation in the first 7 years [42]. Other enamel defects that can be associated to CD are enamel pitting, grooving, and partial or complete loss of the enamel. Of note, dental enamel defects can be found in children in the absence of any other symptoms, as documented in a large epidemiological study in Italian children [43], and are therefore a useful screening tool.

Oral aphthae can be present in children and to a lesser extent also in adults with CD. However, oral ulcers are neither characteristic nor specific to CD since they can also be found in some other chronic gastrointestinal inflammatory states such as inflammatory bowel disease and Bechet's disease. However, it should be noted that these ulcers often regress once the patients are on a gluten-free diet [44].

Delayed tooth eruption has been reported in up to a quarter of patients with CD [44]. This nonspecific sign is possibly related to malnutrition.

A recent study in Israel assessed oral health, bacterial colonization, and salivary buffering capacity of children with CD at diagnosis and on a gluten-free diet [45] and confirmed a higher prevalence of enamel hypoplasia (66 %) in celiac children, while plaque index was significantly lower in the group of celiac children on gluten-free diet, which correlated with a better oral health behavior.

Neurologic Manifestations

Although celiac disease has been associated with many neurologic manifestations in the adult population, this is not as prominent in pediatrics. There has been some evidence to support an increased prevalence of chronic headaches, hypotonia, learning disabilities or ADHD, and developmental delay [46]. There has also been question as to whether an association exists between celiac disease and autism; however, there has been no evidence to support such an association [47, 48]. There is currently no indication to test asymptomatic children with autism for CD [49]. There remains controversy around whether gluten itself can help exacerbate autistic features, although a double-blinded, placebo controlled study done on a small sample of patients indicated no statistically significant differences or findings [50, 51].

Diagnosis

Who to Screen

See Table 13.2. CD should be considered in the differential diagnosis of children with persisting GI symptoms, including especially diarrhea, but also recurrent abdominal pain, vomiting, and even constipation. It should also be a high diagnostic priority for children presenting with failure to thrive. In addition, extra-intestinal symptoms, such as dental enamel defects, short stature, delayed puberty, and refractory iron deficiency anemia should prompt the physician to test for celiac disease. Less commonly, older children and teenagers would also present with dermatitis herpetiformis or osteoporosis.

Table 13.2 Children and young adults who should be screened for CD

Subjects with suggestive GI complaints
• Chronic or recurrent diarrhea
• Failure to thrive
• Vomiting
• Anorexia
• Abdominal distention
• Recurrent abdominal pain
• Constipation
Subjects with extra-intestinal manifestations
• Dental enamel dysplasia
• Short stature
• High transaminases
• Fe-deficient anemia (unexplained)
• Fatigue
• Arthritis
Subjects who may be asymptomatic but are at increased risk of CD
• Autoimmune conditions
• Type 1 diabetes
• Autoimmune thyroiditis
• Autoimmune hepatitis
• First-degree relatives of celiac patients
• Down syndrome
• Turner syndrome
• Williams syndrome

Testing is also recommended for asymptomatic children who have conditions associated with CD (type 1 diabetes mellitus, autoimmune thyroiditis, Down syndrome, Turner syndrome, Williams syndrome, and first-degree relatives of celiac patients). It is recommended that testing of asymptomatic children who belong to groups at risk begin around 3 years of age provided they have had an adequate gluten-containing diet for a minimum of 1 year prior to testing [49].

How to Screen

The initial screening test of choice is the IgA antibody to tissue transglutaminase (TTG). Although the IgA antibody to endomysium (EMA) is considered extremely specific, it suffers from a somewhat lower sensitivity, so is not ideal for screening purposes; in addition to being a direct immunofluroscence test, it is labor-intensive and observer dependent and as such subject to both interpretation error and additional cost. The use of the antigliadin IgA and IgG tests is no longer recommended due to their poor sensitivity and specificity. Table 13.3 outlines the accuracy of

Table 13.3 Sensitivity and specificity ranges for celiac disease serology tests in pediatric patients[a]

Test	Sensitivity (%)	Specificity (%)
IgA AGA	60.9–96	79.4–93.8
IgA EMA	82.6–100	94.7–100
IgA TTG	73.9–100	77.8–100
IgA DGP	80.7–95.1	86.3–93.1
IgG DGP	80.1–98.6	86–96.9

[a]Adapted from [52]

diagnostic screening tests based on a meta-analysis evaluating evidence from 2004 to September 2009 [52]. All individuals with a positive TTG should then be referred to a pediatric gastroenterologist for intestinal biopsy [49].

Endoscopy

The gold standard for diagnosis for CD is small bowel biopsy and histological changes, which correlate with CD. It had been recommended that all children with a positive TTG screen should undergo an upper endoscopy with biopsies to confirm the diagnosis. However, recent guidelines from the European Society for Pediatric Gastroenterology Hepatology and Nutrition (ESPGHAN) now state that a child with a history consistent with CD, who has a TTG >10× above the upper limit of normal a genetic test compatible with celiac disease and positive EMA testing, can bypass the biopsies, as there is no differential diagnosis other than CD [53].

Peculiarity of the Diagnosis in Young Children

The diagnosis of CD in children <2 years old can present a diagnostic dilemma. In this age group, they are more likely to have false negative serology, and the histological changes can be more commonly due to other causes such as cow's milk-sensitive enteropathy, post-enteric syndrome, Giardia infection, autoimmune enteropathy, and common variable immune deficiency. For these reasons, previous diagnostic criteria by ESPGHAN recommended repeating the biopsies before and after a gluten challenge when these children were older. Recently, a study [54] utilizing the old, native anti-gliadin antibodies (AGA) concluded that the second and the third biopsies (before and after the gluten challenge) may also be avoided when diagnosing CD in children younger than 2 years provided that the child, at the time of presentation, has positive anti-endomysial antibodies and villous atrophy on the initial small bowel biopsy. A gluten challenge should be still considered in all other children younger than 2 years. There is also evidence to suggest that in this age group, the anti-deamidated gliadin antibodies may have a higher sensitivity in comparison with both TTG and EMA [55].

IgA Deficiency

A total IgA should be measured in all children at time that serology tests drawn. If they are found to be IgA-deficient (i.e., a serum level of IgA lower than 20 mg/dL), additional testing should be done with IgG-specific antibodies.

Genetic Testing

A child that initially tests negative for celiac disease can develop antibodies and histological changes at any point in the future. This is especially important for patients who have risk factors, such as a first-degree relative with celiac disease, or an associated condition such as type 1 diabetes mellitus. For these patients, it may be worthwhile to consider genetic testing, as either the HLA-DQ2 or HLA-DQ8 haplotype is necessary for the development of CD. Knowledge of the child's haplotype would allow for development of a clinically relevant genetic risk profile. That is, if the genetic testing is negative, no further CD surveillance is needed. However, if the child carries either one of these haplotypes, careful monitoring is required [56].

Associated Conditions

Type 1 Diabetes Mellitus

CD has been associated with several other conditions. One of the most notable, and especially relevant in children and young adults, is with type 1 diabetes mellitus (T1D). There have been multiple studies looking at the prevalence of CD in T1D, and the value has ranged from 3 % to 16 % with a mean prevalence of 8 % [57–60]. A multicenter study also showed a significant percentage of patients (12.2 %) with T1D will have *potential* celiac disease; whether or not these patients should also be put on a gluten-free diet is unclear, with some advising for keeping them on a gluten-containing diet while closely monitoring both clinically and with antibody testing [60, 61]. Current recommendations by the North American Society for Pediatric Gastroenterology, Hepatology and Nutrition (NASPGHAN) include screening all children with T1D for CD. This recommendation is supported by studies, which do show improvement in children with T1D and CD who are put on a gluten-free diet in terms of clinical symptoms, body mass index, and HbA1C [62–65]. However, for children with T1D who otherwise have no symptoms attributable to celiac disease, there is little evidence to support that a gluten-free diet will improve their diabetic control in the short term, and long-term effects are unknown [49].

Genetic Disorders

There is strong evidence for an association between Down syndrome and CD, and the prevalence has been studied several times. One study showed a prevalence of 4.6 %; 69 % of these patients had a classical presentation, 11 % with asymptomatic, and 20 % with silent disease. In those patients with symptoms, the mean time to diagnosis was 3.8 years [66]. A nationwide case-control study in Sweden done from 1973 to 2008 found that patients with Down syndrome had a sixfold increased risk of developing CD compared to the general population [67]. Likewise, females with Turner syndrome have an increased propensity to develop autoimmune conditions such as CD, thyroiditis, and type 1 diabetes mellitus [68]. The prevalence of CD ranges from 2.8 % to 7.9 % in various studies [68–73]. Finally, the prevalence of CD in Williams syndrome is thought to be comparable to that in Down syndrome and Turner syndrome. A study done in Italy found the prevalence of CD to be 9.5 % in patients with Williams syndrome compared to 0.54 % of the healthy control group [74].

The current recommendation is to screen all asymptomatic children with Down, Turner, or Williams syndrome for CD and to consider repeat testing at intervals.

Thyroid Disease

Autoimmune thyroid disease (ATD) can co-occur with CD. Studies have shown prevalence rates ranging from 2.3 % to 7.8 % in children and adolescents diagnosed with autoimmune thyroid disease [75, 76]. However, the reverse has not been shown to be true; that is, it is not proven that children with CD are at increased risk for developing ATD. One study looked at 545 pediatric patients diagnosed with CD and who were following a gluten-free diet; the results showed no significant association with the development of ATD [77]. In spite of the lack of overt autoimmune thyroiditis, however, celiac children show a higher prevalence of antithyroid antibodies. Ansaldi et al. [78] found that 26.2 % of the patients with CD vs. 10 % of the control group had such organ-specific autoantibodies. Of them, 69 % were following a gluten-free diet [78]. The positive predictive value of the antithyroid antibodies in children with CD is, however, low: Cassio et al. showed, in fact, that 74 % of the patients with positive antibody titers remained euthyroid throughout follow-up (8.9 ± 4.0 years) [79]. Current recommendations are to screen all children with ATD for CD, regardless of symptoms [49].

Hepatitis

An increased prevalence of CD has also been shown in patients with autoimmune hepatitis (AIH). This may be because the two disorders share a combination of genes coding for class II human leukocyte antigens. In one study, 47 patients with AIH (6.4 %) were found to have positive serologies (TTG and EMA) and histological findings consistent with CD [80]. In the cohort of patients who have both AIH and CD, a higher percentage achieves treatment-free sustained remission when compared to those who have AIH without a co-existing diagnosis of CD, suggesting that the gluten-free diet does have a long-term adjuvant benefit [81].

Treatment

The treatment for CD is lifelong adherence to a gluten-free diet. This requires complete elimination of wheat, barley, and rye from the diet. Adherence to diet can be difficult. Younger age at diagnosis, being currently a teenager, and current presence of symptoms have been associated with non-compliance to the diet [82]. Of note, it appears that if children were diagnosed with CD at <4 years of age, their subsequent compliance with a gluten-free diet was significantly improved [83]. Noncompliant patients were found to be less likely to have regular visits with their pediatric gastroenterologist, highlighting the importance of adequate follow-up and education [84].

Psychosocial Impact

Having CD can have a major impact on the psychosocial developmental aspects of adolescents as well as social relationship with their peers. For example, dining out with friends can be a difficult experience; although the availability of food choices is certainly on the rise almost worldwide, lack of detailed knowledge about the food preparation can cause concern for cross-contamination. This may also cause embarrassment about not being able to eat the same foods as their friends. Such experiences may affect the rate of compliance with the diet during such social situations. It is important to promote continued education of adolescents to foster compliance with the diet in these types of social situations. Even then, knowledge of the risks associated with noncompliance does not guarantee sustained compliance [85–87]. Another study found that dilemmas arose around food situations at work, during purchases, when travelling, in relation to meals at home and meals outside the home. Emotions, relationships, and the management of daily life were the three main categories of conflict that emerged through the analysis. Specifically, isolation, shame, fear of becoming contaminated by gluten, and worries about being a bother were expressed by the participants [88].

It is also important to remember that strict compliance with a gluten-free diet can be vital to obtaining optimal quality of life. Adolescents with poor compliance report a lower quality of life, more physical problems, a higher burden of illness, more family problems, and more problems in leisure time than adolescents who are compliant with a gluten-free diet. These patients also reported a higher problem of anticipation and higher feelings of "ill-being." Therefore, psychosocial support should be offered to those adolescents who are having a difficult time in adhering to a gluten-free diet [89].

References

1. Ivarsson A, Myleus A, Norstrom F, van der Pals M, Rosen A, Hogberg L, et al. Prevalence of childhood celiac disease and changes in infant feeding. Pediatrics. 2013;131(3):e687–94.
2. Vader W, Kooy Y, Van Veelen P, De Ru A, Harris D, Benckhuijsen W, et al. The gluten response in children with celiac disease is directed toward multiple gliadin and glutenin peptides [Research Support, Non-U.S. Gov't]. Gastroenterology. 2002;122(7):1729–37.
3. Greco L, Romino R, Coto I, Di Cosmo N, Percopo S, Maglio M, et al. The first large population based twin study of coeliac disease [Research Support, Non-U.S. Gov't Twin Study]. Gut. 2002;50(5):624–8.
4. D'Amico MA, Holmes J, Stavropoulos SN, Frederick M, Levy J, DeFelice AR, et al. Presentation of pediatric celiac disease in the United States: prominent effect of breastfeeding. Clin Pediatr (Phila). 2005;44(3):249–58.
5. Akobeng AK, Ramanan AV, Buchan I, Heller RF. Effect of breast feeding on risk of coeliac disease: a systematic review and meta-analysis of observational studies [Meta-Analysis Review]. Arch Dis Child. 2006;91(1):39–43.
6. Auricchio S, Follo D, de Ritis G, Giunta A, Marzorati D, Prampolini L, et al. Does breast feeding protect against the development of clinical symptoms of celiac disease in children? [Comparative Study]. J Pediatr Gastroenterol Nutr. 1983;2(3):428–33.
7. Greco L, Auricchio S, Mayer M, Grimaldi M. Case control study on nutritional risk factors in celiac disease [Research Support, Non-U.S. Gov't]. J Pediatr Gastroenterol Nutr. 1988;7(3):395–9.
8. Peters U, Schneeweiss S, Trautwein EA, Erbersdobler HF. A case-control study of the effect of infant feeding on celiac disease [Research Support, Non-U.S. Gov't]. Ann Nutr Metab. 2001;45(4):135–42.
9. Sollid LM. Breast milk against coeliac disease. Gut. 2002;51(6):767–8.
10. Verhasselt V. Neonatal tolerance under breastfeeding influence [Research Support, Non-U.S. Gov't Review]. Curr Opin Immunol. 2010;22(5):623–30.
11. Ivarsson A, Hernell O, Stenlund H, Persson LA. Breast-feeding protects against celiac disease [Research Support, Non-U.S. Gov't]. Am J Clin Nutr. 2002;75(5):914–21.
12. Myleus A, Hernell O, Gothefors L, Hammarstrom ML, Persson LA, Stenlund H, et al. Early infections are associated with increased risk for celiac disease: an incident case-referent study. BMC Pediatr. 2012;12:194.
13. Stene LC, Honeyman MC, Hoffenberg EJ, Haas JE, Sokol RJ, Emery L, et al. Rotavirus infection frequency and risk of celiac disease autoimmunity in early childhood: a longitudinal study [Research Support, N.I.H., Extramural Research Support, Non-U.S. Gov't]. Am J Gastroenterol. 2006;101(10):2333–40.
14. Troncone R, Auricchio S. Rotavirus and celiac disease: clues to the pathogenesis and perspectives on prevention [Editorial]. J Pediatr Gastroenterol Nutr. 2007;44(5):527–8.
15. Newton KP, Singer SA. Celiac disease in children and adolescents: special considerations [Review]. Semin Immunopathol. 2012;34(4):479–96.
16. Bethune MT, Khosla C. Parallels between pathogens and gluten peptides in celiac sprue [Research Support, N.I.H., Extramural Review]. PLoS Pathog. 2008;4(2):e34.
17. Bach JF. Infections and autoimmune diseases [Review]. J Autoimmun. 2005;25(Suppl):74–80.
18. Jabri B, Sollid LM. Tissue-mediated control of immunopathology in coeliac disease [Research Support, N.I.H., Extramural Research Support, Non-U.S. Gov't Review]. Nat Rev Immunol. 2009;9(12):858–70.
19. Myleus A, Stenlund H, Hernell O, Gothefors L, Hammarstrom ML, Persson LA, et al. Early vaccinations are not risk factors for celiac disease [Research Support, Non-U.S. Gov't]. Pediatrics. 2012;130(1):e63–70.
20. Tanpowpong P, Broder-Fingert S, Katz AJ, Camargo Jr CA. Age-related patterns in clinical presentations and gluten-related issues among children and adolescents with celiac disease. Clin Transl Gastroenterol. 2012;3:e9.

21. Kochhar R, Jain K, Thapa BR, Rawal P, Khaliq A, Bhadada S, et al. Clinical presentation of celiac disease among pediatric compared to adolescent and adult patients [Comparative Study]. Indian J Gastroenterol. 2012;31(3):116–20.
22. McGowan KE, Castiglione DA, Butzner JD. The changing face of childhood celiac disease in north america: impact of serological testing [Research Support, Non-U.S. Gov't]. Pediatrics. 2009;124(6):1572–8.
23. Ravikumara M, Tuthill DP, Jenkins HR. The changing clinical presentation of coeliac disease. Arch Dis Child. 2006;91(12):969–71.
24. Tosco A, Salvati VM, Auricchio R, Maglio M, Borrelli M, Coruzzo A, et al. Natural history of potential celiac disease in children [Research Support, Non-U.S. Gov't]. Clin Gastroenterol Hepatol. 2011;9(4):320–5; quiz e36.
25. Lionetti E, Castellaneta S, Pulvirenti A, Tonutti E, Francavilla R, Fasano A, et al. Prevalence and natural history of potential celiac disease in at-family-risk infants prospectively investigated from birth. J Pediatr. 2012;161(5):908–14.
26. Greco L, Tipo V, Di Donato F, Mayer M. Pulsatile growth pattern during catch-up growth in childhood coeliac disease. Acta Paediatr. 1994;83(7):724–9.
27. Giovenale D, Meazza C, Cardinale GM, Sposito M, Mastrangelo C, Messini B, et al. The prevalence of growth hormone deficiency and celiac disease in short children [Multicenter Study]. Clin Med Res. 2006;4(3):180–3.
28. Bottaro G, Cataldo F, Rotolo N, Spina M, Corazza GR. The clinical pattern of subclinical/silent celiac disease: an analysis on 1026 consecutive cases [Multicenter Study]. Am J Gastroenterol. 1999;94(3):691–6.
29. Fisgin T, Yarali N, Duru F, Usta B, Kara A. Hematologic manifestation of childhood celiac disease. Acta Haematol. 2004;111(4):211–4.
30. Mora S, Barera G, Ricotti A, Weber G, Bianchi C, Chiumello G. Reversal of low bone density with a gluten-free diet in children and adolescents with celiac disease. Am J Clin Nutr. 1998;67(3):477–81.
31. Kavak US, Yuce A, Kocak N, Demir H, Saltik IN, Gurakan F, et al. Bone mineral density in children with untreated and treated celiac disease. J Pediatr Gastroenterol Nutr. 2003;37(4): 434–6.
32. Karkoszka H, Kalita B, Wiecek A, Slimok M, Sikora A, Kokot F, et al. [Influence of gluten free diet on bone mineral density (BMD) in children with celiac disease] [Clinical Trial Controlled Clinical Trial]. Przegl Lek. 2000;57(6):330–3.
33. Mora S, Barera G, Beccio S, Menni L, Proverbio MC, Bianchi C, et al. A prospective, longitudinal study of the long-term effect of treatment on bone density in children with celiac disease [Clinical Trial]. J Pediatr. 2001;139(4):516–21.
34. Mora S, Barera G, Beccio S, Proverbio MC, Weber G, Bianchi C, et al. Bone density and bone metabolism are normal after long-term gluten-free diet in young celiac patients. Am J Gastroenterol. 1999;94(2):398–403.
35. Farre C, Esteve M, Curcoy A, Cabre E, Arranz E, Amat LL, et al. Hypertransaminasemia in pediatric celiac disease patients and its prevalence as a diagnostic clue. Am J Gastroenterol. 2002;97(12):3176–81.
36. Vajro P, Paolella G, Maggiore G, Giordano G. Meta-analysis: pediatric celiac disease, cryptogenic hypertransaminasemia, and autoimmune hepatitis. J Pediatr Gastroenterol Nutr. 2013;56(6):663–70.
37. Pastore L, Carroccio A, Compilato D, Panzarella V, Serpico R, Lo Muzio L. Oral manifestations of celiac disease. J Clin Gastroenterol. 2008;42(3):224–32.
38. Wierink CD, van Diermen DE, Aartman IH, Heymans HS. Dental enamel defects in children with coeliac disease. Int J Paediatr Dent. 2007;17(3):163–8.
39. Avsar A, Kalayci AG. The presence and distribution of dental enamel defects and caries in children with celiac disease. Turk J Pediatr. 2008;50(1):45–50.
40. Acar S, Yetkiner AA, Ersin N, Oncag O, Aydogdu S, Arikan C. Oral findings and salivary parameters in children with celiac disease: a preliminary study. Med Princ Pract. 2012;21(2): 129–33.

41. Rashid M, Zarkadas M, Anca A, Limeback H. Oral manifestations of celiac disease: a clinical guide for dentists. J Mich Dent Assoc. 2011;93(10):42–6.
42. Cheng J, Malahias T, Brar P, Minaya MT, Green PH. The association between celiac disease, dental enamel defects, and aphthous ulcers in a United States cohort. J Clin Gastroenterol. 2010;44(3):191–4.
43. Martelossi S, Zanatta E, Del Santo E, Clarich P, Radovich P, Ventura A. Dental enamel defects and screening for coeliac disease. Acta Paediatr Suppl. 1996;412:47–8.
44. Campisi G, Di Liberto C, Iacono G, Compilato D, Di Prima L, Calvino F, et al. Oral pathology in untreated coeliac [corrected] disease. Aliment Pharmacol Ther. 2007;26(11–12):1529–36.
45. Shetyer E, Berson T, Lachmanovitz O, Hidas A, Wilschanski M, Menachem M, et al. Oral health status and salivary properties in relation to gluten free diet in children with celiac disease. J Pediatr Gastroenterol Nutr. 2013;57(1):49–52.
46. Zelnik N, Pacht A, Obeid R, Lerner A. Range of neurologic disorders in patients with celiac disease. Pediatrics. 2004;113(6):1672–6.
47. Batista IC, Gandolfi L, Nobrega YK, Almeida RC, Almeida LM, Campos Junior D, et al. Autism spectrum disorder and celiac disease: no evidence for a link. Arq Neuropsiquiatr. 2012;70(1):28–33.
48. Pavone L, Fiumara A, Bottaro G, Mazzone D, Coleman M. Autism and celiac disease: failure to validate the hypothesis that a link might exist. Biol Psychiatry. 1997;42(1):72–5.
49. Hill ID, Dirks MH, Liptak GS, Colletti RB, Fasano A, Guandalini S, et al. Guideline for the diagnosis and treatment of celiac disease in children: recommendations of the North American Society for Pediatric Gastroenterology, Hepatology and Nutrition [Guideline Practice Guideline]. J Pediatr Gastroenterol Nutr. 2005;40(1):1–19.
50. Elder JH, Shankar M, Shuster J, Theriaque D, Burns S, Sherrill L. The gluten-free, casein-free diet in autism: results of a preliminary double blind clinical trial [Randomized Controlled Trial Research Support, N.I.H., Extramural]. J Autism Dev Disord. 2006;36(3):413–20.
51. El-Chammas K, Danner E. Gluten-free diet in nonceliac disease [Review]. Nutr Clin Pract. 2011;26(3):294–9.
52. Giersiepen K, Lelgemann M, Stuhldreher N, Ronfani L, Husby S, Koletzko S, et al. Accuracy of diagnostic antibody tests for coeliac disease in children: summary of an evidence report [Evaluation Studies Meta-Analysis Research Support, Non-U.S. Gov't Review]. J Pediatr Gastroenterol Nutr. 2012;54(2):229–41.
53. Husby S, Koletzko S, Korponay-Szabo IR, Mearin ML, Phillips A, Shamir R, et al. European Society for Pediatric Gastroenterology, Hepatology, and Nutrition guidelines for the diagnosis of coeliac disease [Practice Guideline]. J Pediatr Gastroenterol Nutr. 2012;54(1):136–60.
54. Misak Z, Hojsak I, Jadresin O, Kekez AJ, Abdovic S, Kolacek S. Diagnosis of coeliac disease in children younger than 2 years. J Pediatr Gastroenterol Nutr. 2013;56(2):201–5.
55. Barbato M, Maiella G, Di Camillo C, Guida S, Valitutti F, Lastrucci G, et al. The anti-deamidated gliadin peptide antibodies unmask celiac disease in small children with chronic diarrhoea. Dig Liver Dis. 2011;43(6):465–9.
56. Piccini B, Vascotto M, Serracca L, Luddi A, Margollicci MA, Balestri P, et al. HLA-DQ typing in the diagnostic algorithm of celiac disease [Evaluation Studies]. Rev Esp Enferm Dig. 2012;104(5):248–54.
57. Al-Hussaini A, Sulaiman N, Al-Zahrani M, Alenizi A, El Haj I. High prevalence of celiac disease among Saudi children with type 1 diabetes: a prospective cross-sectional study [Research Support, Non-U.S. Gov't]. BMC Gastroenterol. 2012;12:180.
58. Kota SK, Meher LK, Jammula S, Modi KD. Clinical profile of coexisting conditions in type 1 diabetes mellitus patients. Diabetes Metab Syndr. 2012;6(2):70–6.
59. Aktay AN, Lee PC, Kumar V, Parton E, Wyatt DT, Werlin SL. The prevalence and clinical characteristics of celiac disease in juvenile diabetes in Wisconsin. J Pediatr Gastroenterol Nutr. 2001;33(4):462–5.
60. Volta U, Tovoli F, Caio G. Clinical and immunological features of celiac disease in patients with Type 1 diabetes mellitus [Review]. Expert Rev Gastroenterol Hepatol. 2011;5(4):479–87.

61. Franzese A, Iafusco D, Spadaro R, Cavaliere O, Prisco F, Auricchio R, et al. Potential celiac disease in type 1 diabetes: a multicenter study [Multicenter Study]. Diabetes Res Clin Pract. 2011;92(1):53–6.
62. Amin R, Murphy N, Edge J, Ahmed ML, Acerini CL, Dunger DB. A longitudinal study of the effects of a gluten-free diet on glycemic control and weight gain in subjects with type 1 diabetes and celiac disease [Comparative Study]. Diabetes Care. 2002;25(7):1117–22.
63. Hansen D, Brock-Jacobsen B, Lund E, Bjorn C, Hansen LP, Nielsen C, et al. Clinical benefit of a gluten-free diet in type 1 diabetic children with screening-detected celiac disease: a population-based screening study with 2 years' follow-up [Research Support, Non-U.S. Gov't]. Diabetes Care. 2006;29(11):2452–6.
64. Sanchez-Albisua I, Wolf J, Neu A, Geiger H, Wascher I, Stern M. Coeliac disease in children with Type 1 diabetes mellitus: the effect of the gluten-free diet. Diabet Med. 2005;22(8):1079–82.
65. Acerini CL, Ahmed ML, Ross KM, Sullivan PB, Bird G, Dunger DB. Coeliac disease in children and adolescents with IDDM: clinical characteristics and response to gluten-free diet [Research Support, Non-U.S. Gov't]. Diabet Med. 1998;15(1):38–44.
66. Bonamico M, Mariani P, Danesi HM, Crisogianni M, Failla P, Gemme G, et al. Prevalence and clinical picture of celiac disease in italian down syndrome patients: a multicenter study [Multicenter Study]. J Pediatr Gastroenterol Nutr. 2001;33(2):139–43.
67. Marild K, Stephansson O, Grahnquist L, Cnattingius S, Soderman G, Ludvigsson JF. Down syndrome is associated with elevated risk of celiac disease: a nationwide case-control study. J Pediatr. 2013;163(1):237–42.
68. Mortensen KH, Cleemann L, Hjerrild BE, Nexo E, Locht H, Jeppesen EM, et al. Increased prevalence of autoimmunity in Turner syndrome–influence of age [Research Support, Non--U.S. Gov't]. Clin Exp Immunol. 2009;156(2):205–10.
69. Dias Mdo C, Castro LC, Gandolfi L, Almeida RC, Cordoba MS, Pratesi R. Screening for celiac disease among patients with Turner syndrome in Brasilia, DF, midwest region of Brazil [Research Support, Non-U.S. Gov't]. Arq Gastroenterol. 2010;47(3):246–9.
70. Frost AR, Band MM, Conway GS. Serological screening for coeliac disease in adults with Turner's syndrome: prevalence and clinical significance of endomysium antibody positivity. Eur J Endocrinol. 2009;160(4):675–9.
71. Sagodi L, Solyom E, Tamasi K, Minik K. [Prevalence of celiac disease in Turner syndrome]. Orv Hetil. 2006;147(25):1185–8.
72. Bonamico M, Pasquino AM, Mariani P, Danesi HM, Culasso F, Mazzanti L, et al. Prevalence and clinical picture of celiac disease in Turner syndrome [Multicenter Study Research Support, Non-U.S. Gov't]. J Clin Endocrinol Metab. 2002;87(12):5495–8.
73. Ivarsson SA, Carlsson A, Bredberg A, Alm J, Aronsson S, Gustafsson J, et al. Prevalence of coeliac disease in Turner syndrome [Research Support, Non-U.S. Gov't]. Acta Paediatr. 1999;88(9):933–6.
74. Giannotti A, Tiberio G, Castro M, Virgilii F, Colistro F, Ferretti F, et al. Coeliac disease in Williams syndrome. J Med Genet. 2001;38(11):767–8.
75. Sattar N, Lazare F, Kacer M, Aguayo-Figueroa L, Desikan V, Garcia M, et al. Celiac disease in children, adolescents, and young adults with autoimmune thyroid disease [Comparative Study]. J Pediatr. 2011;158(2):272-5 e1.
76. Larizza D, Calcaterra V, De Giacomo C, De Silvestri A, Asti M, Badulli C, et al. Celiac disease in children with autoimmune thyroid disease. J Pediatr. 2001;139(5):738–40.
77. Diamanti A, Ferretti F, Guglielmi R, Panetta F, Colistro F, Cappa M, et al. Thyroid autoimmunity in children with coeliac disease: a prospective survey. Arch Dis Child. 2011;96(11):1038–41.
78. Ansaldi N, Palmas T, Corrias A, Barbato M, D'Altiglia MR, Campanozzi A, et al. Autoimmune thyroid disease and celiac disease in children [Multicenter Study]. J Pediatr Gastroenterol Nutr. 2003;37(1):63–6.
79. Cassio A, Ricci G, Baronio F, Miniaci A, Bal M, Bigucci B, et al. Long-term clinical significance of thyroid autoimmunity in children with celiac disease. J Pediatr. 2010;156(2):292–5.

80. Villalta D, Girolami D, Bidoli E, Bizzaro N, Tampoia M, Liguori M, et al. High prevalence of celiac disease in autoimmune hepatitis detected by anti-tissue tranglutaminase autoantibodies. J Clin Lab Anal. 2005;19(1):6–10.
81. Nastasio S, Sciveres M, Riva S, Filippeschi IP, Vajro P, Maggiore G. Celiac disease-associated autoimmune hepatitis in childhood: long term response to treatment. J Pediatr Gastroenterol Nutr. 2013;56(6):671–4.
82. Kurppa K, Lauronen O, Collin P, Ukkola A, Laurila K, Huhtala H, et al. Factors associated with dietary adherence in celiac disease: a nationwide study. Digestion. 2012;86(4):309–14.
83. Hogberg L, Grodzinsky E, Stenhammar L. Better dietary compliance in patients with coeliac disease diagnosed in early childhood [Research Support, Non-U.S. Gov't]. Scand J Gastroenterol. 2003;38(7):751–4.
84. Jadresin O, Misak Z, Sanja K, Sonicki Z, Zizic V. Compliance with gluten-free diet in children with coeliac disease. J Pediatr Gastroenterol Nutr. 2008;47(3):344–8.
85. Olsson C, Hornell A, Ivarsson A, Sydner YM. The everyday life of adolescent coeliacs: issues of importance for compliance with the gluten-free diet. J Hum Nutr Diet. 2008;21(4):359–67.
86. Arnone J, Fitzsimons V. Adolescents with celiac disease: a literature review of the impact developmental tasks have on adherence with a gluten-free diet [Review]. Gastroenterol Nurs. 2012;35(4):248–54.
87. Olsson C, Lyon P, Hornell A, Ivarsson A, Sydner YM. Food that makes you different: the stigma experienced by adolescents with celiac disease [Research Support, Non-U.S. Gov't]. Qual Health Res. 2009;19(7):976–84.
88. Sverker A, Hensing G, Hallert C. 'Controlled by food'-lived experiences of coeliac disease [Research Support, Non-U.S. Gov't]. J Hum Nutr Diet. 2005;18(3):171–80.
89. Wagner G, Berger G, Sinnreich U, Grylli V, Schober E, Huber WD, et al. Quality of life in adolescents with treated coeliac disease: influence of compliance and age at diagnosis [Research Support, Non-U.S. Gov't]. J Pediatr Gastroenterol Nutr. 2008;47(5):555–61.

Chapter 14
Novel and Experimental Therapies on the Horizon

Ikram Nasr, Joachim Messing, and Paul J. Ciclitira

Introduction

Celiac disease (CD) is a chronic, systemic, autoimmune disorder in genetically predisposed individuals in response to ingestion of toxic gluten. It affects approximately 1 % of the population in Europe and the United States. Gluten proteins belong to the superfamily of prolamins that have diverged among cereals and are unique to the subfamily of Pooideae that include wheat, barley, and rye. They can trigger an autoimmune injury to the gut, skin, liver, joints, uterus, and other organs [1]. Of the individuals with CD, 5–10 % may be sensitive to oats because some people have small-intestinal T cells that react to oat avenins [2]. The resultant lesion in the mucosa of the small intestine is villous atrophy with crypt hyperplasia and intraepithelial lymphocytosis. Villous atrophy is identified on small bowel biopsy, which is considered the gold standard for diagnosing this condition. False negative small bowel histology can be expected due to patchy small bowel mucosal changes [1]. Untreated CD is associated with significant mortality. Undiagnosed CD is associated with a nearly fourfold increased risk of death [3].

I. Nasr, M.D.
Gastroenterology Department, St. Thomas' Hospital, London, UK

J. Messing, Dr. rer. Nat.
Waksman Institute of Microbiology, Rutgers University, Piscataway, NJ, USA

P.J. Ciclitira, M.D. (✉)
Rayne Institute, Gastroenterology Department, St. Thomas' Hospital, Westminster Bridge Road, London SE1 7EH, UK
e-mail: paul.ciclitira@kcl.ac.uk

S.D. Rampertab and G.E. Mullin (eds.), *Celiac Disease*, Clinical Gastroenterology,
DOI 10.1007/978-1-4614-8560-5_14,

Novel Therapies for Celiac Disease

The mainstay of treatment for CD is lifelong avoidance of foods containing gluten. CD, like type 1 diabetes, rheumatoid arthritis, and multiple sclerosis, has a chronic nature where particular HLA alleles are overrepresented among the patients [4]. Most patients go into complete remission when they are put on a gluten-free diet, and they relapse when gluten is reintroduced into the diet. CD is in this respect unique among the chronic inflammatory HLA-associated diseases in that a critical environmental factor has been identified [5].

Although GFD is an effective treatment for CD, it does have its limitations. This is due to its cost, side effects including constipation and weight gain, and the difficulty to maintain a strict GFD. This results in poor dietary compliance. In addition, patients with high-level gluten sensitivity are affected by trace amounts of gluten in foods that are declared gluten-free [6]. These limitations and the insight in the pathogenesis have lead to development of new diagnostics and encouraged investigating into possible novel treatments [7]. Potential therapies involve manipulating the dietary gluten, rendering it less toxic, degrading the enzymes that process gluten, decreasing intestinal permeability, blocking the gluten by inhibiting tissue transglutaminase 2, inhibiting binding of gluten to HLA-DQ with the use of inhibitory peptides, shifting the Th1 to Th2 inflammatory response, proinflammatory cytokine inhibitors, enhancing the immune system, inducing gluten tolerance, gluten vaccines, or preventing or reversing mucosal damage in response to inflammation [8]. Despite the potential treatments that show positive results in theory or ex vivo, the effectiveness, safety, drug delivery, and cost effectiveness of the treatment in vivo need to be taken into account.

See Table 14.1 for a list of experimental therapy, mechanisms of actions, and results.

Avoidance of Toxic Dietary Gluten

Consumption of Gluten with Low Immunogenicity

Selecting products that lack toxic gluten but remain palatable and retains the baking qualities of wheat could be seen as an alternative to the commercially available gluten-free products. Wheat and grains with low immunogenicity have been studied in the management of CD. Certain wheat accessions contain low levels of T-cell stimulatory molecules. By breeding wheat species with low or absent levels of harmful gluten proteins, grains with low or no immunogenicity in celiac patients can be produced. However, a major challenge is the alpha-gliadin gene family, which varies in copy number among wheat cultivars and those that are expressed at different levels (manuscript in preparation). Previously, it has been reported that the immunodominant 33mer encoded by alpha-gliadin genes on wheat chromosome 6D

Table 14.1 Experimental therapy, mechanisms of actions, results, and citation

Experimental therapy	Mechanisms of action	Results	Citation
1. Avoidance of toxic dietary gluten			
1. Consumption of gluten with low immunogenicity	Breeding wheat species with low or absent levels of harmful gluten proteins *Triticum monoccum* and tetraploid *Triticum turgidum* pasta wheat Wheat-free sorghum products	Can achieve products with low toxicity levels Alpha-gliadin gene copy is variable which makes avoiding toxic peptides	[9–11]
2. Modified pretreated gluten	Gluten hydrolysis by lactobacilli	Good but slow fermentation and altered baking outcome	[12]
	Removing alpha-gliadin from *Triticum aestivum*	Reduced T-cell response. Compromised baking quality	[13]
	Removing omega- and gamma-gliadin and LMW-GS foci	Lower immune response. Good baking qualities	
	Genetically altering alpha2-gliadin	Eliminated T-cell response	[14]
2. Gluten detoxification			
3. Oral enzyme therapy			
1. Prolyl endopeptidases (PEP)	Degrade gluten ex vivo	Requires prolonged incubation. An immune response cannot be avoided	[15, 16]
2. Cystatins	Degradation of immunogenic T cells by cystatins in germinating wheat seeds	Good results but poor baking quality	
3. ALV003-treated wheat	Combines both germinating barley and PEP	Reduced IFN-gamma ELISpot to gliadin. No change in symptoms. Phase IIa trial	[17]
4. Probiotics	VSL#3 predigested gliadins	Reduction in zonulin release from intestinal epithelial cells	[18]
	Orally ingested IgG	Potentially good results. Phase 1 clinical trials expected	[19]

(continued)

Table 14.1 (continued)

Experimental therapy	Mechanisms of action	Results	Citation
3. Inhibition of intestinal permeability			
5. Larazotide (AT-1001)	Tight-junction regulatory peptide that inhibits the opening of tight junctions in epithelial cells in the small intestine	Well tolerated. Intestinal epithelial damage may still occur. Phase II study	[20–22]
4. Tissue transglutaminase blockade			
1. Cystamine 2. 2-[(2-oxopropyl) thio]imidazolium inhibitors (L682777 or R283)	Prevents T-cell activation by inhibition of tissue transglutaminase 2 (TG2) and subsequently interfering with gliadin binding to HLA-DQ2/DQ8	In vitro studies promising Effects in vivo are unknown	Pasternack R, Hils M, Zedira Company, Darmstadt, Germany, personal communication, September 2009
5. Th1 to Th2 shift			
1. Decapeptide from durum wheat (sequence QQPQDAVQPF)	The 10mer can inhibit the abnormal immune response triggered by gliadin	Downregulation of IFN-gamma and upregulation of IL-10 (immunomodulator) and a shift from Th1 to Th2 response	[23–26]
6. HLA-DQ groove blockade	Blocks immune activation Amino acid substitution of gliadin rendering it unable to lie within HLA molecule		[14, 27–30]
7. Proinflammatory cytokines inhibition			
1. IL-10	Suppresses Th1 cells IL-10	Works ex vivo. No effect in Crohn's patients. The advances in the field of celiac disease are limited due to the low acceptability of side effects from these drugs	[31–33]
10. Anti-IFN-gamma	IFN-gamma blockade	Prevents histologic damage to healthy mucosa in celiac patients. Disappointing results in Crohn's disease phase I/II trials	[34–37]

(continued)

Table 14.1 (continued)

Experimental therapy	Mechanisms of action	Results	Citation
11. IL-15 inhibitor	Inhibiting the inflammatory response to IL-15	Promising in celiac disease. HuMax-IL-15 has acceptable side effects in rheumatoid arthritis	[38, 39]
12. Anti-TNF-alpha	Management of refractory celiac disease	Small study group. Slow mucosal recovery	[40, 41]
8. Induction of gluten tolerance			
1. Intranasal administration of gliadin peptides in transgenic DQ8 mice	Induction of immune tolerance to gluten and prevents the immune-mediated response to gluten	Lowering T-cell proliferation and the immune response to gliadin The response may be variable in individual patients	[42–44]
9. Gluten peptide vaccine	Gluten vaccination containing three select immunogenic 16mer peptides derived from alpha-gliadin, omega-gliadin, and hordein and injected subcutaneously in transgenic mice	Suppression of CD4 T-cell proliferation and IL-2 and IFN-gamma production and increased the expression of T-reg by splenic CD4 cells in response to a gluten challenge	[45]
10. Pathogenic CD4+ Th cells inhibition	Gliadin-specific Tr1 cell clones suppressed proliferation of pathogenic Th0 cells	Numbers of Tr1 not enough to offer a therapeutic option	[46]
11. Anti-adhesion therapy			
1. Integrin-a4 antagonist: Natalizumab Alemtuzumab AJM300 15. Integrin-a4b7 Vedolizumab (MLN02) Etrolizumab	Inhibit leukocyte adhesion to intestinal mucosa and prevent the migration of leukocytes into inflamed tissue	Not studied in celiac disease. Some have conflicting efficacy data. Large cohort studies are required to conclude the potential safety and efficacy of these drugs in celiac disease	[47–56]
Intestino-trophic mitogens	R-spondin 1 (Rspo1) stimulates the growth of small and large bowel mucosa	Stimulate growth of crypt cells in mouse models of colitis and resort intestinal architecture. No human studies	

is absent in the diploid einkorn, also known as *Triticum monoccum* (gene AA), and the tetraploid *Triticum turgidum* (gene AABB) pasta wheat [9]. On the other hand, hexaploid wheat is needed for bread making. Still, there is a reduction in toxicity observed in vitro with two varieties of bread wheat, one poor in alpha- and beta-gliadins and the other poor in alpha-, beta-, gamma-, and omega-gliadins, which have been tested [10]. Sorghum is a grain that is closely related to maize. Wheat-free sorghum products are safe and palatable in individuals with CD [11].

Modified or Pretreated Gluten

Certain lactobacilli added to sourdough for fermentation hydrolyze the gluten peptide and render them less immunotoxic. This process requires prolonged fermentation, resulting in alteration in the size of the dough, so less fermentation time and mixing with 30 % fermented wheat flour was necessary for better baking results as demonstrated in one study [12]. Patients were challenged for 2 days in this pilot study so long-term safety of this method remains unknown.

Removing alpha-gliadin from *Triticum aestivum* (Chinese Spring) present in chromosome 6 of D-genome (6DS) led to a significant reduction in T-cell stimulatory epitopes but compromised the baking quality of bread. Genetically deleting omega-gliadin, gamma-gliadin, and LMW-GS loci from the short arm of chromosome 1 of the D-genome (1DS) produced a lowering of the immune response to exposure to the wheat with the added benefit of retaining the baking qualities [13]. Another method of detoxifying gluten involves genetically altering the alpha2-gliadin residue by replacing antigenic amino acids with alanine residue, leading to elimination of the T-cell activity [14].

Gluten Detoxification

Oral Enzyme Therapy

Proline residues in some gliadin peptides are resistant to enzymatic degradations in the digestive system leaving them available for abnormal immune response in celiac patients. Enzymatic degradation of this gluten with prolyl endopeptidases (PEP) prevents these peptides from reaching the lamina propria and allows the smaller substrates to be processed by the intestinal brush border enzymes. Microorganisms such as *Flavobacterium meningosepticum*, *Sphingomonas capsulata*, and *Myxococcus xanthus* are able to cleave the immunodominant proline-rich regions [6]. Pyle et al. demonstrated the benefit of PEP in a study when a 2-week gluten challenge with PEP showed no evidence of malabsorption of celiac antibodies [15]. In another study, PEP was reported to require 3 h incubation with the protein in order to degrade it and prevent gluten-related toxicity. This concludes that the ingestion of PEP with diet is unlikely to avoid immune response to gluten [15].

In germinating wheat seeds, gliadin is under the control of intrinsic cystatins. This protease can degrade immunogenic T cell, making it possible to create flour based on germinating wheat safe for celiac individuals but with compromised baking quality.

ALV003 is a mixture of two glutenases, an endoprotease that has the advantage of combining both germinating barley and PEP. Tye-Din et al. tested ALV003-treated wheat flour on celiac patients [17]. The group found no change in symptoms experienced by patients but a reduced IFN-g ELISpot to gliadin in patients consuming the treated flour compared to placebo controls. Further work will help to evaluate the value of this, and a phase IIa trial is currently recruiting in Finland to assess the safety and efficiency of ALV003 in a larger cohort of celiac patients (NCT1255696).

Probiotics

De Angelis et al. showed that VSL#3 predigested gliadins caused a less pronounced reorganization of the intracellular F-actin, which was mirrored by an attenuated effect on intestinal mucosa permeability. The release of zonulin from intestinal epithelial cells treated with gliadins was considerably lower when digested with VSL#3 [18].

Orally ingested IgG is highly resistant to gastric acidity, and approximately 50 % of neutralizing activity survives when reaching the terminal ileum [19]. In view of the low cost and ease of production of cow's milk antibodies, large-scale production of neutralizing gluten antibodies is potentially easy, safe to use, and cost effective. A clinical phase I trial in the USA is expected [6].

Inhibition of Intestinal Permeability

An important factor contributing to the influx of gluten to the lamina propria is increased intestinal permeability through open epithelial tight junctions. Gluten activates zonulin signaling in tight junctions between epithelial cells of patients with CD, leading to increased intestinal permeability to macromolecules. Larazotide (AT-1001) is an oral tight-junction regulatory peptide that acts locally to inhibit the opening of tight junctions in epithelial cells in the small intestine. The treatment appears to be well tolerated, but it does not prevent small-intestinal epithelial damage upon exposure to gluten [20, 21]. The primary end point of the phase II study on AT1001 has not been reached, and conclusions from other phase I and II studies on the clinical trial register have been performed and are not yet available (NCT362856, NCT492960, NCT 620451, NCT 889473) [22].

Tissue Transglutaminase Blockade

Tissue transglutaminase 2 (TG2) stimulates the process of gliadin binding to HLA-DQ2/DQ8 leading to T-cell activation. TG2 inhibition could possibly prevent the selective deamidation of gluten peptides and blocking the binding to the HLA molecules and preventing or reversing the process of T-cell activation and cell damage [5, 6].

Preclinical tests in vitro on small-intestinal samples from a celiac patient demonstrated inhibition of TG2 by cystamine, a competitive inhibitor, and 2-[(2-oxopropyl) thio]imidazolium inhibitors (L682777 or R283). The consequences of TG2 inhibitors in vivo and the effect of inhibiting all transglutaminase action are unknown [6]. Pasternak et al. demonstrated that TG inhibitors based on a high-affinity thiol binding group displayed a very high specificity for TG2 in vitro, which is very promising [6] (Pasternack R, Hils M, Zedira Company, Darmstadt, Germany, personal communication, September 2009).

Th1 to Th2 Shift

In CD, dietary gluten triggers Th1-type immune response leading to enteropathy. A decapeptide (sequence QQPQDAVQPF) isolated from durum wheat prevents the activation of peripheral lymphocytes in CD. This 10mer is isolated by affinity chromatography and gel filtration from alcohol-soluble protein fraction of durum wheat [23, 24]. Silano et al. [25] demonstrated the antagonist effect of this decamer and its ability to inhibit the abnormal immune response triggered by gliadin. The intestinal T lymphocytes derived from eight children with CD were incubated with deamidated gliadin peptide alone and simultaneously with the 10mer. The results revealed that the incubation of celiac intestinal T cells with deamidated gliadin peptides resulted in a significant increase in cell proliferation and IFN-gamma release. The 10mer caused a downregulation of IFN-gamma and upregulation of IL-10, which has an immunomodulatory role, leading to a shift from Th1 to Th2 lymphocyte response [26].

HLA-DQ Groove Blockade

Inhibitors of HLA-DQ2 that present gliadin peptides have been studied to prevent the activation of the inflammatory cascade in CD following exposure to toxic gluten. Attempts to block immune activation were investigated in other immune-mediated conditions such as rheumatoid arthritis, multiple sclerosis, and type 1 diabetes mellitus. Part of the reason for the lack of success in these experiments was achieving effective drug delivery [27, 28]. However, in CD the DQ2 inhibitor will need to reach the small intestine directly via the oral route either before or with gluten ingestion.

Amino acid substitution of gliadin can convert the epitope to an agonist or antagonist and affects in turn the inflammatory process [29]. Alanine amino acid substitution at key positions (3, 8, and 10) in the immunodominant peptide in residues 62–75 of a-2-gliadin in wheat abolishes the immunogenicity of the peptide when tested against T-cell clones [14]. Thc ncutral alanine amino acid present in the peptide affected the capability of the peptide itself to lie within the cleft of the HLA-DQ molecules. Anderson et al. substituted an alanine or lysine amino acid in the immunodominant a-gliadin peptide sequence p57–73 QE65. The substitution to the gliadin peptides could abolish their capacity to stimulate IFN-g production from CD4 T cells and also have anti-inflammatory or protective effects in HLA-DQ2+ CD [30].

Proinflammatory Cytokines Inhibition

Various cytokine therapies are being developed for chronic inflammatory conditions. The advances in the field of CD are limited due to the low acceptability of side effects from these drugs.

IL-10 from regulatory T cells suppresses Th1 cells and likely acts as a mildly counter-regulatory cytokine [31]. IL-10 ex vivo suppresses gluten-dependent T-cell activation in cultured celiac small-intestinal mucosa [32]. But another study tested recombinant IL-10 in Crohn's disease was discontinued due to lack of effect [33].

In CD, the main cytokine produced by the gliadin-specific T-cell clones is IFN-gamma [34]. IFN-g blocking antibody can prevent histologic damage to healthy mucosa in celiac patients [35]. Studies in Crohn's disease revealed disappointing results of phase I/II trials. The drop in Crohn's disease activity index (CDAI) in a small cohort did not reach statistical significance due to an unusually high drop in CDAI in the placebo group [36]. Whereas Reinisch et al. found in a larger cohort of Crohn's disease patients, there was a significant decrease in CRP levels. However, this failed to translate into a clinical response [37]. Such studies may encourage research on testing anti-TNF in CD based on the studies undertaken so far in other inflammatory conditions.

Interleukin-15 (IL-15) is a key proinflammatory, innate response cytokine that plays an important role in several autoimmune diseases. IL-15 inhibitors could be used as a promising therapeutic strategy in CD. Baslund et al. demonstrated that HuMax-IL-15, which is a human IgG1 anti-IL-15 monoclonal antibody, had acceptable side effects in rheumatoid arthritis [38]. Another study investigated the effects of treatment with an IL-15 antagonist (CRB-15) that decreased the incidence and severity of collagen-induced arthritis [39]. More studies need to be conducted to observe the effects in CD in clinical practice.

Anti-TNF-a treatment has been instigated in studies on treatment of refractory CD [40]. Reports demonstrate slow mucosal recovery following treatment with regular anti-TNF-a infusions at 8 weekly intervals [41], or a single dose TNF-a followed by azathioprine maintenance [40]. These studies were on a small group with selection bias so more studies need to be undertaken for accurate conclusions to be drawn.

Induction of Gluten Tolerance

CD is an immune-mediated response to ingested gluten. Induction of immune tolerance to gluten, if successful, could prevent this process from occurring. Intranasal administration of gliadin peptides in transgenic DQ8 mice resulted in lowering the T-cell proliferative response to gliadin and dampening of the inflammatory cascade [42–44]. However, there could be enormous variation in the response by individual patients, making this approach less robust.

Gluten Peptide Vaccine

Another strategy used a gluten vaccination containing three select immunogenic 16mer peptides derived from alpha-gliadin, omega-gliadin, and hordein that account for 60 % of the overall gluten T-cell response. The vaccination was given subcutaneously to gliadin-specific TCR/DQ2 transgenic mice. The result was a suppression of CD4 T-cell proliferation and IL-2 and IFN-g production and increased the expression of T-reg by splenic CD4 cells in response to a gluten challenge. Tye-Din et al. [45] demonstrated that the same 16mer peptides are recognized by the majority of HLA-DQ2-positive, gluten-positive peripheral blood T cells. A patented vaccine continuing the 16mer has finished recruiting for a phase I clinical trial. HLA-DQ8, on the other hand, has a different immunodominant epitope and will not respond to the vaccine. In addition, as the innate immune system plays a role in activating the immune system, celiac patients have different response to the same antigen stimulus [45].

Pathogenic CD4+ Th Cells Inhibition

Gliadin-specific type 1 regulatory T (Tr1) cells are found in the intestinal mucosa of individuals with CD. Gianfrani et al. [46] reported that gliadin-specific Tr1 cell clones suppressed proliferation of pathogenic Th0 cells. Methods to boost the numbers of Tr1 to offer a therapeutic measure need to be sought.

Anti-adhesion Therapy

Chronic inflammatory diseases exhibit leukocyte migration and retention. Adhesion molecules regulate the influx of leukocytes in normal and inflamed gut, local lymphocyte stimulation, and antigen presentation in intestinal mucosal cells. MadCAM-1 is an adhesion molecule specific to the gut. In inflammatory bowel disease (IBD), most of the adhesion molecules are upregulated in inflammatory bowel disease [47]. Inhibiting leukocyte adhesion will prevent the migration of leukocytes into inflamed tissue, which could be a promising treatment for CD. These inhibitory molecules are being studied in IBD so far. There are two humanized antibodies under evaluation for IBD. The first is INTEGRIN-a4 antagonist and includes natalizumab, which is an antibody used in multiple sclerosis and IBD [48, 49], and alemtuzumab, which has been studied in the treatment of refractory CD with conflicting efficacy data [50]. A trail in IBD patients failing anti-TNF-a treatment reported improvement with natalizumab infusion (clinical trial NCT00801125). However, Ananthakrishnan et al. [51] demonstrated that in patients with moderate to severe CD failing two TNF-antagonists, using a third TNF-antagonist therapy appears to be a cost-effective strategy compared to using natalizumab as a third-line therapy without significantly compromising treatment efficacy. Natalizumab is associated with 0.1 % risk of developing progressive multifocal leukoencephalopathy (PML) [52].

AJM300, which is an orally active small molecule, also antagonizes INTEGRIN-a4. Studies in a small cohort of Crohn's disease patients demonstrated reduction in CDAI but no difference compared to placebo [53].

The second humanized antibody targets the adhesion molecule INTEGRIN-a4b7 expressed by gut T cells. Molecules in this group include vedolizumab (MLN02), which demonstrated in phase II trials the capacity to induce remission in ulcerative colitis [54, 55], and etrolizumab, which appears to be well tolerated in moderate to severe ulcerative colitis, but phase II studies are warranted to observe clinical improvement [56].

Overall, large cohort studies are required to conclude the potential safety and efficacy of these drugs in CD.

Intestinotrophic Mitogens

Intestinotrophic mitogens prevent intestinal damage. R-spondin 1 (Rspo1) is a novel epithelial mitogen that stimulates the growth of small and large bowel mucosa. Zhao et al. [57] demonstrated in mouse models of colitis that Rspo1 is able to stimulate the growth of crypt cells, which will hasten mucosal regeneration. This in turn restores the intestinal architecture. The effect of Rspo1 in humans is unknown and studies are yet to be conducted.

Conclusion

While there have been a number of new approaches developed over the years to prevent the onset of the disease in CD patients, they do not have reached a level that would permit abolishing a gluten-free diet for them. Furthermore, most studies rely on the use of synthetic peptides to analyze the immune response rather than intact proteins to predict what is toxic or not. A new approach is therefore needed where intact proteins can be tested in the future.

References

1. Rewers MJ. Epidemiology of celiac disease: what are the prevalence, incidence, and progression of celiac disease? Bethesda, MD: National Institutes of Health; 2004.
2. Lundin KE, Nilsen EM, Scott HG, Løberg EM, Gjøen A, Bratlie J, et al. Oats induced villous atrophy in celiac disease. Gut. 2003;52:1649–52.
3. Rubio-Tapia A, Kyle RA, Kaplan EL, Johnson DR, Page W, Erdtmann F, et al. Increased prevalence and mortality in undiagnosed celiac disease. Gastroenterology. 2009;137(1):88–93.
4. Thorsby E. Invited anniversary review: HLA associated diseases. Hum Immunol. 1997;53:1–11.
5. Sollid LM. Molecular basis of celiac disease. Annu Rev Immunol. 2000;18:53–81.
6. Schuppan D, Junker Y, Barisani D. Celiac disease: from pathogenesis to novel therapies. Gastroenterology. 2009;137:1912–33.
7. Sollid LM, Lundin KE. Diagnosis and treatment of celiac disease. Mucosal Immunol. 2009;2:3–7.
8. Lerner A. New therapeutic strategies for celiac disease. Autoimmun Rev. 2010;9(3):144–7.
9. Molberg O, Uhlen AK, Jensen T, Flaete NS, Fleckenstein B, Arentz-Hansen H, et al. Mapping of gluten T-cell epitopes in the bread wheat ancestors: implications for celiac disease. Gastroenterology. 2005;128(2):393–401.
10. Frisoni M, Corazza GR, Lafiandra D, De Ambrogio E, Filipponi C, Bonvicini F, et al. Wheat deficient in gliadins: promising tool for treatment of celiac disease. Gut. 1995;36:375–8.
11. Ciacci C, Maiuri L, Caporaso N, Bucci C, Del Giudice L, Rita Massardo D, et al. Celiac disease: in vitro and in vivo safety and palatability of wheat-free sorghum food products. Clin Nutr. 2007;26:799–805.
12. Di Cagno R, De Angelis M, Lavermicocca P, De Vincenzi M, Giovannini C, Faccia M, et al. Proteolysis by sourdough lactic acid bacteria: effects on wheat flour protein fractions and gliadin peptides involved in human cereal intolerance. Appl Environ Microbiol. 2002;68:623–33.
13. van den Broeck HC, van Herpen TW, Schuit C, Salentijn EM, Dekking L, Bosch D, et al. Removing celiac disease-related gluten proteins from bread wheat while retaining technological properties: a study with Chinese Spring deletion lines. BMC Plant Biol. 2009;9:41.
14. Ellis HJ, Pollock EL, Engel W, Fraser JS, Rosen-Bronson S, Wieser H, et al. Investigation of the putative immunodominant T cell epitopes in celiac disease. Gut. 2003;52:212–17.
15. Pyle GC, Paaso B, Anderson BE, Allen DD, Marti T, Li Q, et al. Effect of pre-treatment of food gluten with prolyl endopeptidase on gluten-induced malabsorption in celiac sprue. Cell Mol Life Sci. 2007;64:345–55.
16. Matysiak-Budnik T, Candalh C, Cellier C, Dugave C, Namane A, Vidal-Martinez T, et al. Limited efficiency of prolyl-endopeptidase in the detoxification of gliadin peptides in celiac disease. Gastroenterology. 2005;129:786–96.

17. Tye-Din JA, Anderson RP, French RA, Brown GJ, Hodsman P, Siegel M, et al. The effects of ALV003 pre-digestion of gluten on immune response and symptoms in celiac disease in vivo. Clin Immunol. 2010;134:289–95.
18. De Angelis M, Rizzello CG, Fasano A, Clemente MG, De Simone C, Silano M, et al. VSL#3 probiotic preparation has the capacity to hydrolyse gliadin polypeptides responsible for celiac sprue. Biochim Biophys Acta. 2006;1762:80–93.
19. Warny M, Fatimi A, Bostwick EF, Laine DC, Lebel F, LaMont JT, et al. Bovine immunoglobulin concentrate-clostridium difficile retains C difficile toxin neutralizing activity after passage through the human stomach and small intestine. Gut. 1999;44:212–17.
20. Paterson BM, Lammers KM, Arrienta MC, Fasano A, Meddings JB. The safety, tolerance, pharmacokinetic and pharmacodynamic effects of single doses of AT-1001 in celiac disease subjects: a proof of concept study. Aliment Pharmacol Ther. 2007;26:757–66.
21. Kelly CP, Green PH, Murray JA, et al. Intestinal permeability of larazotide acetate in celiac disease: results of a phase IIB 6-week gluten-challenge clinical trial (abstr). Gastroenterology. 2009;136 Suppl 1:M2048.
22. Donnelly SC, Ellis HJ, Ciclitira PJ. Pharmacotherapy and management strategies for celiac disease. Expert Opin Pharmacother. 2011;12(11):1731–44.
23. De Vincenzi M, Gasbarrini G, Silano V. A small peptide from durum wheat gliadin prevents cell agglutination induced by prolamin-peptides toxic in celiac disease. Toxicology. 1997;120:207–13.
24. De Vincenzi M, Luchetti R, Giovannini C, Pogna NE, Saponaro C, Galterio G, et al. In vitro toxicity testing of alcohol-soluble proteins from diploid wheat Triticum monococcum in celiac disease. Biochem Toxicol. 1996;11:313–8.
25. Silano M, Di Benedetto R, Maialetti F, De Vincenzi A, Calcaterra R, Trecca A, et al. A 10-residue peptide from durum wheat promotes a shift from a Th1-type response toward a Th2-type response in celiac disease. Am J Clin Nutr. 2008;87(2):415–23.
26. Silano M, Di Benedetto R, Trecca A, Arrabito G, Leonardi F, De Vincenzi M. A decapeptide from durum wheat prevents celiac peripheral blood lymphocytes from activation by gliadin peptides. Pediatr Res. 2007;61:67–71.
27. Falcioni F, Ito K, Vidovic D, Belunis C, Campbell R, Berthel SJ, et al. Peptidomimetic compounds that inhibit antigen presentation by autoimmune disease-associated class II major histocompatibility molecules. Nat Biotechnol. 1999;17:562–7.
28. Ishioka GY, Adorini L, Guery JC, Gaeta FC, LaFond R, Alexander J, et al. Failure to demonstrate long-lived MHC saturation both in vitro and in vivo. Implications for therapeutic potential of MHC-blocking peptides. J Immunol. 1994;152:4310–19.
29. Silano M, Vincentini O, Iapello A, Mancini E, De Vincenzi M. Antagonist peptides of the gliadin T-cell stimulatory sequences: a therapeutic strategy for celiac disease. J Clin Gastroenterol. 2008;42(Suppl 3 Pt 2):S191–2.
30. Anderson RP, van Heel DA, Tye-Din JA, Jewell DP, Hill AV, et al. Antagonists and non toxic variants of the dominant wheat gliadin T cell epitope in celiac disease. Gut. 2006;55:485–91.
31. Forsberg G, Hernell O, Melgar S, Israelsson A, Hammarström S, Hammarström ML. Paradoxical coexpression of proinflammatory and down-regulatory cytokines in intestinal T cells in childhood celiac disease. Gastroenterology. 2002;123:667–78.
32. Salvati VM, Mazzarella G, Gianfrani C, Levings MK, Stefanile R, De Giulio B, et al. Recombinant human IL-10 suppresses gliadin dependant T-cell activation in ex vivo cultured celiac intestinal mucosa. Gut. 2005;54:46–53.
33. Colombel JF, Rutgeerts P, Malchow H, Jacyna M, Nielsen OH, Rask-Madsen J, et al. Interleukin-10 (Tenovil) in the prevention of postoperative recurrence of Crohn's disease. Gut. 2001;49:42–6.
34. Nissen EM, Lundin KE, Krajci P, Scott H, Sollid LM, Brandtzaeg P. Gluten specific, HLA-DQ restricted T cells from celiac mucosa produce cytokines with Th1 or Th0 profile dominated by interferon gamma. Gut. 1995;37:766–76.

35. Przemioslo RT, Lundin KE, Sollid LM, Nelufer J, Ciclitira PJ. Histological changes in small bowel mucosa induced by gliadin sensitive T lymphocytes can be blocked by anti-interferon gamma antibody. Gut. 1995;36:874–9.
36. Hommes DW, Mikhajlova TL, Stoinov S, Stimac D, Vucelic B, Lonovics J, et al. Fontolizumab, a humanised anti-interferon gamma antibody, demonstrates safety and clinical activity in patients with moderate to severe Crohn's disease. Gut. 2006;55:1131–7.
37. Reinisch W, de Villiers W, Bene L, Simon L, Rácz I, Katz S, et al. Fontolizumab in moderate to severe Crohn's disease: a phase 2, randomized, double-blind, placebo-controlled, multiple-dose study. Inflamm Bowel Dis. 2010;16:233–42.
38. Baslund B, Tvede N, Danneskiold-Samsoe B, Larsson P, Panayi G, Petersen J, et al. Targeting interleukin-15 in patients with rheumatoid arthritis: a proof-of-concept study. Arthritis Rheum. 2005;52:2686–92.
39. Ferrari-Lacraz S, Zanelli E, Neuberg M, Donskoy E, Kim YS, Zheng XX, et al. Targeting IL-15 receptor-bearing cells with an antagonist mutant IL-15/Fc protein prevents disease development and progression in murine collagen-induced arthritis. J Immunol. 2004;173:5818–26.
40. Gillet HR, Arnot ID, McIntyre M, Campbell S, Dahele A, Priest M, et al. Successful infliximab treatment for steroid-refractory celiac disease: a case report. Gastroenterology. 2002;122:800–5.
41. Costantino G, della Torre A, Lo Presti MA, Caruso R, Mazzon E, Fries W. Treatment of life-threatening type 1 refractory celiac disease with long-term infliximab. Dig Liver Dis. 2008;40:74–7.
42. Maurano F, Siciliano RA, De Giulio B, Luongo D, Mazzeo MF, Troncone R, et al. Intranasal administration of one alpha gliadin can downregulate the immune response to whole gliadin in mice. Scand J Immunol. 2001;53:290–5.
43. Rossi M, Maurano F, Caputo N, Auricchio S, Sette A, Capparelli R, et al. Intravenous or intranasal administration of gliadin is able to down-regulate the specific immune response in mice. Scand J Immunol. 1999;50:177–82.
44. Senger S, Luongo D, Maurano F, Mazzeo MF, Siciliano RA, Gianfrani C, et al. Intranasal administration of a recombinant alpha-gliadin down-regulates the immune response to wheat gliadin in DQ8 transgenic mice. Immunol Lett. 2003;88:127–34.
45. Tye-Din JA, Stewart JA, Dromey JA, Beissbarth T, van Heel DA, Tatham A, et al. Comprehensive, quantitative mapping of T cell epitopes in gluten in celiac disease. Sci Transl Med. 2010;2:41ra51.
46. Gianfranci C, Levings MK, Sartirana C, Mazzarella G, Barba G, Zanzi D, et al. Gliadin-specific type 1 regulatory cells from the intestinal mucosa of treated celiac patients inhibit pathogenic T cells. J Immunol. 2006;177:4178–86.
47. Van Assche G, Rutgeerts P. Antiadhesion molecule therapy in inflammatory bowel disease. Inflamm Bowel Dis. 2002;8(4):291–300.
48. Arulanandam T. Biological characteristics of anti-alpha4 integrin monoclonal antibody (natalizumab) a selective adhesion molecule (SAM) inhibitor for the treatment of multiple sclerosis and Crohn's disease [SA23]. Inflamm Res. 2004;53:3.
49. Ghosh S, Panaccione R. Anti-adhesion molecule therapy for inflammatory bowel disease. Ther Adv Gastroenterol. 2010;3:239–58.
50. Verbeek WH, Mulder CJ, Zweegman S. Alemtuzumab for refractory celiac disease. N Engl J Med. 2006;355:1396–7.
51. Ananthakrishnan AN, Hur C, Korzenik JR. Certolizumab pegol compared to natalizumab in patients with moderate to severe Crohn's disease: results of a decision analysis. Dig Dis Sci. 2012 Feb;57(2):472–80.
52. Ransohoff RM. Natalizumab and PML. Nat Neurosci. 2005;8:1275.
53. Takazoe M, Watanabe M, Kawaguchi T, et al. Oral alpha-4 integrin inhibitor (AJM300) in patients with active Crohn's disease: a randomised double-blind, placebo-controlled trial. Gastroenterology. 2009;136(Suppl):S1066.

54. Behm BW, Bickston SJ. Humanized antibody to the alpha4beta7 integrin for induction of remission in ulcerative colitis. Cochrane Database Syst Rev. 2009;1, CD007571. doi:10.1002/14651858.CD007571.
55. Feagan BG, Greenberg GR, Wild G, Fedorak RN, Paré P, McDonald JW, et al. Treatment of ulcerative colitis with a humanized antibody to the alpha4beta7 integrin. N Engl J Med. 2005;352:2499–507.
56. Rutgeerts PJ, Fedorak RN, Hommes DW, Sturm A, Baumgart DC, Bressler B, et al. A randomised phase I study of etrolizumab (rhuMAb β7) in moderate to severe ulcerative colitis. Gut. 2012;61:918–32.
57. Zhao J, de Vera J, Narushima S, Beck EX, Palencia S, Shinkawa P, et al. R-spondin1, a novel intestinotropic mitogen, ameliorates experimental colitis in mice. Gastroenterology. 2007;132:1331–43.

Chapter 15
Morbidity and Mortality Associated with Celiac Disease

Nina Ruth Lewis and Geoffrey K.T. Holmes

Introduction

Previously regarded as a rare disorder, it is now appreciated that celiac disease (CD) is a common healthcare problem affecting 1 % of the general population [1]. Recent and population-based studies have provided more robust estimates of risks traditionally associated with clinically diagnosed CD. They have also begun to explore morbidity and mortality associated with undetected CD. Some of these studies have also demonstrated other morbidity factors and, indeed, some benefits from having CD, such as reduced risk of breast cancer in female celiac patients [2–8] and lower total cholesterol [1–9] in comparison to the general population.

Before the morbidity and mortality associated with CD can be described, the limitations of the studies on which this review is based need to be acknowledged. Firstly, the distinction between clinically diagnosed and undetected CD needs to be reiterated. Despite the development of highly sensitive and specific serological tests allowing noninvasive and large-scale screening of the general population to identify individuals with CD [10, 11], an increased awareness of the condition, and an active case-finding strategy adopted by some centers, there remains a substantial gap between the number of adults with clinically diagnosed CD to those with undetected CD (ratio of undetected CD to diagnosed disease is approximately 8:1 at present in England [12, 13] and 3:1 in Finland [14, 15]). Other than a few population-based screening studies [1, 16–20], reported morbidity and mortality associated

N.R. Lewis, B.Med. Sci, B.M.B.S., M.R.C.P., M.Sc., Ph.D.
Nottingham Digestive Diseases Centre, Queen's Medical Centre, Nottingham University Hospital, Nottingham, Nottinghamshire, UK

G.K.T. Holmes, M.D., Ph.D., F.R.C.P. (✉)
Department of Gastroenterology, Royal Derby Hospital, Uttoxeter Road, Derby, Derbyshire DE22 3NE, UK

25 Whitaker Road, Derby, Derbyshire DE23 6AQ, UK
e-mail: geoffreyholmes@compuserve.com

S.D. Rampertab and G.E. Mullin (eds.), *Celiac Disease*, Clinical Gastroenterology,
DOI 10.1007/978-1-4614-8560-5_15,

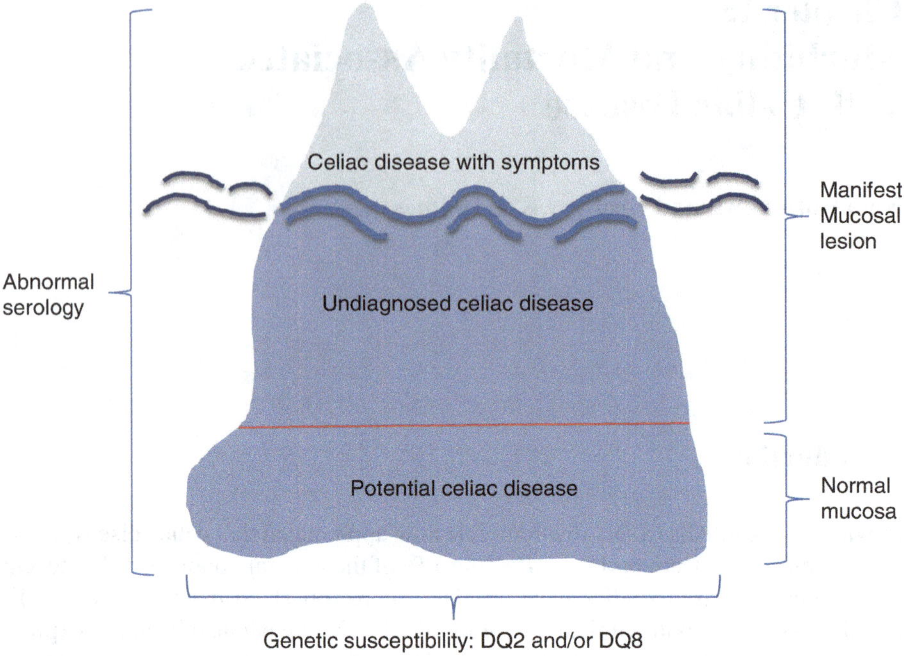

Fig. 15.1 The celiac iceberg. For each patient with CD diagnosed on clinical grounds, there are many others that remain undiagnosed, shown by the submerged part of the iceberg, because of an atypical presentation, lack of symptoms, or the potential stage of the disease

with CD in the literature is based on clinically diagnosed disease that only accounts for the minority or tip of the celiac iceberg [21] (Fig. 15.1). Population-based screening studies are beginning to explore [1, 16–20], but it remains unknown whether people with undetected CD lying below the waterline of the celiac iceberg and accounting for the majority of cases of the condition share similar risks of morbidity to that of clinically diagnosed CD. The population-based screening studies [1, 16–20] are limited because of misclassification bias, relying on the performance of the serological test to define undetected CD. They also lack information on whether any of the participants were diagnosed on clinical grounds with CD and therefore received treatment after serum was submitted for serological testing. Secondly, because CD is so common, it follows that many diseases will occur in association. For the purposes of this review, some of the morbidities will be regarded as complications of CD. Others will be regarded as associations or simply as occurring by chance.

Further limitations to the published studies include:

- Selection biases such as choice and nature of population studied, continued participation in the study, and nonparticipation in the study

- Information biases such as recall of events, collection of data by the study investigators, and measurement of outcomes of interest
- Ascertainment biases such as incidental detection of CD while undergoing tests for another condition and vice versa
- Confounding such as absence of smoking data or treatment with adherence to a gluten-free diet and CD morbidity

Are Celiac Pathogenic Factors Implicated in the Morbidity?

The mechanisms of the intestinal immune-mediated response in CD are not completely clear, but the pathogenesis is thought to involve a complex interplay of immunological factors including tissue transglutaminase (TTG), intraepithelial lymphocytes, cytotoxic T cells, adaptive and innate immune responses, and autoimmunity [22–24]. Such pathogenic factors may predispose celiacs to developing other conditions. Autoantibodies directed against tissue transglutaminase are present in the liver and other extraintestinal tissues such as the thyroid in CD, raising the possibility of a pathogenic role for the humoral-mediated immune responses in the hepatocyte and thyroid injuries observed [25, 26]. Increased intestinal permeability [27] resulting from the intestinal immune-mediated response to gluten may facilitate the entrance of toxins, antigens, and proinflammatory mediators such as interleukins and gamma interferon into the circulation with subsequent tissue insult, which may be of importance in provoking autoimmune disorders and lymphoma.

There may be a shared immunogenetic susceptibility to developing immune dysregulation [28–31]. For example, IDDM1 candidate allelic loci identified for type 1 diabetes located on chromosome 6q21 is found at the exact same position as loci for CD (marker HLA-DQ2) [32]. TTG is ubiquitously expressed and may be critical in other autoimmune diseases, including type 1 diabetes, because it may be expressed within islets [23]. Posttranslational modification of exogenous antigen by an endogenous enzyme may be the link to antienzyme or anti-modified autoantigen antibodies found in several autoimmune diseases such as antibodies to deamidated gliadin in CD [33], citrullinated antigens in rheumatoid arthritis [34, 35], and GAD65 in type 1 diabetes [36]. Monoclonal intraepithelial lymphocytes are implicated in the development of enteropathy-associated T-cell lymphoma and ulcerative jejunitis [37].

Autoimmune Diseases

Recent studies have demonstrated an increased prevalence of CD in some autoimmune disorders including type 1 diabetes, thyroid, and liver disorders.

Diabetes Mellitus

Type 1 diabetes mellitus is the most common and best researched association and precedes the diagnosis of CD in about 90 % of patients [38]. Screening studies have shown that the prevalence among children is about 4.5 % (26 studies) [39], but higher figures of 12.3 % [40] and 10 % [41] have been reported. In adults the prevalence is approximately 3.5 % (eight studies) [38]. Before the age of 20 years, those with established CD have a two- to threefold increased risk of developing type 1 diabetes [42]. It is not surprising that these disorders are associated because both are linked not only to the major compatibility complex class II antigen DQ2 encoded by the alleles DQA1*501 and DQB1*201 but also to the non-HLA loci RGS1, IL18RAP, and TAGAP on chromosomes 1q31, 2q12, and 6q25, respectively [43]. In addition, it has been demonstrated that some children with diabetes have anti-tissue transglutaminase antibodies in the small intestinal mucosa, suggesting that these patients are sensitive to gluten [44]. These findings raise the intriguing possibility that dietary antigens might be of etiological importance in both conditions.

In reports there is divergence in the number of patients with symptoms and signs which probably reflects how carefully these were sought [38]. More recent studies illustrate this point. Of 33 children with diabetes and CD, all interviewed by a doctor, 28 (85 %) had symptoms or biochemical features of CD and in four, the symptoms were only recognized retrospectively after the introduction of a gluten-free diet [40]. In other studies, 13 of 17 children (76 %) had gastrointestinal symptoms [45] and 18 of 68 (26 %) had symptoms including growth retardation, weight loss, failure to gain weight, and gastrointestinal problems [46]. There is evidence that having a diagnosis of CD for longer than 10 years is a risk factor for diabetic retinopathy in type 1 diabetes [47]. Patients with type 1 diabetes and CD have significantly greater carotid intima-media thickness than either those with diabetes or CD alone, and this could be of importance in accelerating cardiovascular disease [48].

Whether or not to screen patients with diabetes for CD remains controversial, but a case can be made for a screening program when the high frequency of the association is considered. In addition, patients may have symptoms, and a gluten-free diet can improve health and prevent complications. There is support for screening children and adolescents with type 1 diabetes [40, 41, 49], and in practice, screening is being increasingly undertaken [50]. What the interval between screening tests should be has been debated, but since diabetics are kept under annual review, screening is easily arranged. In one study most diagnoses of CD were made within 2–3 years, with a cumulative prevalence of 10 % at 5 years [41]. Adult patients, parents or guardians of children, and, where possible, children themselves should be fully involved at all stages of the screening, diagnostic, and treatment process and be advised by sympathetic doctors and dietitians skilled in the gluten-free diet.

The commencement of a gluten-free diet results in improvement in health, height, and weight and a reduction in hypoglycemic episodes in some series but not all [40, 49, 51, 52]. Those who regard themselves as asymptomatic should be offered a gluten-free diet because it may improve health, and if it does not, it is likely to be abandoned by patients themselves.

Thyroid Disease

Of 184 patients with CD attending an outpatient clinic in the Netherlands, based on thyroid biochemistry, 3.8 % (95 % CI 1.8–7.6) had subclinical hypothyroidism, 12 % (95 % CI 8–16) had overt hypothyroidism, while 2 % (95 % CI 0.8–5.0) had Graves' disease. Conversely, 4.8 % (95 % CI 0.7–8.9) of outpatients with Hashimoto's thyroiditis were diagnosed with CD. In this study, the observed prevalence of thyroid disease was compared with that reported in American cohorts. The prevalence of overt hypothyroidism was at least 10 times more common in celiacs than in the general population, while Graves' disease had approximately the same frequency [53]. Thyroid disease occurred three times more commonly in adults with newly diagnosed CD than controls drawn from such as medical and nursing staff, blood donors, and patients attending for endoscopy [54]. Employing the Swedish In-Patient Registry, CD was found to be associated with hypothyroidism (hazard ratio [HR] 4.4 [95 % CI 3.4–5.6]), thyroiditis (HR 3.6 [95 % CI: 1.9–6.7]), and hyperthyroidism (HR 2.9 [95 % CI 2.0–4.2]) [55]. The highest risk estimates for thyroid disease were observed in children and have raised the question whether children with CD should be screened for thyroid disease [56, 57]. Autoimmune thyroiditis may arise when children are on a gluten-free diet, which suggests that thyroid disturbance is independent of gluten [56]. However, gluten withdrawal in adults may normalize thyroid tests in those with subclinical hypothyroidism [54]. There are implications for the treatment of hypothyroidism in those with untreated CD in that increased doses of levothyroxine may be required to maintain the euthyroid state. Following the institution of a gluten-free diet when small bowel absorption becomes more efficient, a reduction in the dose may be required. The presence of CD should be suspected if patients with hypothyroidism require greater than expected doses of replacement therapy [58].

It is important to be aware of these associations because those with CD may have symptoms such as weight loss, lethargy, and diarrhea attributed to CD in relapse because of lax adherence to a gluten-free diet, rather than to the presence of thyroid disease.

Liver Disease

A number of liver conditions have been reported to be associated with CD [59, 60]. Recent population-based data using the General Practice Research Database and Swedish In-Patient Registry observed a fourfold increased risk of having an autoimmune liver disease, HR 3.6 [95 % CI 1.5–9.0] for primary biliary cirrhosis, and HR 4.5 [95 % CI 2.5–8.0] for primary sclerosing cholangitis in people with CD in comparison to general population controls [61, 62]. In contrast to the reported 0.2 % prevalence of autoimmune liver disease in CD, the most common hepatic injury to affect celiacs is of an isolated hypertransaminasemia, observed to affect

10 % of adults newly diagnosed with CD in a recent population-based cohort [63]. The observed hypertransaminasemia has been coined "gluten" or "celiac hepatitis" [64]. The hepatic injury is reputed to be characterized by absence of serum autoantibodies (other than endomysial and tissue transglutaminase antibodies), elevated transaminases, the presence of mild lobular and portal tract inflammation, and steatosis that is reversible on treatment with a gluten-free diet [64]. With significant reduction in transaminases and the transaminase result normalizing in 86 % of those with an abnormal result at diagnosis of CD following a year of treatment with a gluten-free diet, it suggests that investigations for liver disease should only be initiated in those celiacs with persistent hypertransaminasemia despite gluten-free diet or if otherwise indicated.

Other Autoimmune Diseases

A population-based study found an 11-fold increased risk (HR 11.4 [95 % CI 4.4–29.6]) of Addison's disease developing in those with CD, and conversely, those with established Addison's disease had a ninefold increased risk of developing CD (odds ratio [OR] 8.6 [95 % CI 3.4–21.8]) [65]. A Swedish study revealed an increased risk of uveitis (HR 1.32 [95 % CI 1.10–1.58]), which persisted 5 years after the diagnosis of CD (HR 1.31 [95 % CI 1.04–1.64]) [66] and may respond to a gluten-free diet. A positive association between CD and immune thrombocytopenia has been reported irrespective of which disorder came first [67].

The relationship between CD and psoriasis is well established. In one study a threefold increase was observed in comparison with age- and sex-matched controls (OR 2.7 [95 % CI 1.7–4.5]) [68]. In a more recent nationwide investigation from Sweden, those with CD were at increased risk of developing psoriasis before (HR 1.72 [95 % CI 1.54–1.92]) and after (OR 1.91 [95 % CI 1.58–2.31]) the diagnosis of CD. Children with CD were also at increased risk of developing psoriasis later in life (HR 2.05 [95 % CI 1.62–2.60]) [69].

When systemic lupus erythematosus was defined as having at least two records of the diagnosis in the Swedish Patient Register, a threefold increased risk among individuals with CD was observed (HR 2.87 [95 % CI 1.97–4.17]) [70]. A study reporting an increased risk of primary hyperparathyroidism in CD (HR 1.91 [95 % CI 1.44–2.52]) had some weaknesses such as misclassification and lack of biochemical information with regard to hyperparathyroidism as the authors accepted [71]. The prevalence of rheumatoid arthritis was not increased in CD in a study that had some limitations [72], but mortality from rheumatoid arthritis was elevated in a Swedish cohort (SMR 7.3 [95 % CI 2.7–15.9]) [73]. Sjögren's syndrome [74], hypoparathyroidism [75], hypopituitarism [76], dermatomyositis [77], scleroderma [78], alopecia areata [79], and myasthenia gravis [80] have all been described in association with CD but only in small series or case reports.

Vascular Diseases

Like in the general population, vascular disease is the most important single cause of mortality in diagnosed CD, accounting for 39 % of all deaths [73]. However, the possibility that CD might afford some protection from vascular disease mortality was first raised by Whorwell and colleagues in 1976 who observed a reduced risk of death from ischemic heart disease in men (but not women) with diagnosed CD [81] and further supported by studies in Scotland [2] and Italy [82]. However, Peters, using data from the Swedish In-Patient Registry, observed patients with diagnosed CD (n = 10,032) had 50 % increased mortality risk from ischemic heart disease (standardized mortality ratio [SMR] 1.5 [95 % CI 1.3–1.8]) and 40 % increased mortality risk from cerebrovascular disease (SMR 1.4 [95 % CI 1.1–1.9]) in comparison to the Swedish general population [73]. In contrast, there were no differences in rates of cardiovascular deaths in longitudinal cohorts of diagnosed celiacs in Scotland [7] or in England [83] relative to the general population.

On examining risk of cardiovascular mortality in the presence of villous atrophy within the Swedish In-Patient Registry celiac cohort, 19 % (HR 1.19 [95 % CI 1.11–1.28]) increased risk of death was observed compared to general population controls [84]. Cardiovascular mortality rates were similar, however, in serology-positive "undetected" CD and serology-negative controls in American [20] and British [85] general population screening studies.

A Swedish hospital-based cohort study of 13,358 people with CD observed people with CD were at increased risk of myocardial infarction (HR 1.27 [95 % CI 1.09–1.48]) and angina pectoris (HR 1.46 [95 % CI 1.25–1.70]) [86]. In an updated analysis with over twice the original cohort size and longer follow-up period, the risk of ischemic heart disease remained greater in people with CD relative to the general population (HR 1.19 [95 % CI 1.11–1.28]) [87]. In contrast, no differences were observed in the risk of neither myocardial infarction (HR 0.85 [95 % CI 0.63–1.13]) nor stroke (HR 1.29 [95 % CI 0.98–1.70]) in people with treated CD in comparison to general population controls in a British population-based cohort study [88]. Such differences in vascular morbidity and mortality risks may be due to differences in smoking patterns and socioeconomic exposures between countries.

A total of 367 celiac patients identified by presence of positive celiac serology or characteristic changes on small bowel histology had no increased risk of cardiovascular disease events such as myocardial infarction (unadjusted HR 1.10 [95 % CI 0.62–1.92]) in comparison to 5,537 controls who had negative celiac serology [89].

Recent studies have found some evidence of a favorable vascular risk profile in CD. Adults newly diagnosed with CD have lower total cholesterol levels than the general population, with the reduction greater in men (21 %; −1.09 mmol/L [95 % CI −0.97, −1.21]) than in women (9 %; −0.46 mmol/L [95 % CI −0.24, −0.68]) [9]. While no increase in total cholesterol following a year's treatment with a gluten-free diet was observed, there was a significant increase in HDL cholesterol [9]. In a cross-sectional population screening study, people with positive endomysial antibodies "undetected" CD had an 8 % (0.5 mmol/L) reduction in total cholesterol and a 2.4 mmHg lower diastolic blood pressure in comparison to antibody-negative controls [1]. Adults with treated CD are reported to be less likely to have a diagnosis of hypertension (OR 0.68 [95 % CI 0.60–0.76]) and have a lower reported antihypertensive medication use in comparison to age- and sex-matched general population controls [88]. Routine and systematic collection of smoking history is lacking in most studies. CD appears to be associated with nonsmoking in small and selected case–control studies although it is unclear whether this is a causal association [90–92]. In contrast, smoking was more common in pregnant women with diagnosed CD than those without CD using data combined from national birth registers and Swedish In-Patient Registry [93].

In contrast, other studies have reported CD is associated with an adverse vascular profile. Homocysteine concentrations were significantly higher in newly diagnosed adult celiacs than in controls, though the concentrations were not longitudinally assessed in these 35 celiacs to determine if there was any change with exposure to a gluten-free diet [94]. Carotid intima-media thickness and high-sensitivity C-reactive protein, a systemic marker of inflammation, were significantly higher in diagnosed celiacs maintained on a gluten-free diet for at least 1 year compared to age- and sex-matched controls [48].

Further work is warranted to explore the pathophysiological mechanisms involved in the atherosclerosis process in CD or clarify if other processes particular to people with CD change the vascular risk. We also need to explore whether there is an altering, attenuating effect on the vascular risk profile by treatment with a gluten-free diet to help support or refute general population screening for CD.

Though suggested by Fonager using the Danish National Registry [95], no association between CD and cardiomyopathy nor myocarditis or pericarditis was observed in the Swedish hospital-based cohort of celiacs compared to controls [96]. In a further large Swedish population-based cohort study, patients with CD were at a nonsignificantly increased risk of idiopathic cardiomyopathy (HR 1.73 [CI 95 % 1.00–3.00]) [97]. The two conditions may be linked through inflammation and autoimmune mechanisms. The small increased risk of atrial fibrillation in CD (HR 1.34 [95 % CI 1.24–1.44]) [98] may also be associated with these mechanisms.

Malignancy

The association between lymphoma, other malignancies, and CD has been known for 50 years [99]. Early studies were limited in their ability to provide precise estimates of the malignancy risks because of deficiencies such as small sample size and the selection of patients from specialist celiac centers. As a consequence the risks were often overestimated. With the advent of larger population-based studies, modest increased risks for lymphoma were found at around fivefold [3–5, 100–106]. The increased risk for small intestinal lymphoma 2 years after the diagnosis of CD is about 40 times [5]. An analysis of 31 series of patients with gluten sensitivity diagnosed using serology with or without biopsy or where there was an entry in the medical notes that the diagnosis had been made, gave a relative risk for non-Hodgkin lymphoma of 4.42 [95 % CI 3.72–5.26] [107]. A recent meta-analysis has calculated the risk of any malignancy and lymphoid malignancy developing in CD [108]. Diagnosed and undiagnosed patients with CD were considered together, which might be regarded as a shortcoming of the study [109]. There was no association between CD and the risk of any malignancy (OR 1.07 [95 % CI 0.89–1.29]), although the risk for non-Hodgkin lymphoma was as expected increased (OR 2.61 [95 % CI 2.04–3.33]). For T-cell non-Hodgkin lymphoma, the risk was high (OR 15.84 [95 % CI 7.85–31.94]). Others have also demonstrated no association between CD and any malignancy [4, 5, 103, 104, 110–112]. Some of these studies have importantly excluded the first 1–2 years of follow-up to minimize bias [4, 5, 104, 110]. It seems that the increased risk conferred by non-Hodgkin lymphoma is possibly balanced out by a reduction in the risk of some other cancers. Breast cancer, the leading cause of cancer in women in the general population, appears to be less common in those diagnosed with CD [2–8]. Reasons for this are unclear, though a population-based survey of 7,416 women with CD suggests there are potentially adverse as well as favorable breast cancer risk profile features in CD in comparison with the general population [113]. With body mass index and height similar to the general population this study [113] suggests that anthropomorphic exposures may not be responsible [114]. Endometrial (HR 0.60 [95 % CI 0.41–0.86]) and ovarian cancer (HR 0.89 [95 % CI 0.59–1.34]) are both reported as reduced in CD [8]. Data on CD and the risk of lung cancer are contradictory with some studies showing a negative [4, 111, 115] and some a positive association [5]. However, a recent large Swedish study has shown a neutral risk [116].

It is important to note that lymphoproliferative malignancy is an uncommon complication of CD when absolute numbers of tumors are considered. For example, the risk beyond 1 year of the diagnosis of CD is about 1 in 1,200 person years [4]. In addition, approximately 20 small bowel lymphomas, 12 small bowel adenocarcinomas, and 12 esophageal carcinomas would be encountered each year in the whole population of the United Kingdom [117]. Studies have shown that the overall risk of cancer decreases over time and after 10–15 years ceases [3, 118]. This observation may be linked to the protective effect of a gluten-free diet [119].

Enteropathy-associated T-cell lymphoma (EATL) is a type of lymphoma linked to CD. With an annual incidence of 0.5–1.0 per million of the population in Western countries, it is rare and accounts for about 5 % of all lymphomas [120] and 10–16 % of all lymphomas of the gastrointestinal tract [121]. Recent studies have indicated that EATL comprises two disorders EATL 1 and EATL 2 that are morphologically and genetically distinct [122]. EATL 1 is typically found in Western countries, comprising about 80 % of cases and is strongly associated with CD, while EATL 2 is the predominant type in Asia representing over 90 % of cases [120]. In one study, four (27 %) of 15 patients with EATL 2 had a clinical history of CD [12], but none of 38 cases reported from Asia had a history of CD, and although in some mucosa adjacent to the tumors showed villous atrophy and crypt hyperplasia, this was not regarded as indicative of CD [121]. It has to be conceded that the relationship of

EATL 2 to CD is unclear. CD56 is more commonly found in EATL 2, 73 % [120] and 91 % [121], than EATL 1, 30 % [120], and might be a useful marker.

Patients with either type have similar clinical features, and the prognosis is poor with a median overall survival of 10 months. Having CD worsens the outlook. A survey of small bowel malignancy in the United Kingdom showed a poor prognosis for lymphoma associated with CD, with a survival of only 13 % at 30 months [117]. For those without CD, the corresponding figure was 52 %. The poor outlook in those with CD is probably due to the adverse effects of malabsorption [117]. Urgent new treatments are required. High-dose ifosfamide, etoposide, and epirubicin/methotrexate followed by autologous stem cell transplantation improve outlook, but this might reflect patients in better condition to tolerate this intensive regime [123].

Celiac disease is not only associated with EATL but with a wide variety of other lymphomas. Of 56 non-Hodgkin lymphomas that occurred in CD, only 19 were EATL, the majority being of non-intestinal B-cell and T-cell type. Sixteen NHL were of B-cell lineage which more than doubled the risk (SIR 2.0 [95 % CI 1.3–3.6]) [101]. Those with B-cell lymphomas have a better prognosis that their T-cell counterparts [124].

Increased risks of oropharyngeal cancer; esophageal cancer; colon, liver, pancreatic, and small intestinal adenocarcinoma; and papillary cancer of the thyroid have been demonstrated [3, 125, 126], but in contrast to lymphomas where there is evidence that a gluten-free diet will reduce the risk [82, 119], for these malignancies, there is no evidence at present that a gluten-free diet will reduce their occurrence. In the British survey, of 175 adenocarcinomas of the small bowel encountered, 23 (13 %) were associated with CD. Overall survival at 30 months was 58 % and was not affected by the presence of CD [117]. An increased risk for tumors in the right and transverse colon occurs but not in the descending colon or rectum [3]. It is tempting to speculate that in celiac patients, gluten residues may enter the proximal colon and so provoke cancerous change. The increase in liver cancer might simply reflect the presence of disorders associated with CD that are risk factors for liver malignancy, e.g., primary biliary cirrhosis [3].

The development of EATL may be heralded by clinical relapse after a period of good response to gluten-free diet although EATL and CD can be diagnosed at the same time. In a subgroup of patients, there is progressive deterioration in the context of a refractory form of CD. Of those with EATL, common presentations are intestinal obstruction (49 %) and perforation (37 %), and a laparotomy is required to establish the diagnosis in about three quarters of patients. Of patients with small bowel adenocarcinoma, most present with intestinal obstruction (77 %) [117].

Malignancy in Undetected Celiac Disease

The increased risk of malignancy in CD has been the force calling for population screening studies to be undertaken. However, the number of cancers arising is small. This was evident from some early studies but often overlooked. For example, in a

British survey of malignancy in CD involving about 20 centers interested in CD, 133 lymphomas, 19 adenocarcinomas of the small bowel, and 10 esophageal cancers were encountered [115]. The average number of tumors seen at each center was low and equated to 6.7, 0.95, and 0.5, respectively. Emphasis was placed too often on relative risks rather than absolute numbers of tumors.

Three European case–control studies of similar design have attempted to ascertain the risk of non-Hodgkin lymphoma in undetected CD [100, 102, 127]. A total of 2,397 patients with non-Hodgkin lymphoma were included with the presence of CD in cases and controls determined by endomysial antibody testing. One of the investigations was unable to find an increased risk [127], while another observed a threefold increased risk confined to CD diagnosed clinically before the study but not in CD detected by screening [102]. In the third study the risk was threefold but the diagnosis of CD preceded the onset of non-Hodgkin lymphoma in four of the six cases [100]. In a population-based Finnish cohort study of 8,000 people gathered between 1978 and 1980 and observed for 20 years with reliance on the Finnish Cancer Registry for the detection of cancers (99 % complete for incident cancers), no increase in risk of malignancy was found in tissue transglutaminase-positive cases ($n = 202$; RR 0.91 [95 % CI 0.60–1.37]) or in endomysial antibody-positive participants ($n = 73$; RR 0.67 [95 % CI 0.28–1.61]) compared with serology-negative controls [128]. Only three non-Hodgkin lymphomas were found, one each in the groin and lower extremities, one in the tonsil, and one involving the skin. There were no enteropathy-associated T-cell lymphomas. Other studies of undetected CD have not shown any increase in cancer in undetected CD, (RR 0.73 [95 % CI 0.30–1.77]) [18], (OR 1.29 [95 % CI 0.77–2.15]) [20], (HR 1.27 [95 % CI 0.57–2.85]) [85], and (HR 0.97 [95 % CI 0.44–2.14]) [106]. Since these studies show that the risk of malignancy in undetected CD is not different to that observed in the general population, the fear of malignancy should not be used as an argument for early detection or screening for CD.

Refractory Celiac Disease

Nonresponsive CD is regarded as failure to respond to a strict gluten-free diet given for 6–12 months and can be regarded as primary, the patient has never responded to diet, or secondary, response is lost after an initial improvement with return of symptoms. Depending on study design and study population selected, the prevalence is about 7–30 % [129, 130]. Most cases of nonresponsive CD are related to continuing ingestion of gluten either deliberately or inadvertently, and this should be checked by a skilled dietitian [131]. Serological tests and repeat small bowel biopsies will help in the assessment. Having confirmed the index diagnosis of CD is correct and established adherence to a gluten-free diet, other causes of deterioration need excluding. These include conditions associated with CD such as overt intestinal lymphoma, pancreatic insufficiency, small bowel bacterial overgrowth, microscopic colitis, irritable bowel syndrome, inflammatory bowel disease, lactose intolerance, and thyroid dysfunction [129, 130]. Some of these are mentioned in this review and amenable to treatment. There are a few rare conditions with villous atrophy not related to CD such as common variable immunodeficiency and autoimmune enteropathy.

Patients are described as having refractory CD (RCD) when symptoms and villous atrophy persist (primary) or recur (secondary) despite adherence to a strict gluten-free diet and when other causes of nonresponse have been excluded. RCD can be subdivided in types 1 and 2 [132]. In three recent European series, RCD 2 forms 54 % [133], 28 % [134], and 75 % [135] of the total group. These different frequencies might represent differences in patient selection and methods used to determine the type.

Type 1 has a phenotypically normal T-cell population on duodenal histology and carries a good prognosis. Steroids and azathioprine are effective and the 5-year survival is over 90 %. In type 2 RCD there is an aberrant intraepithelial T-cell population that carries intracytoplasmic but not surface CD3, usually lacks CD8, and has clonal rearrangements of the T-cell receptor-γ gene. It thus resembles a low-grade lymphoma. Prognosis for those with type 2 RCD is poor, with no satisfactory treatments [136]. Transition to EATL is common [132–135]. The 5-year survival in type 1 was 96 % but in type 2 was 58 %, falling to 8 % in 26 (52 %) patients who developed EATL [133]. EATL can arise directly from aberrant intraepithelial T-cell lymphocytes or after passing through a stage of refractory CD that manifests as chronic ulcerative jejunoileitis.

The prevalence of RCD is unknown. High figures from specialist referral centers are unrepresentative of the diagnosis at large. Recently more representative data have been provided. Of 528 patients with CD actually diagnosed at an American referral center, only 8 (1.5 %) had RCD and of these 8, 5 (0.9 %) had type 1 RCD, 2 (0.4 %) had type 2 RCD, and in one the status was unknown [137]. Among 204 celiacs residing in Olmsted County, Minnesota, USA, identified over a 56-year period, only two developed type 1 RCD and one type 2 RCD [138]. These results accord with those from our center which show that only 5 (0.7 %) of 713 nonreferred patients with CD had type 2 RCD. These results indicate that RCD is rare. It has been speculated that RCD might be more common and more severe in Europe than the USA, but only studies using agreed diagnostic criteria will clarify this [139].

For clinicians the challenge is to identify these entities and distinguish them from poor adherence to a gluten-free diet. Recent weight loss is a predictor of RCD [130], and severe malnutrition, malabsorption, and hypoalbuminemia are typical presenting features [140]. Tests that can be carried out include endoscopy and enteroscopy to assess the small bowel mucosa and biopsy suspicious areas and imaging techniques such as barium follow-through, MRI, CT, PET, and capsule endoscopy to look for bowel ulcerations, lymphoma, and other malignancy. The phenotype of intraepithelial lymphocytes in the small intestinal mucosa should be determined by immunohistochemistry and/or flow cytometry and clonal T-cell receptor rearrangements assessed [135, 138, 139, 141].

Metabolic Bone Disease and Fracture

Meta-analysis of published studies suggests that there is a modest increase in the risk of fracture in CD (any fracture relative risk 1.38 [95 % CI 1.14–1.68]) [142]. Although osteoporosis is just one of many factors predisposing to fracture, it is appreciated that the risk of sustaining an osteoporotic fracture doubles with each standard deviation decrease in bone mineral density (BMD) [143]. For example, a 50-year-old woman with T-score −2 at the femoral neck has 9.2 % 10-year probability of sustaining a hip, vertebral, or wrist fracture in comparison to the 5.9 % probability in a woman of the same age with T-score −1. Though osteoporosis can be reliably assessed by measurement of BMD using noninvasive dual-energy X-ray absorptiometry (DEXA), the real issue is identifying which celiacs are at particular risk of reduced BMD and thus rationalizing referrals for DEXA screening. Meta-analysis of published studies suggests there is a moderate reduction of BMD in untreated CD with weighted mean T-scores at the lumbar spine and hip of −1.7 and −1.4 (osteopenia defined as T-score −1 to −2.4) [142]. Observational studies have suggested that a gluten-free diet improves BMD in people with symptomatic CD. For example, Valdimarsson observed a median 3 % (interquartile range 1–7) increase in BMD at the lumbar spine in 62 celiacs following 12 months treatment with a gluten-free diet [144], whereas McFarlane observed a 6.6 % [95 % CI 3.1–10.1] absolute increase in the lumbar spine over an identical time period of treatment in 21 celiacs [145]. A systematic review of those risk factors for fracture in the general population which are probably related to a low BMD identified high risk factors (relative risk or odds ratio of >2.0) such as age over 70 years, previous osteoporotic fracture, weight loss greater than 10 %, and low body weight as reflected by body mass index (<20 kg/m^2 or weight <40 kg) [146]. DEXA screening for osteoporosis should therefore be offered to untreated celiacs with these features, to those celiacs with persisting symptoms despite adherence with at least a year's treatment with a gluten-free diet, and those celiacs with poor adherence to a gluten-free diet [142].

Studies observing prevalence of osteomalacia in newly diagnosed CD involved patients that had particular reasons for measuring different elements of bone profile so are likely to be limited by ascertainment. Elevated alkaline phosphatase is a useful biochemical test to screen for osteomalacia in celiacs as it is in the general population [63, 147, 148]. Elevated alkaline phosphatase is also independently associated with clinical features of malabsorption in adults newly diagnosed with CD [63]. The observed reduction in alkaline phosphatase with treatment of CD [144, 149, 150] supports the importance of gluten withdrawal to help treat any underlying osteomalacia [144, 149, 150]. Normalization of an isolated elevated alkaline phosphatase with treatment of CD may also remove the need for further invasive investigations such as a bone biopsy.

Neurological and Psychiatric Disorders

The true prevalence of these complications of CD is unknown because of variable definitions of the disorders that have been used and that results have often been based on small groups of patients from specialist referral centers which skews the figures [151]. Furthermore, it is not certain which results, if any, are specific for CD. In a large population-based study from Sweden using the In-Patient Registry examining the risk of neurological disease in 14,000 celiacs and 70,000 age- and sex-matched controls, celiacs were only at increased risk of polyneuropathy (HR 3.4 [95 % CI 2.3–5.1]) [152]. However, even here, ascertainment bias probably influenced the results because the cohort was assembled on the basis of admitted patients. Retrospective data from the celiac clinic in Derby, United Kingdom, which is not a referral center, found 160 neurological and 103 psychiatric problems among 620 patients (some had more than one disorder) [153]. The most common three conditions were depression, epilepsy, and migraine.

Depression

It might be expected that those with a chronic debilitating condition, especially if the diagnosis is delayed and the treatment is a restrictive diet that limits social interaction [154], will lead to depression. Depression in CD can be severe to the point where patients may attempt and succeed in suicide [7, 155]. However, whether depression is more common among celiac patients is disputed, with some finding a positive association and some not. Most investigations have included only small numbers of patients, but a large population-based cohort study from Sweden using the In-Patient Registry observed an increased risk of depression after the diagnosis of CD was made (HR 1.8 [95 % CI 1.6–2.2]) [156]. Those with a history of prior depression were at increased risk of a subsequent diagnosis of CD (OR 2.3 [95 % CI 2.0–2.81]), and it was suggested that this may be due to screening for CD among those with mood disorders. An American study of 600 patients with CD, 200 with irritable bowel syndrome, and 200 healthy controls found the prevalence of depression similar in all three groups at 17.2 %, 18.5 %, and 16 %, respectively [157]. A significant increase in depression in celiac patients with coexistent type 1 diabetes was found at 37 %, compared to 16 % with CD alone. It appears that having two chronic diseases is sufficient to tip the balance in favor of depression. However, even these large studies had methodological problems. For example, in the American investigation, psychiatric records could not be accessed, while in the Swedish one, celiac patients with mood disorders were identified through a hospital-based register, raising the possibility that these were more severely affected than average patients. A recent meta-analysis has shown that depression is more common in CD than in healthy adults but anxiety levels are similar [158]. Patients with CD are prone to sleep disorders that are related to depression, anxiety, and fatigue [159].

A gluten-free diet improves depression and anxiety in some but not all cases [158, 160, 161]. Vitamin B supplementation as well as a gluten-free diet is recommended to improve mood [162]. Impaired availability of tryptophan may be important in depressive and behavioral disorders in CD [160].

Epilepsy

Whether patients with CD have an increased risk of epilepsy is still not clear, because some studies have shown an association [163] and others have not [164, 165]. The association, even if it exists, is likely to be weak. A combination of CD, bilateral occipital calcifications, and epilepsy has been reported mainly from Italy [166]. In some of these patients, a gluten-free diet may control the seizures [166, 167]. A link between gluten sensitivity and temporal lobe epilepsy with hippocampal sclerosis has been shown [168].

Migraine

Migraine may occur in CD and improve or is cured by a gluten-free diet [169, 170].

Other Neurological Conditions

Many other conditions are encountered in patients with CD but only rarely even in large celiac clinics [153]. These include spinocerebellar and cerebellar disorders, peripheral neuropathy, myelopathy, brainstem encephalitis, and chronic progressive leukoencephalopathy. Whether there is a link between schizophrenia and CD has been debated over the last 50 years. Two more recent surveys found an increased risk [171] and no risk [172], so this issue remains controversial. Dementia and cognitive impairment occur in CD [173, 174], but only 13 patients with the onset of cognitive decline within 2 years of the symptomatic onset or a severe exacerbation of CD could be identified over a 35-year period from the Mayo Clinic (MN, USA) [175]. Although in some patients cognitive decline and gastrointestinal symptoms occurred simultaneously and a gluten-free diet halted or improved cognitive impairment, the strength of this association merits further study. There is no firm link between autism and CD. The association between CD and multiple sclerosis has not been convincingly demonstrated, but a recent study of 72 cases found CD to be present in eight although only mild abnormalities were present in the duodenal mucosa [176]. Gluten-free diet may stabilize those with sensory ganglionopathy [177].

It has to be concluded that a neurological or psychiatric disorder specific for CD has not been identified. Most are likely to be chance associations, apart from perhaps some forms of epilepsy and neuropathy.

Malabsorption does not satisfactorily explain how these disorders arise because vitamin supplementation is rarely helpful and hypovitaminosis is not always present. Moreover, no neurological abnormalities may occur in the presence of severe vitamin deficiency. While heredity, infection, toxins, altered immunity, vasculitis, and a direct neurotoxic effect of gluten have been implicated in causing these, there is still much to be unraveled.

The effect of a gluten-free diet in these patients ranges from reversal of dysfunction, as seen in some patients with epilepsy and cerebral calcifications, to stabilization of the illness, as may occur in cognitive decline, to making little or no difference. Vitamin deficiencies should be corrected, and this may benefit some patients with cerebellar ataxia (vitamin E) and depression (pyridoxine). Steroids and immunosuppression in general are of no value.

Gluten Ataxia and Neuropathy

In 1996 gluten sensitivity was reported in patients with neurological disorders of unknown cause based on the presence of serum antigliadin antibodies; the majority of patients had ataxia or peripheral neuropathy [178]. The terms gluten ataxia and gluten neuropathy were coined to describe these entities. Duodenal biopsy showed CD to be present in only one third of patients [179, 180]. Supporting evidence for gluten ataxia continues to accumulate, such as the association with HLA-DQ2 and DQ8, the presence of circulating Purkinje cell antibodies, and the presence of anti-tissue transglutaminase antibody in the gut and brain [180]. In addition, 60 % of patients have evidence of cerebellar atrophy on MRI scanning [180]. Proton MR spectroscopy may be abnormal indicating atrophy or abnormal cerebellar function not necessarily associated with cell death [181]. Of importance is the observation that these conditions may be improved by gluten-free diet [180].

The reason why some patients develop neurological problems could revolve around a newly identified tissue transglutaminase, transglutaminase 6 [182]. This work extends the concept of gluten sensitivity beyond the bowel (CD) and skin (dermatitis herpetiformis) to involve the nervous system [183].

Reproductive Problems

Previous studies have raised concern about reduced fertility and increased adverse pregnancy-related outcomes in women with CD [184]. Some authors have accepted that infertility is a complication of CD [185–187]. Reported associations between

CD and miscarriage have also added to the concern, though most of the studies have used small, selected populations and have been limited in their ability to adjust for potential confounders [184, 188–193]. However, a population-based cohort study using the General Practice Research Database observed that although rates of miscarriage were significantly higher in women with CD in comparison to the general population (rate ratio 1.31 [95 % CI 1.06–1.61]), there was no difference in risk of stillbirth, nor was there any difference in fertility rates in women with CD ($n = 1{,}521$) compared to general population controls (fertility rate ratio 1.01 [95 % CI 0.90–1.14]) [194]. Age-specific rates showed that female celiacs had lower fertility when younger but higher fertility when older when compared to general population controls [194]. Fertility rate ratios of incident and prevalent female celiacs were similar to the overall analysis, and there was no difference between the prevalent and incident groups [194]. It was speculated that together with the increase in cesarean section risk among celiacs, the age shift in fertility could be reflective of socioeconomic advantages in women with CD [194]. A recent population-based cohort study based on 7,416 female celiacs provided further evidence that female celiacs have no difference in fertility in comparison to general population controls [195]. Others have also found that overall there is no association between CD and fertility [196, 197]. There was also no difference in the proportion of celiacs with one or more live births (87.8 % vs. 87.6 %; p-value = 0.82) or the number of stillbirths (19.05 stillbirths reported per 1,000 total number of reported live births and stillbirths) compared with the general population [198]. Women with untreated CD are at greater risk of delivering small babies than those without CD [198].

Hyposplenism

Since splenic macrophages have a major role in phagocytosing bacteria and the spleen is the principal producer of antibodies, hyposplenic (functional or anatomic) persons have an increased susceptibility to serious infections caused by encapsulated bacteria and other pathogens such as pneumococcal septicemia [199, 200]. Hyposplenism, which may be a complication of chronic folate deficiency, the result of excessive loss of lymphocytes through the damaged gastrointestinal tract or related to the mucosal lesion [201], is a well-documented complication of CD in historical case series [202–213]. Hyposplenism appears to be much less common in children with CD [203, 208, 209, 212] with duration of exposure to gluten, a significant factor for the prevalence and severity of the hyposplenism [204]. Adherence to a gluten-free diet was associated with a decrease in pitted red cells suggesting hyposplenism may be reversible [202], but this observation is not supported by other investigators [213]. Higher pitted red cell counts were also observed in those with more severe duodenal histology [209] or with complicated CD such as jejunoileitis [206].

Risk of Infection in Celiac Disease

Using the Swedish In-Patient Registry linked to death registration data, a population-based cohort study observed people with CD ($n = 10{,}032$) had a sevenfold increased risk of death from septicemia (SMR 7.1 [95 % CI 1.9–18.2]) and threefold increased risk of death from infection (SMR 2.9 [95 % CI 1.5–3.0]) and pneumonia (SMR 2.9 [95 % CI 2.1–3.8]) in comparison to general population controls [73]. Using the same In-Patient Registry, a recent population-based cohort study observed people with CD ($n = 15{,}325$) had a twofold increased risk of infection (HR 1.6 [95 % CI 1.2–1.9]) and a fourfold increased risk of pneumococcal infection (HR 2.5 [95 % CI 1.2–5.1]) [214]. However, no increased risk of infection from meningococcus was observed. There was no difference in risk estimates for sepsis between celiacs diagnosed in childhood as opposed to in adulthood [214].

Although studies link overwhelming infection with hyposplenism in the general population [199, 200] and that large population-based studies describe increased risk of mortality and morbidity from infection in people with CD, the risk of infection in people with CD and hyposplenism is not known nor is the prevalence of hyposplenism in contemporary CD. Since 1992, a 23-valent pneumococcal polysaccharide vaccination (PPV) has been recommended in the United Kingdom by the Department of Health as part of the national immunization program for individuals at risk in the general population, including those with hyposplenia and CD. Despite this recommendation to vaccinate celiacs against pneumococcus being reinforced by primary care groups, recent primary care data suggests only the minority of British celiacs have received pneumococcal vaccination [215]. Annual influenza vaccination is also appropriate as this reduces the frequency of secondary bacterial infection.

Inflammatory Bowel Disease

Ulcerative colitis and Crohn's disease affect patients with CD, but the strength of the association is disputed. Among a group of 455 cases, ulcerative colitis affected five (prevalence ratio 3.56 [95 % CI 1.48–8.56]) and Crohn's disease, five (8.49 [95 % CI 3.53–20.42]) [216]. The prevalence of inflammatory bowel disease comprising five patients with ulcerative colitis and five with lymphocytic colitis was ten times higher in the celiac group (10 of 305; 3.3 %) than in the control group (2 of 601; 0.33 %) [217]. If only ulcerative colitis were considered, the result still remained higher (OR 4.99 [95 % CI 1.0–25.9]). The prevalence of CD in inflammatory bowel disease did not differ from the control group. No cases of Crohn's disease were identified among the celiac patients and in 90 % of instances CD was diagnosed first. A multicenter study found no increased risk of CD in inflammatory bowel disease but when an association does occur ulcerative colitis is more common than Crohn's disease [218]. Microscopic colitis is more common in CD with a prevalence in one series of 44 out of 1,009 patients (4.3 %) [219]. The results of such studies are affected by referral bias, the different study populations, and criteria for diagnosing the conditions. While the links may be nonexistent or weak, these additional diagnoses need to be considered in patients with CD who do not show the expected responses to a gluten-free diet or unaccountably deteriorate, particularly with regard to bowel disturbance because specific treatments will be required to restore good health.

Other Gastrointestinal Disorders

Symptoms such as abdominal bloating, diarrhea, and constipation are common to the irritable bowel syndrome and CD, so the two conditions are easily confused. A meta-analysis of five case–control studies employing biopsy diagnosis of CD found a fourfold increase among patients with irritable bowel syndrome meeting the Rome II criteria (34 of 952) compared with controls (12 of 1,798) (OR 4.34 [95 % CI 1.78–10.6]) [220]. This supports a search for CD among irritable bowel patients who may be benefited by a gluten-free diet. However, this strategy has been challenged by a recent American study that found a similar prevalence of CD in non-constipated irritable bowel syndrome compared to controls [221]. On the evidence some will choose to screen all patients or be more selective, targeting those where the diagnosis of CD seems likely (e.g., those with a family history of CD, anemia, osteoporosis, or a linked associated disease such as diabetes) [221]. The incidence of eosinophilic esophagitis appears to be increased in CD [222]. Intussusception affects adults with CD and may occur at the site of an adenocarcinoma of the small bowel [223]. Children may also be affected [224].

CD is associated with an increased risk of pancreatitis as shown by studies using the Swedish In-Patient Registry. The risk of any pancreatitis developing within 5 years of the diagnosis of CD is almost threefold (HR 2.76 [95 % CI 2.36–3.22]) [225]. CD and noncirrhotic intrahepatic hypertension may occur together but the reasons are unknown [59].

Enamel defects and recurrent aphthous ulcers are observed in CD but prevalence figures vary widely [226]. Enamel hypoplasia had the same frequency in celiac patients and controls [226], but a higher prevalence in patients has been reported [227, 228]. Conversely, CD was found to be more common in those with enamel defects [229]. Recurrent aphthous ulcers occur more commonly in CD in some series [226, 228], but not all [230]. CD occurs more commonly in those with aphthous ulcers than in the general population with a threefold increase although small bowel histological changes may be mild [231]. A gluten-free diet may be curative [232]. Clinicians need to be aware of these manifestations which include glossitis and angular stomatitis and that they may be the only manifestation of CD. It is difficult to account for the differing prevalences of these conditions, but differences in food consumption by the groups under study may be one explanation. Autoimmune mechanisms may play a part, but not apparently, malabsorption [233].

Pulmonary Disorders

Patients with CD in a nationwide cohort study from Sweden were found to be at a small increased risk of chronic obstructive pulmonary disease before diagnosis of CD (HR 1.22 [95 % CI 1.02–1.46]) which was also evident 5 years after diagnosis (HR 1.17 [95 % CI 1.00–1.37]) [234]. Why this should be is not clear but may be linked to malabsorption and malnutrition [234]. The risk of asthma is increased in CD (HR 1.61 [95 % CI 1.50–1.72]) and persists 5 years after the celiac diagnosis [235]. The risk is also evident before the diagnosis of CD. Shared genetics may play a part in this association. Diffuse lung disease occurs in CD including fibrosing alveolitis, bird fancier's lung, and farmer's lung, but the strength of these associations is not clear.

Miscellaneous Disorders

In a Scandinavian cohort of patients with cystic fibrosis, the prevalence of CD was three times greater (1.2 %, 1:83) than the general prevalence of CD in Norway and Sweden [236]. A study from Poland also found an increased prevalence of cystic fibrosis compared to healthy controls [237]. Both these studies can be criticized: the first on the grounds that the prevalence figures for CD in the general population were low and the second that screened school children were used to make the comparison. Patients with biopsy-verified CD have a twofold risk of tuberculosis (HR 2.0 [95 % CI 1.3–3.0]), and there is also an increased risk before the diagnosis of CD [238]. Ascertainment bias was evident because the risk of tuberculosis was highest in the first year of follow-up. Children with CD were not at increased risk, and the risk disappeared 5 years after the diagnosis of CD. The number of patients developing tuberculosis was low. Vitamin D deficiency might explain this association [238]. An increased risk of venous thromboembolism among adult celiac patients may occur [239]. However, no overall risk was found in a Danish study (OR 1.0 [95 % CI 0.8–1.4]) which corrected for risk factors such as medications and several comorbidities [240]. An increased risk of developing urinary stones has been found in CD before and after the celiac diagnosis [241]. When the first year of follow-up was excluded, the HR was 1.25 [95 % CI 1.10–1.43]. Hyperoxaluria has been proposed as a causative factor and a gluten-free diet may be beneficial [242]. A threefold increased risk of end-stage renal disease has been found in CD (HR 2.87 [95 % CI 2.22–3.71]), although the underlying mechanism is unknown [243]. The risk persists after 5 years of follow-up. Endometriosis may be associated with prior CD possibly due to ongoing inflammation, persisting for more than 5 years after the celiac diagnosis (HR 1.33 [95 % CI 1.00–1.79]) [244]. CD has been linked to sarcoid perhaps through common haplotypes [245–247].

Genetic Disorders

The prevalence of CD is increased in some genetic disorders. Approximately 5 % of children with Down syndrome were affected [248], while 6 of 63 children with Williams syndrome had CD compared with 1 in 184 of the student population [249]. The prevalence in Turner syndrome is 5–8 % [250, 251]. Gastrointestinal symptoms and short stature are often present in patients with these syndromes, and if associated CD is a contributing factor, they may benefit from a gluten-free diet. Screening these groups is recommended [249, 251] and the determination of HLA-DQ2 and HLA-DQ8 to exclude those who do not require screening because of the absence of these markers of CD [248].

Dermatitis Herpetiformis

Dermatitis herpetiformis forms part of the same spectrum of gluten-enteropathy disorders as CD [252]. Although most people with dermatitis herpetiformis have a gluten-sensitive enteropathy, this is usually asymptomatic with primary manifestations usually cutaneous [253, 254]. Earlier hospital-based case series observed people with dermatitis herpetiformis were at increased risk of mortality and malignancy such as lymphoma in keeping with those observations in people with CD [111, 255–259]. However, these studies were limited, based on small numbers of patients typically identified from a hospital specialist clinic and therefore unlikely to be representative of dermatitis herpetiformis in the population. A recent, large population-based study observed people with dermatitis herpetiformis were at no excess risk of death (all-cause mortality hazard ratio 0.93 [95 % CI 0.70–1.23]), malignancy (any malignancy hazard ratio 1.0 [95 % CI 0.73–1.49]), or indeed lymphoma (hazard ratio 1.6 [95 % CI 0.44, 6.06]) in comparison to the general population [260]. No increase in risk of cancer in people with dermatitis herpetiformis was also observed using data from the Swedish In-Patient Registry [3]. With no excess fracture risk also observed in people with dermatitis herpetiformis (any fracture hazard ratio 1.10 [95 % CI 0.77–1.52]) compared with the general population, screening and surveillance of people with dermatitis herpetiformis for decreased bone mineral density seems unwarranted [260].

Mortality in Undetected Celiac Disease

Recent general population screening studies have reported mortality in undetected celiac disease. Though the prevalence of CD in these investigations is approximately 1 %, they are somewhat restricted by the small absolute numbers of celiac serology-positive individuals with limited power. In a British population of adults aged 45 years or older and in an American population of adults aged 50 years or older with undetected CD, no increase in mortality rate was observed [20, 85]. Including younger ages of celiacs, similar findings were observed in another British cohort [16] and a Finnish screening study [18] of no excess risk. Using the Swedish In-Patient Registry, adults with positive celiac serology, though normal duodenal histology, had no increased mortality rates compared with the general population [84]. In contrast, a screening study from Germany reported an increased age-adjusted hazard ratio of 2.53 [95 % CI 1.50–4.25] compared with the general population. With the 1.89 % prevalence of CD in men, concern was raised as to whether there were false positive serological results such as due to liver disease in the cohort [17]. An American study reported a fourfold increase in risk of death in undetected CD though the cohort is unlikely to be representative of contemporary populations with the serum samples taken from Air Force recruits in the 1950s [19].

Mortality in Diagnosed Celiac Disease

In an analysis of ten studies that have addressed mortality in diagnosed CD [261], mortality rates varied from 1.26 in a Finnish report [111] to 3.8 in patients from Italy with a diagnostic delay of 10 years or more after the onset of symptoms [82]. It is unsurprising to find different rates because of the different populations studied. One investigation found the degree of compliance with a gluten-free diet correlates with mortality as do the severity of the clinical presentation and the length of time from onset of symptoms to the diagnosis of CD [82]. Most studies found that the increased risk decreases over time after the celiac diagnosis, but in those diagnosed in childhood, the increased risk may persist for 25 years or more [7]. A recent meta-analysis showed an increased risk for all-cause mortality in CD (OR 1.24 [95 % CI 1.19–1.30]) which, it was suggested, may be partly explained by an increased risk of cardiovascular mortality [108]. In a study of 1,092 celiac patients from a single center, all-cause mortality was increased (SMR 1.37 [95 % CI 1.19–2.13]) [83]. Of interest, mortality had not materially altered over the follow-up period of this study, which covered the pre-and post-serology era. Most excess deaths were from malignancy, digestive disease, and respiratory disease.

Conclusion

Diabetes mellitus was among the earliest disorders to be described in association with CD. The first recorded case in a child appeared in 1925 [262], while the earliest example in an adult was reported in 1956 [263]. Since these early descriptions, the number of recognized comorbidities has mushroomed as evident from this review. It is incumbent on those who care for celiac patients to be aware of these associations so that patients receive optimum management.

References

1. West J, Logan RF, Hill PG, Lloyd A, Lewis S, Hubbard R, et al. Seroprevalence, correlates, and characteristics of undetected coeliac disease in England. Gut. 2003;52(7):960–5.
2. Logan RF, Rifkind EA, Turner ID, Ferguson A. Mortality in CD. Gastroenterology. 1989;97(2):265–71.
3. Askling J, Linet M, Gridley G, Halstensen TS, Ekstrom K, Ekbom A. Cancer incidence in a population-based cohort of individuals hospitalized with CD or dermatitis herpetiformis. Gastroenterology. 2002;123(5):1428–35.
4. West J, Logan RF, Smith CJ, Hubbard RB, Card TR. Malignancy and mortality in people with coeliac disease: population based cohort study. BMJ. 2004;329(7468):716–9.
5. Card TR, West J, Holmes GK. Risk of malignancy in diagnosed coeliac disease: a 24-year prospective, population-based, cohort study. Aliment Pharmacol Ther. 2004;20(7):769–75.
6. Silano M, Volta U, Mecchia AM, Dessi M, Di Benedetto R, De Vincenzi M. Delayed diagnosis of coeliac disease increases cancer risk. BMC Gastroenterol. 2007;7:8.
7. Solaymani-Dodaran M, West J, Logan RF. Long-term mortality in people with CD diagnosed in childhood compared with adulthood: a population-based cohort study. Am J Gastroenterol. 2007;102(4):864–70.
8. Ludvigsson JF, West J, Ekbom A, Stephansson O. Reduced risk of breast, endometrial and ovarian cancer in women with CD. Int J Cancer. 2012;131(3):E244–50.
9. Lewis NR, Sanders DS, Logan RF, Fleming KM, Hubbard RB, West J. Cholesterol profile in people with newly diagnosed coeliac disease: a comparison with the general population and changes following treatment. Br J Nutr. 2009;102(4):509–13.
10. Lewis NR, Scott BB. Systematic review: the use of serology to exclude or diagnose coeliac disease (a comparison of the endomysial and tissue transglutaminase antibody tests). Aliment Pharmacol Ther. 2006;24(1):47–54.
11. Lewis NR, Scott BB. Meta-analysis: deamidated gliadin peptide antibody and tissue transglutaminase antibody compared as screening tests for coeliac disease. Aliment Pharmacol Ther. 2010;31(1):73–81.
12. Holmes GKT. To determine the incidence and prevalence of adult coeliac disease in Derby City. Gut 2009;58(Suppl 2):A409.
13. Hurley JJ, Lee B, Turner JK, Beale A, Jenkins HR, Swift GL. Incidence and presentation of reported coeliac disease in Cardiff and the Vale of Glamorgan: the next 10 years. Eur J Gastroenterol Hepatol. 2012;24(5):482–6.
14. Lohi S, Mustalahti K, Kaukinen K, Laurila K, Collin P, Rissanen H, et al. Increasing prevalence of coeliac disease over time. Aliment Pharmacol Ther. 2007;26(9):1217–25.
15. Collin P, Huhtala H, Virta L, Kekkonen L, Reunala T. Diagnosis of CD in clinical practice: physician's alertness to the condition essential. J Clin Gastroenterol. 2007;41(2):152–6.
16. Johnston SD, Watson RG, McMillan SA, Sloan J, Love AH. Coeliac disease detected by screening is not silent–simply unrecognized. QJM. 1998;91(12):853–60.
17. Metzger MH, Heier M, Maki M, Bravi E, Schneider A, Lowel H, et al. Mortality excess in individuals with elevated IgA anti-transglutaminase antibodies: the KORA/MONICA Augsburg cohort study 1989-1998. Eur J Epidemiol. 2006;21(5):359–65.
18. Lohi S, Maki M, Rissanen H, Knekt P, Reunanen A, Kaukinen K. Prognosis of unrecognized coeliac disease as regards mortality: a population-based cohort study. Ann Med. 2009;41(7):508–15.
19. Rubio-Tapia A, Kyle RA, Kaplan EL, Johnson DR, Page W, Erdtmann F, et al. Increased prevalence and mortality in undiagnosed CD. Gastroenterology. 2009;137(1):88–93.
20. Godfrey JD, Brantner TL, Brinjikji W, Christensen KN, Brogan DL, Van Dyke CT, et al. Morbidity and mortality among older individuals with undiagnosed CD. Gastroenterology. 2010;139(3):763–9.
21. Feighery C. Fortnightly review: coeliac disease. BMJ. 1999;319(7204):236–9.
22. Sollid LM. Molecular basis of CD. Annu Rev Immunol. 2000;18:53–81.

23. Sollid LM, Jabri B. CD and transglutaminase 2: a model for posttranslational modification of antigens and HLA association in the pathogenesis of autoimmune disorders. Curr Opin Immunol. 2011;23(6):732–8.
24. Qiao SW, Iversen R, Raki M, Sollid LM. The adaptive immune response in CD. Semin Immunopathol. 2012;34(4):523–40.
25. Korponay-Szabo IR, Halttunen T, Szalai Z, Laurila K, Kiraly R, Kovacs JB, et al. In vivo targeting of intestinal and extraintestinal transglutaminase 2 by coeliac autoantibodies. Gut. 2004;53(5):641–8.
26. Naiyer AJ, Shah J, Hernandez L, Kim SY, Ciaccio EJ, Cheng J, et al. Tissue transglutaminase antibodies in individuals with CD bind to thyroid follicles and extracellular matrix and may contribute to thyroid dysfunction. Thyroid. 2008;18(11):1171–8.
27. van Elburg RM, Uil JJ, Mulder CJ, Heymans HS. Intestinal permeability in patients with coeliac disease and relatives of patients with coeliac disease. Gut. 1993;34(3):354–7.
28. Trynka G, Wijmenga C, van Heel DA. A genetic perspective on coeliac disease. Trends Mol Med. 2010;16(11):537–50.
29. Zhernakova A, van Diemen CC, Wijmenga C. Detecting shared pathogenesis from the shared genetics of immune-related diseases. Nat Rev Genet. 2009;10(1):43–55.
30. Xavier RJ, Rioux JD. Genome-wide association studies: a new window into immune-mediated diseases. Nat Rev Immunol. 2008;8(8):631–43.
31. Fernando MM, Stevens CR, Walsh EC, De Jager PL, Goyette P, Plenge RM, et al. Defining the role of the MHC in autoimmunity: a review and pooled analysis. PLoS Genet. 2008;4(4):e1000024.
32. Zhong F, McCombs CC, Olson JM, Elston RC, Stevens FM, McCarthy CF, et al. An autosomal screen for genes that predispose to CD in the western counties of Ireland. Nat Genet. 1996;14(3):329–33.
33. Osman AA, Gunnel T, Dietl A, Uhlig HH, Amin M, Fleckenstein B, et al. B cell epitopes of gliadin. Clin Exp Immunol. 2000;121(2):248–54.
34. Girbal-Neuhauser E, Durieux JJ, Arnaud M, Dalbon P, Sebbag M, Vincent C, et al. The epitopes targeted by the rheumatoid arthritis-associated antifilaggrin autoantibodies are post-translationally generated on various sites of (pro)filaggrin by deimination of arginine residues. J Immunol. 1999;162(1):585–94.
35. Schellekens GA, de Jong BA, van den Hoogen FH, van de Putte LB, van Venrooij WJ. Citrulline is an essential constituent of antigenic determinants recognized by rheumatoid arthritis-specific autoantibodies. J Clin Invest. 1998;101(1):273–81.
36. Dunne JL, Overbergh L, Purcell AW, Mathieu C. Posttranslational modifications of proteins in type 1 diabetes: the next step in finding the cure? Diabetes. 2012;61(8):1907–14.
37. Ashton-Key M, Diss TC, Pan L, Du MQ, Isaacson PG. Molecular analysis of T-cell clonality in ulcerative jejunitis and enteropathy-associated T-cell lymphoma. Am J Pathol. 1997;151(2):493–8.
38. Holmes GK. Coeliac disease and Type 1 diabetes mellitus - the case for screening. Diabet Med. 2001;18(3):169–77.
39. Holmes GK. Screening for coeliac disease in type 1 diabetes. Arch Dis Child. 2002;87(6):495–8.
40. Hansen D, Brock-Jacobsen B, Lund E, Bjorn C, Hansen LP, Nielsen C, et al. Clinical benefit of a gluten-free diet in type 1 diabetic children with screening-detected CD: a population-based screening study with 2 years' follow-up. Diabetes Care. 2006;29(11):2452–6.
41. Larsson K, Carlsson A, Cederwall E, Jonsson B, Neiderud J, Lernmark A, et al. Annual screening detects CD in children with type 1 diabetes. Pediatr Diabetes. 2008;9(4 Pt 2):354–9.
42. Ludvigsson JF, Ludvigsson J, Ekbom A, Montgomery SM. CD and risk of subsequent type 1 diabetes: a general population cohort study of children and adolescents. Diabetes Care. 2006;29(11):2483–8.
43. Smyth DJ, Plagnol V, Walker NM, Cooper JD, Downes K, Yang JH, et al. Shared and distinct genetic variants in type 1 diabetes and CD. N Engl J Med. 2008;359(26):2767–77.

44. Maglio M, Florian F, Vecchiet M, Auricchio R, Paparo F, Spadaro R, et al. Majority of children with type 1 diabetes produce and deposit anti-tissue transglutaminase antibodies in the small intestine. Diabetes. 2009;58(7):1578–84.
45. Narula P, Porter L, Langton J, Rao V, Davies P, Cummins C, et al. Gastrointestinal symptoms in children with type 1 diabetes screened for CD. Pediatrics. 2009;124(3):e489–95.
46. Taler I, Phillip M, Lebenthal Y, de Vries L, Shamir R, Shalitin S. Growth and metabolic control in patients with type 1 diabetes and CD: a longitudinal observational case-control study. Pediatr Diabetes. 2012;13(8):597–606.
47. Mollazadegan K, Kugelberg M, Montgomery SM, Sanders DS, Ludvigsson J, Ludvigsson JF. A population-based study of the risk of diabetic retinopathy in patients with type 1 diabetes and CD. Diabetes Care. 2012;36(2):316–21.
48. Pitocco D, Giubilato S, Martini F, Zaccardi F, Pazzano V, Manto A, et al. Combined atherogenic effects of CD and type 1 diabetes mellitus. Atherosclerosis. 2011;217(2):531–5.
49. Goh C, Banerjee K. Prevalence of coeliac disease in children and adolescents with type 1 diabetes mellitus in a clinic based population. Postgrad Med J. 2007;83(976):132–6.
50. Frohlich-Reiterer EE, Hofer S, Kaspers S, Herbst A, Kordonouri O, Schwarz HP, et al. Screening frequency for CD and autoimmune thyroiditis in children and adolescents with type 1 diabetes mellitus–data from a German/Austrian multicenter survey. Pediatr Diabetes. 2008;9(6):546–53.
51. Narula P, Porter L, Langton J, Rao V, Davies P, Cummins C, et al. Gastrointestinal symptoms in children with type 1 diabetes screened for CD. Pediatrics. 2009;124(3):e489–95.
52. Taler I, Phillip M, Lebenthal Y, de Vries L, Shamir R, Shalitin S. Growth and metabolic control in patients with type 1 diabetes and CD: a longitudinal observational case-control study. Pediatr Diabetes. 2012;13(8):597–606.
53. Hadithi M, de Boer H, Meijer JW, Willekens F, Kerckhaert JA, Heijmans R, et al. Coeliac disease in Dutch patients with Hashimoto's thyroiditis and vice versa. World J Gastroenterol. 2007;13(11):1715–22.
54. Sategna-Guidetti C, Volta U, Ciacci C, Usai P, Carlino A, De Franceschi L, et al. Prevalence of thyroid disorders in untreated adult CD patients and effect of gluten withdrawal: an Italian multicenter study. Am J Gastroenterol. 2001;96(3):751–7.
55. Elfstrom P, Montgomery SM, Kampe O, Ekbom A, Ludvigsson JF. Risk of thyroid disease in individuals with CD. J Clin Endocrinol Metab. 2008;93(10):3915–21.
56. Meloni A, Mandas C, Jores RD, Congia M. Prevalence of autoimmune thyroiditis in children with CD and effect of gluten withdrawal. J Pediatr. 2009;155(1):51–5, 55 e1.
57. Sari S, Yesilkaya E, Egritas O, Bideci A, Dalgic B. Prevalence of CD in Turkish children with autoimmune thyroiditis. Dig Dis Sci. 2009;54(4):830–2.
58. Collins D, Wilcox R, Nathan M, Zubarik R. CD and hypothyroidism. Am J Med. 2012;125(3):278–82.
59. Eapen CE, Nightingale P, Hubscher SG, Lane PJ, Plant T, Velissaris D, et al. Non-cirrhotic intrahepatic portal hypertension: associated gut diseases and prognostic factors. Dig Dis Sci. 2011;56(1):227–35.
60. Mounajjed T, Oxentenko A, Shmidt E, Smyrk T. The liver in CD: clinical manifestations, histologic features, and response to gluten-free diet in 30 patients. Am J Clin Pathol. 2011;136(1):128–37.
61. Ludvigsson JF, Elfstrom P, Broome U, Ekbom A, Montgomery SM. CD and risk of liver disease: a general population-based study. Clin Gastroenterol Hepatol. 2007;5(1):63–9 e1.
62. Lawson A, West J, Aithal GP, Logan RF. Autoimmune cholestatic liver disease in people with coeliac disease: a population-based study of their association. Aliment Pharmacol Ther. 2005;21(4):401–5.
63. Lewis NR, Sanders D, Teahon K, Logan RFA, Fleming KM, West J. Prevalence and consequence of hypertransaminaseaemia in incident coeliac disease; how common is it and does it matter? Gut. 2009;58(Suppl 1):A6.
64. Maggiore G, Caprai S. The liver in CD. J Pediatr Gastroenterol Nutr. 2003;37(2):117–9.

65. Elfstrom P, Montgomery SM, Kampe O, Ekbom A, Ludvigsson JF. Risk of primary adrenal insufficiency in patients with CD. J Clin Endocrinol Metab. 2007;92(9):3595–8.
66. Mollazadegan K, Kugelberg M, Tallstedt L, Ludvigsson JF. Increased risk of uveitis in coeliac disease: a nationwide cohort study. Br J Ophthalmol. 2012;96(6):857–61.
67. Olen O, Montgomery SM, Elinder G, Ekbom A, Ludvigsson JF. Increased risk of immune thrombocytopenic purpura among inpatients with coeliac disease. Scand J Gastroenterol. 2008;43(4):416–22.
68. Birkenfeld S, Dreiher J, Weitzman D, Cohen AD. Coeliac disease associated with psoriasis. Br J Dermatol. 2009;161(6):1331–4.
69. Ludvigsson JF, Lindelof B, Zingone F, Ciacci C. Psoriasis in a nationwide cohort study of patients with CD. J Invest Dermatol. 2011;131(10):2010–6.
70. Ludvigsson JF, Rubio-Tapia A, Chowdhary V, Murray JA, Simard JF. Increased risk of systemic lupus erythematosus in 29,000 patients with biopsy-verified CD. J Rheumatol. 2012;39(10):1964–70.
71. Ludvigsson JF, Kampe O, Lebwohl B, Green PH, Silverberg SJ, Ekbom A. Primary hyperparathyroidism and CD: a population-based cohort study. J Clin Endocrinol Metab. 2012;97(3):897–904.
72. Neuhausen SL, Steele L, Ryan S, Mousavi M, Pinto M, Osann KE, et al. Co-occurrence of CD and other autoimmune diseases in celiacs and their first-degree relatives. J Autoimmun. 2008;31(2):160–5.
73. Peters U, Askling J, Gridley G, Ekbom A, Linet M. Causes of death in patients with CD in a population-based Swedish cohort. Arch Intern Med. 2003;163(13):1566–72.
74. Patinen P, Aine L, Collin P, Hietanen J, Korpela M, Enckell G, et al. Oral findings in coeliac disease and Sjogren's syndrome. Oral Dis. 2004;10(6):330–4.
75. Kohler S, Wass JA. Hypoparathyroidism and coeliac disease: a potentially dangerous combination. J R Soc Med. 2009;102(8):311–4.
76. Collin P, Hakanen M, Salmi J, Maki M, Kaukinen K. Autoimmune hypopituitarism in patients with coeliac disease: symptoms confusingly similar. Scand J Gastroenterol. 2001;36(5):558–60.
77. Song MS, Farber D, Bitton A, Jass J, Singer M, Karpati G. Dermatomyositis associated with CD: response to a gluten-free diet. Can J Gastroenterol. 2006;20(6):433–5.
78. Gomez-Puerta JA, Gil V, Cervera R, Miquel R, Jimenez S, Ramos-Casals M, et al. Coeliac disease associated with systemic sclerosis. Ann Rheum Dis. 2004;63(1):104–5.
79. Corazza GR, Andreani ML, Venturo N, Bernardi M, Tosti A, Gasbarrini G. CD and alopecia areata: report of a new association. Gastroenterology. 1995;109(4):1333–7.
80. Freeman HJ, Gillett HR, Gillett PM, Oger J. Adult CD with acetylcholine receptor antibody positive myasthenia gravis. World J Gastroenterol. 2009;15(38):4741–4.
81. Whorwell PJ, Alderson MR, Foster KJ, Wright R. Death from ischaemic heart-disease and malignancy in adult patients with coeliac disease. Lancet. 1976;2(7977):113–4.
82. Corrao G, Corazza GR, Bagnardi V, Brusco G, Ciacci C, Cottone M, et al. Mortality in patients with coeliac disease and their relatives: a cohort study. Lancet. 2001;358(9279):356–61.
83. Grainge MJ, West J, Card TR, Holmes GK. Causes of death in people with CD spanning the pre- and post-serology era: a population-based cohort study from Derby, UK. Am J Gastroenterol. 2011;106(5):933–9.
84. Ludvigsson JF, Montgomery SM, Ekbom A, Brandt L, Granath F. Small-intestinal histopathology and mortality risk in CD. JAMA. 2009;302(11):1171–8.
85. Canavan C, Logan RF, Khaw KT, West J. No difference in mortality in undetected coeliac disease compared with the general population: a UK cohort study. Aliment Pharmacol Ther. 2011;34(8):1012–9.
86. Ludvigsson JF, de Faire U, Ekbom A, Montgomery SM. Vascular disease in a population-based cohort of individuals hospitalised with coeliac disease. Heart. 2007;93(9):1111–5.
87. Ludvigsson JF, James S, Askling J, Stenestrand U, Ingelsson E. Nationwide cohort study of risk of ischemic heart disease in patients with CD. Circulation. 2011;123(5):483–90.

88. West J, Logan RF, Card TR, Smith C, Hubbard R. Risk of vascular disease in adults with diagnosed coeliac disease: a population-based study. Aliment Pharmacol Ther. 2004;20(1):73–9.
89. Wei L, Spiers E, Reynolds N, Walsh S, Fahey T, MacDonald TM. The association between coeliac disease and cardiovascular disease. Aliment Pharmacol Ther. 2008;27(6):514–9.
90. Austin AS, Logan RF, Thomason K, Holmes GK. Cigarette smoking and adult coeliac disease. Scand J Gastroenterol. 2002;37(8):978–82.
91. Patel AH, Loftus Jr EV, Murray JA, Harmsen WS, Zinsmeister AR, Sandborn WJ. Cigarette smoking and celiac sprue: a case-control study. Am J Gastroenterol. 2001;96(8):2388–91.
92. Snook JA, Dwyer L, Lee-Elliott C, Khan S, Wheeler DW, Nicholas DS. Adult coeliac disease and cigarette smoking. Gut. 1996;39(1):60–2.
93. Ludvigsson JF, Montgomery SM, Ekbom A. Smoking and CD: a population-based cohort study. Clin Gastroenterol Hepatol. 2005;3(9):869–74.
94. Dickey W, Ward M, Whittle CR, Kelly MT, Pentieva K, Horigan G, et al. Homocysteine and related B-vitamin status in coeliac disease: effects of gluten exclusion and histological recovery. Scand J Gastroenterol. 2008;43(6):682–8.
95. Fonager K, Sorensen HT, Norgard B, Thulstrup AM. Cardiomyopathy in Danish patients with coeliac disease. Lancet. 1999;354(9189):1561.
96. Elfstrom P, Hamsten A, Montgomery SM, Ekbom A, Ludvigsson JF. Cardiomyopathy, pericarditis and myocarditis in a population-based cohort of inpatients with coeliac disease. J Intern Med. 2007;262(5):545–54.
97. Emilsson L, Andersson B, Elfstrom P, Green PH, Ludvigsson JF. Risk of idiopathic dilated cardiomyopathy in 29,000 patients with CD. J Am Heart Assoc. 2012;1(3):e001594.
98. Emilsson L, Smith JG, West J, Melander O, Ludvigsson JF. Increased risk of atrial fibrillation in patients with coeliac disease: a nationwide cohort study. Eur Heart J. 2011;32(19):2430–7.
99. Catassi C, Bearzi I, Holmes GK. Association of CD and intestinal lymphomas and other cancers. Gastroenterology. 2005;128(4 Suppl 1):S79–86.
100. Catassi C, Fabiani E, Corrao G, Barbato M, De Renzo A, Carella AM, et al. Risk of non-Hodgkin lymphoma in CD. JAMA. 2002;287(11):1413–9.
101. Smedby KE, Akerman M, Hildebrand H, Glimelius B, Ekbom A, Askling J. Malignant lymphomas in coeliac disease: evidence of increased risks for lymphoma types other than enteropathy-type T cell lymphoma. Gut. 2005;54(1):54–9.
102. Mearin ML, Catassi C, Brousse N, Brand R, Collin P, Fabiani E, et al. European multi-center study on coeliac disease and non-Hodgkin lymphoma. Eur J Gastroenterol Hepatol. 2006;18(2):187–94.
103. Anderson LA, McMillan SA, Watson RG, Monaghan P, Gavin AT, Fox C, et al. Malignancy and mortality in a population-based cohort of patients with coeliac disease or "gluten sensitivity". World J Gastroenterol. 2007;13(1):146–51.
104. Goldacre MJ, Wotton CJ, Yeates D, Seagroatt V, Jewell D. Cancer in patients with ulcerative colitis, Crohn's disease and coeliac disease: record linkage study. Eur J Gastroenterol Hepatol. 2008;20(4):297–304.
105. Gao Y, Kristinsson SY, Goldin LR, Bjorkholm M, Caporaso NE, Landgren O. Increased risk for non-Hodgkin lymphoma in individuals with CD and a potential familial association. Gastroenterology. 2009;136(1):91–8.
106. Elfstrom P, Granath F, Ekstrom Smedby K, Montgomery SM, Askling J, Ekbom A, et al. Risk of lymphoproliferative malignancy in relation to small intestinal histopathology among patients with CD. J Natl Cancer Inst. 2011;103(5):436–44.
107. Kane EV, Newton R, Roman E. Non-Hodgkin lymphoma and gluten-sensitive enteropathy: estimate of risk using meta-analyses. Cancer Causes Control. 2011;22(10):1435–44.
108. Tio M, Cox MR, Eslick GD. Meta-analysis: coeliac disease and the risk of all-cause mortality, any malignancy and lymphoid malignancy. Aliment Pharmacol Ther. 2012;35(5):540–51.

109. Ludvigsson JF. Commentary: coeliac disease, mortality and malignancy. Aliment Pharmacol Ther. 2012;35(7):839–40. discussion 40–2.
110. Elfstrom P, Granath F, Ye W, Ludvigsson JF. Low risk of gastrointestinal cancer among patients with CD, inflammation, or latent CD. Clin Gastroenterol Hepatol. 2012;10(1):30–6.
111. Viljamaa M, Kaukinen K, Pukkala E, Hervonen K, Reunala T, Collin P. Malignancies and mortality in patients with coeliac disease and dermatitis herpetiformis: 30-year population-based study. Dig Liver Dis. 2006;38(6):374–80.
112. Green PH, Fleischauer AT, Bhagat G, Goyal R, Jabri B, Neugut AI. Risk of malignancy in patients with CD. Am J Med. 2003;115(3):191–5.
113. Lewis NR, Logan R, Sanders D, Holmes. G, West J. Reproductive and hormonal factors for breast cancer among women with coeliac disease; a population-based questionnaire study. Gut. 2009;58(Suppl 2):A413.
114. Michels KB, Ekbom A. Caloric restriction and incidence of breast cancer. JAMA. 2004;291(10):1226–30.
115. Swinson CM, Slavin G, Coles EC, Booth CC. Coeliac disease and malignancy. Lancet. 1983;1(8316):111–5.
116. Ludvigsson JF, West J, Hubbard R, Card T. Neutral risk of lung cancer in adults with CD - nationwide cohort study. Lung Cancer. 2012;78(3):179–84.
117. Howdle PD, Jalal PK, Holmes GK, Houlston RS. Primary small-bowel malignancy in the UK and its association with coeliac disease. QJM. 2003;96(5):345–53.
118. Grainge MJ, West J, Solaymani-Dodaran M, Card TR, Logan RF. The long-term risk of malignancy following a diagnosis of coeliac disease or dermatitis herpetiformis: a cohort study. Aliment Pharmacol Ther. 2012;35(6):730–9.
119. Holmes GK, Prior P, Lane MR, Pope D, Allan RN. Malignancy in coeliac disease–effect of a gluten-free diet. Gut. 1989;30(3):333–8.
120. Delabie J, Holte H, Vose JM, Ullrich F, Jaffe ES, Savage KJ, et al. Enteropathy-associated T-cell lymphoma: clinical and histological findings from the international peripheral T-cell lymphoma project. Blood. 2011;118(1):148–55.
121. Tse E, Gill H, Loong F, Kim SJ, Ng SB, Tang T, et al. Type II enteropathy-associated T-cell lymphoma: a multicenter analysis from the Asia Lymphoma Study Group. Am J Hematol. 2012;87(7):663–8.
122. Deleeuw RJ, Zettl A, Klinker E, Haralambieva E, Trottier M, Chari R, et al. Whole-genome analysis and HLA genotyping of enteropathy-type T-cell lymphoma reveals 2 distinct lymphoma subtypes. Gastroenterology. 2007;132(5):1902–11.
123. Sieniawski M, Angamuthu N, Boyd K, Chasty R, Davies J, Forsyth P, et al. Evaluation of enteropathy-associated T-cell lymphoma comparing standard therapies with a novel regimen including autologous stem cell transplantation. Blood. 2010;115(18):3664–70.
124. Halfdanarson TR, Rubio-Tapia A, Ristow KM, Habermann TM, Murray JA, Inwards DJ. Patients with CD and B-cell lymphoma have a better prognosis than those with T-cell lymphoma. Clin Gastroenterol Hepatol. 2010;8(12):1042–7.
125. Landgren AM, Landgren O, Gridley G, Dores GM, Linet MS, Morton LM. Autoimmune disease and subsequent risk of developing alimentary tract cancers among 4.5 million US male veterans. Cancer. 2011;117(6):1163–71.
126. Volta U, Vincentini O, Silano M. Papillary cancer of thyroid in CD. J Clin Gastroenterol. 2011;45(5):e44–6.
127. Farre C, Domingo-Domenech E, Font R, Marques T, Fernandez de Sevilla A, Alvaro T, et al. CD and lymphoma risk: a multicentric case–control study in Spain. Dig Dis Sci. 2004;49(3):408–12.
128. Lohi S, Maki M, Montonen J, Knekt P, Pukkala E, Reunanen A, et al. Malignancies in cases with screening-identified evidence of coeliac disease: a long-term population-based cohort study. Gut. 2009;58(5):643–7.
129. Fine KD, Meyer RL, Lee EL. The prevalence and causes of chronic diarrhea in patients with celiac sprue treated with a gluten-free diet. Gastroenterology. 1997;112(6):1830–8.

130. Leffler DA, Dennis M, Hyett B, Kelly E, Schuppan D, Kelly CP. Etiologies and predictors of diagnosis in nonresponsive CD. Clin Gastroenterol Hepatol. 2007;5(4):445–50.
131. Dickey W, Hughes DF, McMillan SA. Disappearance of endomysial antibodies in treated CD does not indicate histological recovery. Am J Gastroenterol. 2000;95(3):712–4.
132. Cellier C, Delabesse E, Helmer C, Patey N, Matuchansky C, Jabri B, et al. Refractory sprue, coeliac disease, and enteropathy-associated T-cell lymphoma. French Coeliac Disease Study Group. Lancet. 2000;356(9225):203–8.
133. Al-Toma A, Verbeek WH, Hadithi M, von Blomberg BM, Mulder CJ. Survival in refractory coeliac disease and enteropathy-associated T-cell lymphoma: retrospective evaluation of single-center experience. Gut. 2007;56(10):1373–8.
134. Daum S, Ipczynski R, Schumann M, Wahnschaffe U, Zeitz M, Ullrich R. High rates of complications and substantial mortality in both types of refractory sprue. Eur J Gastroenterol Hepatol. 2009;21(1):66–70.
135. Malamut G, Afchain P, Verkarre V, Lecomte T, Amiot A, Damotte D, et al. Presentation and long-term follow-up of refractory CD: comparison of type 1 with type 1I. Gastroenterology. 2009;136(1):81–90.
136. Malamut G, Meresse B, Cellier C, Cerf-Bensussan N. Refractory CD: from bench to bedside. Semin Immunopathol. 2012;34(4):601–13.
137. Roshan B, Leffler DA, Jamma S, Dennis M, Sheth S, Falchuk K, et al. The incidence and clinical spectrum of refractory CD in a North American referral center. Am J Gastroenterol. 2011;106(5):923–8.
138. Rubio-Tapia A, Murray JA. Classification and management of refractory coeliac disease. Gut. 2010;59(4):547–57.
139. Malamut G, Cellier C. Is refractory CD more severe in old Europe? Am J Gastroenterol. 2011;106(5):929–32.
140. Meijer JW, Mulder CJ, Goerres MG, et al. Coeliac disease and (extra) intestinal T-cell lymphoma. Scand J Gastroenterol. 2004;S241:78–84.
141. Verbeek WH, Goerres MS, von Blomberg BM, Oudejans JJ, Scholten PE, Hadithi M, et al. Flow cytometric determination of aberrant intra-epithelial lymphocytes predicts T-cell lymphoma development more accurately than T-cell clonality analysis in refractory CD. Clin Immunol. 2008;126(1):48–56.
142. Lewis NR, Scott BB. Guidelines on osteoporosis in coeliac disease and inflammatory bowel disease. Glasgow: British Society of Gastroenterology; 2006.
143. Kanis JA, Johnell O, Oden A, Dawson A, De Laet C, Jonsson B. Ten year probabilities of osteoporotic fractures according to BMD and diagnostic thresholds. Osteoporos Int. 2001;12(12):989–95.
144. Valdimarsson T, Lofman O, Toss G, Strom M. Reversal of osteopenia with diet in adult coeliac disease. Gut. 1996;38(3):322–7.
145. McFarlane XA, Bhalla AK, Robertson DA. Effect of a gluten-free diet on osteopenia in adults with newly diagnosed coeliac disease. Gut. 1996;39(2):180–4.
146. Espallargues M, Sampietro-Colom L, Estrada MD, Sola M, del Rio L, Setoain J, et al. Identifying bone-mass-related risk factors for fracture to guide bone densitometry measurements: a systematic review of the literature. Osteoporos Int. 2001;12(10):811–22.
147. Hodkinson HM, McPherson CK. Alkaline phosphatase in a geriatric inpatient population. Age Ageing. 1973;2(1):28–33.
148. Peach H, Compston JE, Vedi S, Horton LW. Value of plasma calcium, phosphate, and alkaline phosphatase measurements in the diagnosis of histological osteomalacia. J Clin Pathol. 1982;35(6):625–30.
149. Kemppainen T, Kroger H, Janatuinen E, Arnala I, Lamberg-Allardt C, Karkkainen M, et al. Bone recovery after a gluten-free diet: a 5-year follow-up study. Bone. 1999;25(3):355–60.
150. Sategna-Guidetti C, Grosso SB, Grosso S, Mengozzi G, Aimo G, Zaccaria T, et al. The effects of 1-year gluten withdrawal on bone mass, bone metabolism and nutritional status in newly-diagnosed adult coeliac disease patients. Aliment Pharmacol Ther. 2000;14(1):35–43.

151. Holmes GKT. Neurological and psychiatric complications in coeliac disease. In: Epilepsy and other neurological disorders in coeliac disease, Chap. 34. Sydney: John Libbey; p. 251–64.
152. Ludvigsson JF, Olsson T, Ekbom A, Montgomery SM. A population-based study of coeliac disease, neurodegenerative and neuroinflammatory diseases. Aliment Pharmacol Ther. 2007;25(11):1317–27.
153. Pengiran Tengah DS, Wills AJ, Holmes GKT. Neurological complications of coeliac disease. Postgrad Med J. 2002;78(921):393–8.
154. Addolorato G, Mirijello A, D'Angelo C, Leggio L, Ferrulli A, Vonghia L, et al. Social phobia in coeliac disease. Scand J Gastroenterol. 2008;43(4):410–5.
155. Ludvigsson JF, Sellgren C, Runeson B, Langstrom N, Lichtenstein P. Increased suicide risk in coeliac disease–a Swedish nationwide cohort study. Dig Liver Dis. 2011;43(8):616–22.
156. Ludvigsson JF, Reutfors J, Osby U, Ekbom A, Montgomery SM. Coeliac disease and risk of mood disorders–a general population-based cohort study. J Affect Disord. 2007;99(1–3):117–26.
157. Garud S, Leffler D, Dennis M, Edwards-George J, Saryan D, Sheth S, et al. Interaction between psychiatric and autoimmune disorders in coeliac disease patients in the Northeastern United States. Aliment Pharmacol Ther. 2009;29(8):898–905.
158. Smith DF, Gerdes LU. Meta-analysis on anxiety and depression in adult CD. Acta Psychiatr Scand. 2012;125(3):189–93.
159. Zingone F, Siniscalchi M, Capone P, Tortora R, Andreozzi P, Capone E, et al. The quality of sleep in patients with coeliac disease. Aliment Pharmacol Ther. 2010;32(8):1031–6.
160. Pynnonen PA, Isometsa ET, Verkasalo MA, Kahkonen SA, Sipila I, Savilahti E, et al. Gluten-free diet may alleviate depressive and behavioural symptoms in adolescents with coeliac disease: a prospective follow-up case-series study. BMC Psychiatry. 2005;5:14.
161. Roos S, Karner A, Hallert C. Psychological well-being of adult coeliac patients treated for 10 years. Dig Liver Dis. 2006;38(3):177–80.
162. Hallert C, Svensson M, Tholstrup J, Hultberg B. Clinical trial: B vitamins improve health in patients with coeliac disease living on a gluten-free diet. Aliment Pharmacol Ther. 2009;29(8):811–6.
163. Cronin CC, Jackson LM, Feighery C, Shanahan F, Abuzakouk M, Ryder DQ, et al. Coeliac disease and epilepsy. QJM. 1998;91(4):303–8.
164. Pengiran Tengah DS, Holmes GK, Wills AJ. The prevalence of epilepsy in patients with CD. Epilepsia. 2004;45(10):1291–3.
165. Ranua J, Luoma K, Auvinen A, Maki M, Haapala AM, Peltola J, et al. CD-related antibodies in an epilepsy cohort and matched reference population. Epilepsy Behav. 2005;6(3):388–92.
166. Gobbi G, Bouquet F, Greco L, Lambertini A, Tassinari CA, Ventura A, et al. Coeliac disease, epilepsy, and cerebral calcifications. The Italian Working Group on Coeliac Disease and Epilepsy. Lancet. 1992;340(8817):439–43.
167. Johnson AM, Dale RC, Wienholt L, Hadjivassiliou M, Aeschlimann D, Lawson JA. Coeliac disease, epilepsy, and cerebral calcifications: association with TG6 autoantibodies. Dev Med Child Neurol. 2012;55(1):90–3.
168. Peltola M, Kaukinen K, Dastidar P, Haimila K, Partanen J, Haapala AM, et al. Hippocampal sclerosis in refractory temporal lobe epilepsy is associated with gluten sensitivity. J Neurol Neurosurg Psychiatry. 2009;80(6):626–30.
169. Gabrielli M, Cremonini F, Fiore G, Addolorato G, Padalino C, Candelli M, et al. Association between migraine and CD: results from a preliminary case-control and therapeutic study. Am J Gastroenterol. 2003;98(3):625–9.
170. Zelnik N, Pacht A, Obeid R, Lerner A. Range of neurologic disorders in patients with CD. Pediatrics. 2004;113(6):1672–6.
171. Eaton W, Mortensen PB, Agerbo E, Byrne M, Mors O, Ewald H. Coeliac disease and schizophrenia: population based case control study with linkage of Danish national registers. BMJ. 2004;328(7437):438–9.

172. West J, Logan RF, Hubbard RB, Card TR. Risk of schizophrenia in people with coeliac disease, ulcerative colitis and Crohn's disease: a general population-based study. Aliment Pharmacol Ther. 2006;23(1):71–4.
173. Collin P, Pirttila T, Nurmikko T, Somer H, Erila T, Keyrilainen O. CD, brain atrophy, and dementia. Neurology. 1991;41(3):372–5.
174. Casella S, Zanini B, Lanzarotto F, Ricci C, Marengoni A, Romanelli G, et al. Cognitive performance is impaired in coeliac patients on gluten-free diet: a case-control study in patients older than 65 years of age. Dig Liver Dis. 2012;44(9):729–35.
175. Hu WT, Murray JA, Greenaway MC, Parisi JE, Josephs KA. Cognitive impairment and CD. Arch Neurol. 2006;63(10):1440–6.
176. Rodrigo L, Hernandez-Lahoz C, Fuentes D, Alvarez N, Lopez-Vazquez A, Gonzalez S. Prevalence of CD in multiple sclerosis. BMC Neurol. 2011;11:31.
177. Hadjivassiliou M, Rao DG, Wharton SB, Sanders DS, Grunewald RA, Davies-Jones AG. Sensory ganglionopathy due to gluten sensitivity. Neurology. 2010;75(11):1003–8.
178. Hadjivassiliou M, Gibson A, Davies-Jones GA, Lobo AJ, Stephenson TJ, Milford-Ward A. Does cryptic gluten sensitivity play a part in neurological illness? Lancet. 1996;347(8998):369–71.
179. Hadjivassiliou M, Grunewald RA, Kandler RH, Chattopadhyay AK, Jarratt JA, Sanders DS, et al. Neuropathy associated with gluten sensitivity. J Neurol Neurosurg Psychiatry. 2006;77(11):1262–6.
180. Hadjivassiliou M, Sanders DS, Woodroofe N, Williamson C, Grunewald RA. Gluten ataxia. Cerebellum. 2008;7(3):494–8.
181. Hadjivassiliou M, Wallis LI, Hoggard N, Grunewald RA, Griffiths PD, Wilkinson ID. MR spectroscopy and atrophy in Gluten, Friedreich's and SCA6 ataxias. Acta Neurol Scand. 2012;126(2):138–43.
182. Hadjivassiliou M, Aeschlimann P, Strigun A, Sanders DS, Woodroofe N, Aeschlimann D. Autoantibodies in gluten ataxia recognize a novel neuronal transglutaminase. Ann Neurol. 2008;64(3):332–43.
183. Hadjivassiliou M, Sanders DS, Grunewald RA, Woodroofe N, Boscolo S, Aeschlimann D. Gluten sensitivity: from gut to brain. Lancet Neurol. 2010;9(3):318–30.
184. Rostami K, Steegers EA, Wong WY, Braat DD, Steegers-Theunissen RP. Coeliac disease and reproductive disorders: a neglected association. Eur J Obstet Gynecol Reprod Biol. 2001;96(2):146–9.
185. Ozgor B, Selimoglu MA. Coeliac disease and reproductive disorders. Scand J Gastroenterol. 2010;45(4):395–402.
186. Green PH, Jabri B. Coeliac disease. Lancet. 2003;362(9381):383–91.
187. Choi JM, Lebwohl B, Wang J, Lee SK, Murray JA, Sauer MV, et al. Increased prevalence of CD in patients with unexplained infertility in the United States. J Reprod Med. 2011;56(5–6):199–203.
188. Ciacci C, Cirillo M, Auriemma G, Di Dato G, Sabbatini F, Mazzacca G. CD and pregnancy outcome. Am J Gastroenterol. 1996;91(4):718–22.
189. Martinelli P, Troncone R, Paparo F, Torre P, Trapanese E, Fasano C, et al. Coeliac disease and unfavourable outcome of pregnancy. Gut. 2000;46(3):332–5.
190. Meloni GF, Dessole S, Vargiu N, Tomasi PA, Musumeci S. The prevalence of coeliac disease in infertility. Hum Reprod. 1999;14(11):2759–61.
191. Norgard B, Fonager K, Sorensen HT, Olsen J. Birth outcomes of women with CD: a nationwide historical cohort study. Am J Gastroenterol. 1999;94(9):2435–40.
192. Sher KS, Mayberry JF. Female fertility, obstetric and gynaecological history in coeliac disease: a case control study. Acta Paediatr Suppl. 1996;412:76–7.
193. Smecuol E, Maurino E, Vazquez H, Pedreira S, Niveloni S, Mazure R, et al. Gynaecological and obstetric disorders in coeliac disease: frequent clinical onset during pregnancy or the puerperium. Eur J Gastroenterol Hepatol. 1996;8(1):63–89.

194. Tata LJ, Card TR, Logan RF, Hubbard RB, Smith CJ, West J. Fertility and pregnancy-related events in women with CD: a population-based cohort study. Gastroenterology. 2005;128(4):849–55.
195. Lewis NR, Logan R, Sanders D, Holmes G, West J. Fertility and pregnancy related events in women with coeliac disease: a population based questionnaire. Gut. 2009;58(Suppl 2):A412.
196. Zugna D, Richiardi L, Akre O, Stephansson O, Ludvigsson JF. A nationwide population-based study to determine whether coeliac disease is associated with infertility. Gut. 2010;59(11):1471–5.
197. Hogen Esch CE, Van Rijssen MJ, Roos A, Koning F, Dekker FW, Mearin ML, et al. Screening for unrecognized coeliac disease in subfertile couples. Scand J Gastroenterol. 2011;46(12):1423–8.
198. Khashan AS, Henriksen TB, Mortensen PB, McNamee R, McCarthy FP, Pedersen MG, et al. The impact of maternal CD on birthweight and preterm birth: a Danish population-based cohort study. Hum Reprod. 2010;25(2):528–34.
199. Guidelines for the prevention and treatment of infection in patients with an absent or dysfunctional spleen. Working Party of the British Committee for Standards in Haematology Clinical Haematology Task Force. BMJ. 1996;312(7028):430–4.
200. Thomsen RW, Schoonen WM, Farkas DK, Riis A, Jacobsen J, Fryzek JP, et al. Risk for hospital contact with infection in patients with splenectomy: a population-based cohort study. Ann Intern Med. 2009;151(8):546–55.
201. Baker PG, Jones JV, Peacock DB, Read AE. The immune response of phiX 174 in man. III. Evidence for an association between hyposplenism and immunodeficiency in patients with coeliac disease. Gut. 1975;16(7):538–42.
202. Corazza GR, Frisoni M, Vaira D, Gasbarrini G. Effect of gluten-free diet on splenic hypofunction of adult coeliac disease. Gut. 1983;24(3):228–30.
203. Corazza GR, Lazzari R, Frisoni M, Collina A, Gasbarrini G. Splenic function in childhood coeliac disease. Gut. 1982;23(5):415–6.
204. Corazza GR, Zoli G, Di Sabatino A, Ciccocioppo R, Gasbarrini G. A reassessment of splenic hypofunction in CD. Am J Gastroenterol. 1999;94(2):391–7.
205. Croese J, Harris O, Bain B. Coeliac disease. Haematological features, and delay in diagnosis. Med J Aust. 1979;2(7):335–8.
206. Di Sabatino A, Rosado MM, Cazzola P, Riboni R, Biagi F, Carsetti R, et al. Splenic hypofunction and the spectrum of autoimmune and malignant complications in CD. Clin Gastroenterol Hepatol. 2006;4(2):179–86.
207. Marsh GW, Stewart JS. Splenic function in adult coeliac disease. Br J Haematol. 1970;19(4):445–57.
208. McCarthy CF, Fraser ID, Evans KT, Read AE. Lymphoreticular dysfunction in idiopathic steatorrhoea. Gut. 1966;7(2):140–8.
209. O'Grady JG, Stevens FM, Harding B, O'Gorman TA, McNicholl B, McCarthy CF. Hyposplenism and gluten-sensitive enteropathy. Natural history, incidence, and relationship to diet and small bowel morphology. Gastroenterology. 1984;87(6):1326–31.
210. O'Grady JG, Stevens FM, McCarthy CF. Genetic influences on splenic function in coeliac disease. Gut. 1985;26(10):1004–7.
211. Robertson DA, Swinson CM, Hall R, Losowsky MS. Coeliac disease, splenic function, and malignancy. Gut. 1982;23(8):666–9.
212. Robinson PJ, Bullen AW, Hall R, Brown RC, Baxter P, Losowsky MS. Splenic size and function in adult coeliac disease. Br J Radiol. 1980;53(630):532–7.
213. Trewby PN, Chipping PM, Palmer SJ, Roberts PD, Lewis SM, Stewart JS. Splenic atrophy in adult coeliac disease: is it reversible? Gut. 1981;22(8):628–32.
214. Ludvigsson JF, Olen O, Bell M, Ekbom A, Montgomery SM. Coeliac disease and risk of sepsis. Gut. 2008;57(8):1074–80.
215. Pebody RG, Hippisley-Cox J, Harcourt S, Pringle M, Painter M, Smith G. Uptake of pneumococcal polysaccharide vaccine in at-risk populations in England and Wales 1999-2005. Epidemiol Infect. 2008;136(3):360–9.

216. Yang A, Chen Y, Scherl E, Neugut AI, Bhagat G, Green PH. Inflammatory bowel disease in patients with CD. Inflamm Bowel Dis. 2005;11(6):528–32.
217. Leeds JS, Horoldt BS, Sidhu R, Hopper AD, Robinson K, Toulson B, et al. Is there an association between coeliac disease and inflammatory bowel diseases? A study of relative prevalence in comparison with population controls. Scand J Gastroenterol. 2007;42(10):1214–20.
218. Casella G, D'Inca R, Oliva L, Daperno M, Saladino V, Zoli G, et al. Prevalence of CD in inflammatory bowel diseases: an IG-IBD multicenter study. Dig Liver Dis. 2010;42(3): 175–78.
219. Green PH, Yang J, Cheng J, Lee AR, Harper JW, Bhagat G. An association between microscopic colitis and CD. Clin Gastroenterol Hepatol. 2009;7(11):1210–6.
220. Ford AC, Chey WD, Talley NJ, Malhotra A, Spiegel BM, Moayyedi P. Yield of diagnostic tests for CD in individuals with symptoms suggestive of irritable bowel syndrome: systematic review and meta-analysis. Arch Intern Med. 2009;169(7):651–8.
221. Cash BD, Rubenstein JH, Young PE, Gentry A, Nojkov B, Lee D, et al. The prevalence of CD among patients with nonconstipated irritable bowel syndrome is similar to controls. Gastroenterology. 2011;141(4):1187–93.
222. Thompson JS, Lebwohl B, Reilly NR, Talley NJ, Bhagat G, Green PH. Increased incidence of eosinophilic esophagitis in children and adults with CD. J Clin Gastroenterol. 2012;46(1): e6–e11.
223. Gonda TA, Khan SU, Cheng J, Lewis SK, Rubin M, Green PH. Association of intussusception and CD in adults. Dig Dis Sci. 2010;55(10):2899–903.
224. Reilly NR, Aguilar KM, Green PH. Should intussusception in children prompt screening for CD? J Pediatr Gastroenterol Nutr. 2013;56(1):56–9.
225. Sadr-Azodi O, Sanders DS, Murray JA, Ludvigsson JF. Patients with CD have an increased risk for pancreatitis. Clin Gastroenterol Hepatol. 2012;10(10):1136–42 e3.
226. Procaccini M, Campisi G, Bufo P, Compilato D, Massaccesi C, Catassi C, et al. Lack of association between CD and dental enamel hypoplasia in a case-control study from an Italian central region. Head Face Med. 2007;3:25.
227. Avsar A, Kalayci AG. The presence and distribution of dental enamel defects and caries in children with CD. Turk J Pediatr. 2008;50(1):45–50.
228. Cheng J, Malahias T, Brar P, Minaya MT, Green PH. The association between CD, dental enamel defects, and aphthous ulcers in a United States cohort. J Clin Gastroenterol. 2010;44(3):191–4.
229. El-Hodhod MA, El-Agouza IA, Abdel-Al H, Kabil NS, Bayomi KA. Screening for CD in children with dental enamel defects. ISRN Pediatr. 2012;2012:763783.
230. Bucci P, Carile F, Sangianantoni A, D'Angio F, Santarelli A, Lo Muzio L. Oral aphthous ulcers and dental enamel defects in children with coeliac disease. Acta Paediatr. 2006;95(2): 203–7.
231. Shakeri R, Zamani F, Sotoudehmanesh R, Amiri A, Mohamadnejad M, Davatchi F, et al. Gluten sensitivity enteropathy in patients with recurrent aphthous stomatitis. BMC Gastroenterol. 2009;9:44.
232. Campisi G, Di Liberto C, Carroccio A, Compilato D, Iacono G, Procaccini M, et al. Coeliac disease: oral ulcer prevalence, assessment of risk and association with gluten-free diet in children. Dig Liver Dis. 2008;40(2):104–7.
233. Wierink CD, van Diermen DE, Aartman IH, Heymans HS. Dental enamel defects in children with coeliac disease. Int J Paediatr Dent. 2007;17(3):163–8.
234. Ludvigsson JF, Inghammar M, Ekberg M, Egesten A. A nationwide cohort study of the risk of chronic obstructive pulmonary disease in coeliac disease. J Intern Med. 2012;271(5):481–9.
235. Ludvigsson JF, Hemminki K, Wahlstrom J, Almqvist C. CD confers a 1.6-fold increased risk of asthma: a nationwide population-based cohort study. J Allergy Clin Immunol. 2011;127(4): 1071–3.
236. Fluge G, Olesen HV, Gilljam M, Meyer P, Pressler T, Storrosten OT, et al. Co-morbidity of cystic fibrosis and CD in Scandinavian cystic fibrosis patients. J Cyst Fibros. 2009;8(3): 198–202.

237. Walkowiak J, Blask-Osipa A, Lisowska A, Oralewska B, Pogorzelski A, Cichy W, et al. Cystic fibrosis is a risk factor for CD. Acta Biochim Pol. 2010;57(1):115–8.
238. Ludvigsson JF, Sanders DS, Maeurer M, Jonsson J, Grunewald J, Wahlstrom J. Risk of tuberculosis in a large sample of patients with coeliac disease–a nationwide cohort study. Aliment Pharmacol Ther. 2011;33(6):689–96.
239. Ludvigsson JF, Welander A, Lassila R, Ekbom A, Montgomery SM. Risk of thromboembolism in 14,000 individuals with coeliac disease. Br J Haematol. 2007;139(1):121–7.
240. Johannesdottir SA, Erichsen R, Horvath-Puho E, Schmidt M, Sorensen HT. Coeliac disease and risk of venous thromboembolism: a nationwide population-based case-control study. Br J Haematol. 2012;157(4):499–501.
241. Ludvigsson JF, Zingone F, Fored M, Ciacci C, Cirillo M. Moderately increased risk of urinary stone disease in patients with biopsy-verified coeliac disease. Aliment Pharmacol Ther. 2012;35(4):477–84.
242. Ciacci C, Spagnuolo G, Tortora R, Bucci C, Franzese D, Zingone F, et al. Urinary stone disease in adults with CD: prevalence, incidence and urinary determinants. J Urol. 2008;180(3):974–9.
243. Welander A, Prutz KG, Fored M, Ludvigsson JF. Increased risk of end-stage renal disease in individuals with coeliac disease. Gut. 2012;61(1):64–8.
244. Stephansson O, Falconer H, Ludvigsson JF. Risk of endometriosis in 11,000 women with CD. Hum Reprod. 2011;26(10):2896–901.
245. Hwang E, McBride R, Neugut AI, Green PH. Sarcoidosis in patients with CD. Dig Dis Sci. 2008;53(4):977–81.
246. Ludvigsson JF, Wahlstrom J, Grunewald J, Ekbom A, Montgomery SM. Coeliac disease and risk of sarcoidosis. Sarcoidosis Vasc Diffuse Lung Dis. 2007;24(2):121–6.
247. Rutherford RM, Brutsche MH, Kearns M, Bourke M, Stevens F, Gilmartin JJ. Prevalence of coeliac disease in patients with sarcoidosis. Eur J Gastroenterol Hepatol. 2004;16(9):911–5.
248. Wouters J, Weijerman ME, van Furth AM, Schreurs MW, Crusius JB, von Blomberg BM, et al. Prospective human leukocyte antigen, endomysium immunoglobulin A antibodies, and transglutaminase antibodies testing for CD in children with Down syndrome. J Pediatr. 2009;154(2):239–42.
249. Giannotti A, Tiberio G, Castro M, Virgilii F, Colistro F, Ferretti F, et al. Coeliac disease in Williams syndrome. J Med Genet. 2001;38(11):767–8.
250. Frost AR, Band MM, Conway GS. Serological screening for coeliac disease in adults with Turner's syndrome: prevalence and clinical significance of endomysium antibody positivity. Eur J Endocrinol. 2009;160(4):675–9.
251. Sagodi L, Solyom E, Tamasi K, Minik K. [Prevalence of CD in Turner syndrome]. Orv Hetil. 2006;147(25):1185–8.
252. Marks J, Shuster S, Watson AJ. Small-bowel changes in dermatitis herpetiformis. Lancet. 1966;2(7476):1280–2.
253. Shuster S, Watson AJ, Marks J. Coeliac syndrome in dermatitis herpetiformis. Lancet. 1968;1(7552):1101–6.
254. Fry L, McMinn RM, Cowan JD, Hoffbrand AV. Effect of gluten-free diet on dermatological, intestinal, and haematological manifestations of dermatitis herpetiformis. Lancet. 1968;1(7542):557–61.
255. Swerdlow AJ, Whittaker S, Carpenter LM, English JS. Mortality and cancer incidence in patients with dermatitis herpetiformis: a cohort study. Br J Dermatol. 1993;129(2):140–4.
256. Collin P, Pukkala E, Reunala T. Malignancy and survival in dermatitis herpetiformis: a comparison with coeliac disease. Gut. 1996;38(4):528–30.
257. Leonard JN, Tucker WF, Fry JS, Coulter CA, Boylston AW, McMinn RM, et al. Increased incidence of malignancy in dermatitis herpetiformis. Br Med J (Clin Res Ed). 1983;286(6358):16–8.
258. Gawkrodger DJ, Blackwell JN, Gilmour HM, Rifkind EA, Heading RC, Barnetson RS. Dermatitis herpetiformis: diagnosis, diet and demography. Gut. 1984;25(2):151–7.

259. Sigurgeirsson B, Agnarsson BA, Lindelof B. Risk of lymphoma in patients with dermatitis herpetiformis. BMJ. 1994;308(6920):13–5.
260. Lewis NR, Logan RF, Hubbard RB, West J. No increase in risk of fracture, malignancy or mortality in dermatitis herpetiformis: a cohort study. Aliment Pharmacol Ther. 2008;27(11):1140–7.
261. Biagi F, Corazza GR. Mortality in CD. Nat Rev Gastroenterol Hepatol. 2010;7(3):158–62.
262. Poynton FJ, Cole LB. A case of coeliac disease with glycosuria. Br J Childhood Dis. 1925;22:30–6.
263. Finlay JM, Wightman KJR. Modern treatment of the malabsorption syndrome in adults. Ann Intern Med. 1956;45:191–206.

Chapter 16
Refractory Celiac Disease

Georgia Malamut and Christophe Cellier

Introduction

Celiac disease (CD) is a small-intestinal enteropathy induced by gluten in genetically predisposed individuals with HLA DQ2/DQ8 genotype. Its prevalence is 1 % in Europe and the USA. Its clinical presentation is hypervariable, and diagnosis relies on the detection of specific serum antibodies and on the demonstration of intestinal villous atrophy. Treatment relies on a lifelong gluten-free diet (GFD), which prevents bone, autoimmune, and malignant complications. Resistance to a GFD is mainly due to bad observance. Nevertheless, a small subgroup of CD patients may be primarily or secondarily resistant to a GFD due to an authentic refractory celiac disease (RCD).

Poor adherence to a GFD needs to be first excluded accordingly with the fact that less than 50 % of patients are compliant [1]. Persistent symptoms of malabsorption and intestinal villous atrophy after at least 12 months of a strict GFD define RCD. Diagnosis of this condition is made after exclusion of other small bowel diseases such as autoimmune enteropathy [2], tropical sprue [3], or common variable immunodeficiency [4].

RCD has been subdivided into two subgroups:

1. Type 1 RCD (RCDI) is defined by persisting villous atrophy despite a strict GFD associated with an increased number of intraepithelial lymphocytes (IEL) bearing a normal phenotype with surface CD3 and CD8 expression.
2. Type II RCD (RCDII) is characterized by clonal expansion of abnormal IEL lacking surface markers CD3, CD8, and T-cell receptor (TCR) (CD3s-, CD8s-, TCR-) and preserved expression of intracellular CD3 [5, 6].

G. Malamut, M.D., Ph.D. • C. Cellier, M.D., Ph.D. (✉)
Department of Gastroenterology, Hôpital Européen Georges Pompidou, 20 rue Leblanc,
Inserm U989 Université Paris Descartes, Paris 75015, France
e-mail: christophe.cellier@egp.aphp.fr

S.D. Rampertab and G.E. Mullin (eds.), *Celiac Disease*, Clinical Gastroenterology,
DOI 10.1007/978-1-4614-8560-5_16, © Springer Science+Business Media New York 2014

Frequency of RCDI and RCDII remains unknown. In the Derby cohort, West and Holmes report approximately 0.7 % of RCDII patients in a series of 713 celiac patients [7]. In this latest study, diagnosis of RCDII patients was made solely on the basis of ulcerative jejunitis [7], causing possible errors leading to underestimates of RCDII and overestimation of RCDI. A second recent study in a single North American referral center suggests a cumulative incidence of 1.5 % for both RCDI and RCDII among CD patients initially diagnosed in this center [8]. In this study, over 80 % of RCD patients were classified as type 1. A higher frequency of cases of RCDI than of RCDII was also observed in two other studies from the USA [9] and from Germany [10]. In contrast, a higher frequency of RCDII over RCDI was reported in two studies from Holland [11] and from France [12].

Diagnosis

Diagnosis of RCD relies on persistent malabsorption and villous atrophy after 1 year of strict GFD ascertained by a dietitian. Endoscopic assessment includes upper gastrointestinal endoscopy with biopsy. Double-balloon enteroscopy is required in suspicion of RCDII for a better assessment of ulcers, particularly for evidence of ulcerative jejunitis found in roughly 70 % of patients [12, 13].

Capsule endoscopy is useful by giving the extent of lesions. Capsule endoscopy has a superior accuracy in predicting villous atrophy than optical endoscopy [14, 15]. Furthermore, besides the diagnosis of persistent villous atrophy, capsule endoscopy allows the visualization of ulcers all along the intestinal tract, which may suggest RCDII before diagnostic confirmation [16]. Moreover, we experienced three cases of overt lymphoma revealed by capsule endoscopy, which presented with very suspicious intestinal strictures and jejunal ulcers [17]. Double-balloon enteroscopy, reaching the distal small bowel in the three cases, confirmed the capsule findings [15, 17].

Thus, the limitation of capsule endoscopy is the risk of retention, particularly in RCDII patients who are particularly at risk for strictures. It requires preliminary radiological imaging of the small bowel in order to rule out stricturing disease. The second limitation is the need of biopsy during endoscopy for definitive diagnosis.

In RCDI, histological examination is similar to that found in active celiac disease with villous atrophy and increased normal IEL. No other diagnostic criteria have been yet defined for RCDI. In contrast, the hallmark abnormal population, detected by three combined techniques, makes the diagnosis of RCDII more specific: over 25 % of the CD103+ or CD45+ IEL lacking surface CD3-T-cell receptor complexes on flow cytometry or more than 50 % IEL expressing intracellular CD3ε but no CD8 in formalin-fixed sections and/or the presence of a detectable clonal rearrangement of the gamma chain of the TCR in duodenal biopsies [12]. Similar features allow detecting lymphocytic gastritis and colitis containing the same abnormal population in around 50 % and 30 % of RCDII patients, respectively [12] (Table 16.1).

Table 16.1 Main criteria to differentiate RCDI and RCDII

Criteria	RCDI	RCDII
Ulcerative jejunitis	–	+
Abnormal phenotype of intraepithelial lymphocytes	–	+
Clonal rearrangement of TCR	–	+
Very increased risk of EATL	–	+
Poor prognosis (5-year survival of 50 %)	–	+

RCDII may be misdiagnosed when flow cytometry analysis of freshly isolated IEL is lacking. Discrepancies in diagnosis tools are probably involved in differences observed between European and North American countries [8, 9, 18]. Indeed, flow cytometry is commonly used in Europe for the diagnosis of aberrant IEL and is a technique that is more sensitive and more precise than immunohistochemistry [18]. Heterogeneity in detection of the clonal TCR rearrangement may also explain diagnostic differences, and specificity of the PCR product needs to be attested by formation of homoduplexes [12].

Clinical Forms and Prognosis

Primary resistance to a GFD is seen in roughly one-third to one-half of patients with RCDI and RCDII, respectively [12]. Besides the abnormal phenotype of IEL, RCDII has a more severe clinical presentation and is frequently associated with endoscopic ulcerative jejunitis responsible for severe protein loss enteropathy. Symptoms are notably less severe in RCDI, and endoscopic and histological features are similar to those found in active CD [12]. RCDII is associated with poor prognosis with 5-year survival rates of 44–58 % [9, 11, 12]. The more severe malnutrition combined with the higher risk of developing overt lymphoma explains the higher mortality in RCDII when compared to RCDI [12]. Even if the prognosis of RCDI is much better than RCDII, the mortality rate appears higher than in uncomplicated CD [9, 10].

There is as yet no curative treatment for RCD. Immunosuppressive drugs have only a poor effect on the histological response and may predispose to overt lymphoma [19]. Indeed, 33–52 % of RCDII patients develop enteropathy-associated T-cell lymphoma (EATL) within 5 years after diagnosis of RCDII is made [11, 12]. Onset of EATL in RCDI is much lower than in RCDII, with a 5-year rate of 14 % in the more conservative studies [12]. The higher risk of transformation into overt lymphoma in RCDII is due to its state of low-grade intraepithelial lymphoma [6]. Indeed, at this stage, clonal IEL are already engaged in malignant transformation as attested by their clonality, the presence of their chromosomal abnormalities, the recurrent partial trisomy 1q22-q44, and their tendency to disseminate in and outside the intestine [12, 20].

Abnormal IEL may be found in mesenteric lymph nodes, blood, bone marrow, and in different epitheliums such as lung and skin [12]. A high percentage of abnormal cells (up to 92 %) is predictive of abnormal circulating cells in peripheral blood [21]. Diagnosis of extraintestinal RCDII lesions can be performed by evidence of the same clonal TCR γ/δ chain rearrangement that is present in duodenum but also by immunohistochemistry.

EATL may develop in intestinal but also in cutaneous lesions of RCDII, with expression of the same IEL-specific integrin CD103. The clonal filiation between RCDII IEL and EATL is demonstrated by presence of the same TCRγ chain rearrangement [6]. In practice, regular follow-up, including control enteroscopy, computed tomography scan (CT-scan) or MRI small bowel follow-through, and positron emission tomography (PET) scan, is necessary to screen EATL as early as possible. No established interval has been yet defined. Specialized investigations can be reasonably performed every year and 6 months in RCDI and RCDII patients, respectively [12]. PET scan is of particular interest because high intensity is correlated with location of proliferating overt lymphoma cells [22] contrasting with the low intensity of nonproliferating RCDII cells [23]. It can further guide realization of radiological guided biopsy or explorative laparoscopy.

Pathogenesis

It is still debated whether RCD patients have a particular genetic background differentiating them from patients with uncomplicated CD. The small numbers of patients are the main limitations of genetic investigations. It has been reported that severity of celiac disease was correlated with the number of HLA-DQ2 copies: homozygosity for HLA-DQ2 was observed in 25.5 % of RCD I, 44.1 % of RCD II, and 53.3 % of EATL patients versus 20.7 % of uncomplicated CD patients and 2.1 % of controls [24]. Other genes involved in lymphocyte signaling (genes: *SH2B3* (12q34), *PTPN2* (18q11), *RGS1* (1q31)) and associated with celiac disease may be involved in the risk of developing lymphoma [25]. Studies are in progress, and ongoing genome-wide association studies suggest that the known celiac susceptibility variants may be not found in RCDII [26].

Exposure to gluten appears to be an important environmental factor as it increases the risk of autoimmune diseases and malignancies [27]. Risk of lymphomatous complications was reported to be four times higher in patients without observance to a GFD than compliant patients [28]. The amount of gluten consumption could be responsible for the differences in terms of severity of CD. A recent study reports a more severe outcome of CD in South compared to North Europe in relationship to a higher gluten intake [29]. The scientific rationale may rely on more intense production, under gluten exposure, of the cytokine IL-15, now known to play a key role in the progression of lymphoma associated with CD [30].

Infections, particularly viral infections, may constitute another environmental factor favoring emergence of RCD. Epidemiological factors argue that viral infections such as rotavirus infection may increase the risk of CD in genetically predisposed individuals [31]. We can hypothesize that viral infection triggers inflammation and autoimmunity by hyperproduction of IL-15. Indeed, IL-15 is induced by a variety of intracellular pathogens [32]. We observed hepatitis B or C at onset of refractoriness in 20 % and 10 % of RCDI and RCDII patients, respectively [12].

The role of viruses in the pathogenesis of chronic inflammatory and autoimmune diseases is a popular hypothesis supported by a large number of studies. More than a specific virus, it is rather suspected that components of the antiviral responses and notably type 1 interferons might promote the onset of chronic inflammatory disorders (reviewed in [33]). Type 1 interferon may notably stimulate the survival and proliferation of CD8+ T cells and NK cells [34] either directly or via the induction of IL-15 [35]. We can hypothesize that such a mechanism may occur in RCDI, helping the immunological reaction initiated by gluten to evolve toward autoimmunity. Accordingly, symptoms improve under immunosuppressive treatments [11, 12]. However, mechanisms of RCDI are largely unknown and remain to be substantiated.

More progress has been performed recently in the understanding of the pathogenesis of RCDII. The phenotype is now well defined with accumulation of small clonal IEL without proliferation but with apoptosis defect [30]. In active CD and RCDII, IL-15 is produced in excess by enterocytes and lamina propria mononuclear cells. IELs are, in CD and RCD, enriched in cytolytic proteins (perforin, granzymes, Fas ligand) and produce large amounts of interferon gamma (IFN-γ), indicating their likely contribution to the prominent apoptosis observed in the flattened-surface epithelium [30, 36, 37]. The granzyme-perforin cytotoxicity accounts for the severe epithelial lesions observed in RCDII. Moreover, IL-15 exerts potent antiapoptotic effects that prevent the elimination of activated IELs and promote their massive accumulation [30]. Survival signal delivered by IL-15 requires, through the receptor of IL-15, IL-15Rβγ, activation of Jak3, STAT5, and the antiapoptotic factor Bcl-xL. Human anti-IL-15 antibodies inhibit ex vivo the IL-15-driven signaling pathway in intestinal organotypic cultures of RCDII patients. In vivo, treatment of mice overexpressing human IL-15 in the small bowel with this antibody wiped out the IEL hyperplasia observed in these mice [38].

Treatments

It has not yet been possible to design an effective treatment for RCD I or II. Steroids improved clinical symptoms in most patients with either type of RCD. Yet a histological response was observed only in 30–40 % of cases [12]. Steroid dependence and/or resistance requires trials of immunosuppressive agents such as azathioprine, cyclosporine, or anti-TNF-α with transient clinical response but rare mucosal improvement [12]. In RCDI, no scientific rationale has yet been established to treat specifically RCDI patients with targeted therapy.

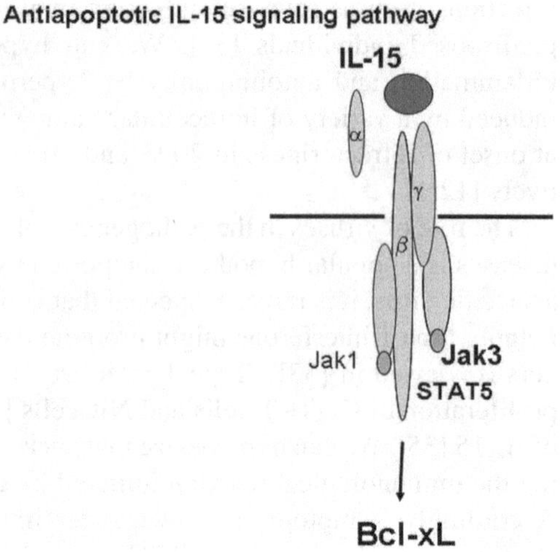

Fig. 16.1 Antiapoptotic IL-15 signaling pathway

In RCDII immunosuppressive drugs have, as could be expected, no impact on the abnormal clonal IEL population and could enhance the risk of overt lymphoma as observed with azathioprine and anti-CD52 [12, 19]. The bad prognosis of RCDII led to more aggressive treatments such as chemotherapy. Contrary to EATL which expressed Ki67, RCDII is characterized by onset of IEL with abnormal phenotype which massively accumulated without in situ detectable proliferation [30]. The non-proliferative RCDII cells are thus difficult to eradicate by regular chemotherapy [12] and may represent a reservoir of cells susceptible to more aggressive transformation.

Purine analogues such as pentostatine or cladribine (2CDA) showed moderate clinical, histological, and hematological efficacies [39, 40]. In our retrospective study of RCDII patients [12], 2CDA induced clinical and histological response. However, explosive onset of overt lymphoma was observed in the two treated patients within 3–8 weeks after treatment, precluding further use of these drugs inasmuch as enhanced risk of transformation into overt lymphoma has been previously observed in a series of 17 RCDII patients treated with 2CDA [40].

One possible alternative strategy is the use of the autologous hematopoietic stem cell transplantation which induced clinical and histological response, but no sustained reduction of abnormal IEL in the 13 treated patients [41, 42]. The use of chemotherapy before autologous hematopoietic stem cell transplantation may probably increase hematological response, and we are currently evaluating this strategy in a prospective phase II trial. Setting up targeted strategy appears necessary to complete the therapeutic armory to treat RCDII and to prevent overt lymphoma, whose prognosis is even worse than RCDII. Only 20 % of patients are alive 5 years after the diagnosis of lymphoma [43–45].

Targeted therapy blocking IL-15 signalling appears the treatment of choice in RCDII but needs to be tested in clinical trials [38] (Fig. 16.1). The recent development of a humanized anti-IL-15 antibody which has already been used without any major side effects in a phase I–II trial in rheumatoid arthritis suggests the feasibility of this therapeutic approach [46]. Another possibility is to block the downstream molecules activated by IL-15. JAK3 inhibitor, currently used in treating rheumatoid arthritis [47], is another interesting drug to treat RCDII [48]. Treatment of RCDII will probably combine, in the near future, conventional chemotherapy agents and targeted therapy by anti-IL-15 antibodies or inhibitors of downstream activated molecules.

Conclusion

In conclusion, RCD refers to two distinct entities. On one hand, RCDI is indistinguishable from uncomplicated active CD except its autonomy toward gluten exposure, which probably relies on self-perpetuated autoimmune mechanisms. On the other hand, RCDII is a low-grade lymphoma characterized by clonal expansion of small aberrant IEL. Small bowel investigations (enteroscopy, videocapsule endoscopy) and specialized techniques of IEL analyses (immunohistochemistry, molecular biology, flow cytometry) are necessary for diagnosis of both forms of RCD. Prognosis of RCDII is very poor due to incurable malnutrition and very high risk of overt lymphoma. Survival of RCDI is better than in RCDII but inferior to CD survival [9, 12]. Recent advances in dissecting the pathogenesis of CD and RCD intend to hope next efficient treatments for these rare but severe diseases.

Acknowledgments We thank Nadine Cerf-Bensussan and Bertrand Meresse (Inserm U989, Université Paris Descartes) for collaboration for the figure.

References

1. Vahedi K, Mascart F, Mary JY, Laberenne JE, Bouhnik Y, Morin MC, et al. Reliability of antitransglutaminase antibodies as predictors of gluten-free diet compliance in adult celiac disease. Am J Gastroenterol. 2003;98(5):1079–87.
2. Akram S, Murray JA, Pardi DS, Alexander GL, Schaffner JA, Russo PA, et al. Adult autoimmune enteropathy: Mayo Clinic Rochester experience. Clin Gastroenterol Hepatol. 2007;5(11):1282–90.
3. Khokhar N, Gill ML. Tropical sprue: revisited. J Pak Med Assoc. 2004;54(3):133–4.
4. Malamut G, Verkarre V, Suarez F, Viallard JF, Lascaux AS, Cosnes J, et al. The enteropathy associated with common variable immunodeficiency: the delineated frontiers with celiac disease. Am J Gastroenterol. 2010;105(10):2262–75.
5. Cellier C, Patey N, Mauvieux L, Jabri B, Delabesse E, Cervoni JP, et al. Abnormal intestinal intraepithelial lymphocytes in refractory sprue. Gastroenterology. 1998;114(3):471–81.
6. Cellier C, Delabesse E, Helmer C, Patey N, Matuchansky C, Jabri B, et al. Refractory sprue, coeliac disease, and enteropathy-associated T-cell lymphoma. French Coeliac Disease Study Group. Lancet. 2000;356(9225):203–8.
7. West J. Celiac disease and its complications: a time traveller's perspective. Gastroenterology. 2009;136(1):32–4.

8. Roshan B, Leffler DA, Jamma S, Dennis M, Sheth S, Falchuk K, et al. The incidence and clinical spectrum of refractory celiac disease in a North American referral center. Am J Gastroenterol. 2011;106(5):923–8.
9. Rubio-Tapia A, Kelly DG, Lahr BD, Dogan A, Wu TT, Murray JA. Clinical staging and survival in refractory celiac disease: a single center experience. Gastroenterology. 2009;136(1):99–107.
10. Daum S, Ipczynski R, Schumann M, Wahnschaffe U, Zeitz M, Ullrich R. High rates of complications and substantial mortality in both types of refractory sprue. Eur J Gastroenterol Hepatol. 2009;21(1):66–70.
11. Al-Toma A, Verbeek WH, Hadithi M, von Blomberg BM, Mulder CJ. Survival in refractory coeliac disease and enteropathy associated T cell lymphoma: retrospective evaluation of single center experience. Gut. 2007;56:1373–8.
12. Malamut G, Afchain P, Verkarre V, Lecomte T, Amiot A, Damotte D, et al. Presentation and long-term follow-up of refractory celiac disease: comparison of type 1 with type II. Gastroenterology. 2009;136(1):81–90.
13. Daum S, Cellier C, Mulder CJ. Refractory coeliac disease. Best Pract Res. 2005;19(3):413–24.
14. Murray JA, Rubio-Tapia A, Van Dyke CT, Brogan DL, Knipschield MA, Lahr B, et al. Mucosal atrophy in celiac disease: extent of involvement, correlation with clinical presentation, and response to treatment. Clin Gastroenterol Hepatol. 2008;6(2):186–93.
15. Malamut G, Murray JA, Cellier C. Refractory celiac disease. Gastrointest Endosc Clin N Am. 2012;22(4):759–72.
16. Daum S, Wahnschaffe U, Glasenapp R, Borchert M, Ullrich R, Zeitz M, et al. Capsule endoscopy in refractory celiac disease. Endoscopy. 2007;39(5):455–8.
17. Barret M, Malamut G, Rahmi G, Samaha A, Edery J, Verkarre V, Macintyre E, Lenain E, Châtellier G, Cerf-Bensussan N, Cellier C. Diagnostic yield of capsule endoscopy in refractory celiac disease. Am J Gastroenterol. 2012;107(10):1546–53.
18. Malamut G, Cellier C. Is refractory celiac disease more severe in old Europe? Am J Gastroenterol. 2013;106(5):929–32.
19. Goerres MS, Meijer JW, Wahab PJ, Kerckhaert JA, Groenen PJ, Van Krieken JH, et al. Azathioprine and prednisone combination therapy in refractory coeliac disease. Aliment Pharmacol Ther. 2003;18(5):487–94.
20. Verkarre V, Romana SP, Cellier C, Asnafi V, Mention JJ, Barbe U, et al. Recurrent partial trisomy 1q22-q44 in clonal intraepithelial lymphocytes in refractory celiac sprue. Gastroenterology. 2003;125(1):40–6.
21. Malamut G, Verkarre V, Meresse B, Macintyre E, Brousse N, Cerf-Bensussan N, Cellier C. High rate of abnormal intestinal intraepithelial lymphocytes is predictive of extra-digestive diffusion in refractory coeliac disease [Abstract]. Gut. 2008;57(suppl II):A30.
22. Malamut G, Chandesris O, Verkarre V, Meresse B, Callens C, Macintyre E, et al. Enteropathy associated T cell lymphoma in celiac disease: a large retrospective study. Dig Liver Dis. 2013;45(5):377–84.
23. Hoffmann M, Vogelsang H, Kletter K, Zettinig G, Chott A, Raderer M. 18F-fluoro-deoxyglucose positron emission tomography (18F-FDG-PET) for assessment of enteropathy-type T cell lymphoma. Gut. 2003;52(3):347–51.
24. Al-Toma A, Goerres MS, Meijer JW, Pena AS, Crusius JB, Mulder CJ. Human leukocyte antigen-DQ2 homozygosity and the development of refractory celiac disease and enteropathy-associated T-cell lymphoma. Clin Gastroenterol Hepatol. 2006;4(3):315–9.
25. Smyth DJ, Plagnol V, Walker NM, Cooper JD, Downes K, Yang JH, et al. Shared and distinct genetic variants in type 1 diabetes and celiac disease. N Engl J Med. 2008;359(26):2767–77.
26. Wijmenga C. Genetic and risk for associated autoimmune disorders and refractory coeliac disease (abstract). Mastering the coeliac condition, 2012, Florence, Italy.

27. Askling J, Linet M, Gridley G, Halstensen TS, Ekstrom K, Ekbom A. Cancer incidence in a population-based cohort of individuals hospitalized with celiac disease or dermatitis herpetiformis. Gastroenterology. 2002;123(5):1428–35.
28. Holmes GK, Prior P, Lane MR, Pope D, Allan RN. Malignancy in coeliac disease–effect of a gluten free diet. Gut. 1989;30(3):333–8.
29. Biagi F, Corazza GR. Mortality in celiac disease. Nat Rev Gastroenterol Hepatol. 2011;7(3):158–62.
30. Mention JJ, Ben Ahmed M, Begue B, Barbe U, Verkarre V, Asnafi V, et al. Interleukin 15: a key to disrupted intraepithelial lymphocyte homeostasis and lymphomagenesis in celiac disease. Gastroenterology. 2003;125(3):730–45.
31. Stene LC, Honeyman MC, Hoffenberg EJ, Haas JE, Sokol RJ, Emery L, et al. Rotavirus infection frequency and risk of celiac disease autoimmunity in early childhood: a longitudinal study. Am J Gastroenterol. 2006;101(10):2333–40.
32. Waldmann TA, Tagaya Y. The multifaceted regulation of interleukin-15 expression and the role of this cytokine in NK cell differentiation and host response to intracellular pathogens. Annu Rev Immunol. 1999;17:19–49.
33. Foxman EF, Iwasaki A. Genome-virome interactions: examining the role of common viral infections in complex disease. Nat Rev Microbiol. 2011;4:254–64.
34. Gough DJ, Messina NL, Clarke CJ, Johnstone RW, Levy DE. Constitutive type 1 interferon modulates homeostatic balance through tonic signaling. Immunity. 2012;36(2):166–74.
35. Colpitts SL, Stoklasek TA, Plumlee CR, Obar JJ, Guo C, Lefrancois L. Cutting edge: the role of IFN-alpha receptor and MyD88 signaling in induction of IL-15 expression in vivo. J Immunol. 2012;188(6):2483–7.
36. Ciccocioppo R, Di Sabatino A, Parroni R, Muzi P, D'Alo S, Ventura T, et al. Increased enterocyte apoptosis and Fas-Fas ligand system in celiac disease. Am J Clin Pathol. 2001;115(4):494–503.
37. Di Sabatino A, Ciccocioppo R, D'Alo S, Parroni R, Millimaggi D, Cifone MG, et al. Intraepithelial and lamina propria lymphocytes show distinct patterns of apoptosis whereas both populations are active in Fas based cytotoxicity in coeliac disease. Gut. 2001;49(3):380–6.
38. Malamut G, El Machhour R, Montcuquet N, Martin-Lanneree S, Dusanter-Fourt I, Verkarre V, et al. IL-15 triggers an antiapoptotic pathway in human intraepithelial lymphocytes that is a potential new target in celiac disease-associated inflammation and lymphomagenesis. J Clin Invest. 2010;120(6):2131–43.
39. Dray X, Joly F, Lavergne-Slove A, Treton X, Bouhnik Y, Messing B. A severe but reversible refractory sprue. Gut. 2006;55(8):1210–1.
40. Al-Toma A, Goerres MS, Meijer JW, von Blomberg BM, Wahab PJ, Kerckhaert JA, et al. Cladribine therapy in refractory celiac disease with aberrant T cells. Clin Gastroenterol Hepatol. 2006;4(11):1322–7.
41. Al-Toma A, Visser OJ, van Roessel HM, von Blomberg BM, Verbeek WH, Scholten PE, et al. Autologous hematopoietic stem cell transplantation in refractory celiac disease with aberrant T-cells. Blood. 2007;109(5):2243–9.
42. Tack GJ, Wondergem MJ, Al-Toma A, Verbeek WH, Schmittel A, Machado MV, et al. Auto-SCT in refractory celiac disease type II patients unresponsive to cladribine therapy. Bone Marrow Transplant. 2011;46(6):840–6.
43. Egan LJ, Walsh SV, Stevens FM, Connolly CE, Egan EL, McCarthy CF. Celiac-associated lymphoma. A single institution experience of 30 cases in the combination chemotherapy era. J Clin Gastroenterol. 1995;21(2):123–9.
44. Gale J, Simmonds PD, Mead GM, Sweetenham JW, Wright DH. Enteropathy-type 1ntestinal T-cell lymphoma: clinical features and treatment of 31 patients in a single center. J Clin Oncol. 2000;18(4):795–803.

45. Daum S, Ullrich R, Heise W, Dederke B, Foss HD, Stein H, et al. Intestinal non-Hodgkin's lymphoma: a multicenter prospective clinical study from the German Study Group on Intestinal non-Hodgkin's Lymphoma. J Clin Oncol. 2003;21(14):2740–6.
46. Waldmann TA. Targeting the interleukin-15 system in rheumatoid arthritis. Arthritis Rheum. 2005;52(9):2585–8.
47. Fleischmann R, Cutolo M, Genovese MC, Lee EB, Kanik KS, Sadis S, et al. Phase IIb dose-ranging study of the oral JAK inhibitor tofacitinib (CP-690,550) or adalimumab monotherapy versus placebo in patients with active rheumatoid arthritis with an inadequate response to disease-modifying antirheumatic drugs. Arthritis Rheum. 2012;64(3):617–29.
48. Yokoyama S, Perera PY, Waldmann TA, Hiroi T, Perera LP. Tofacitinib, a janus kinase inhibitor demonstrates efficacy in an IL-15 transgenic mouse model that recapitulates pathologic manifestations of celiac disease. J Clin Immunol. 2013;33(3):586–94.

Chapter 17
Celiac Disease: Dispelling Misconceptions and Myths

Erica Boettcher and Sheila E. Crowe

Misconception #1: Celiac Disease Is Rare

Once considered an uncommon disease, the prevalence of CD is now estimated in the range of 1:100 to 1:300 in genetically susceptible populations [1–6]. Variability exists both across and within countries, likely reflecting true population differences in the risk of CD as well as differences in study design and screening strategy [1, 7]. It is estimated that only 10–15 % of current cases of celiac disease have been diagnosed in the USA [5, 8] compared to some other countries where rates of diagnosis are greater than 50 % [6].

A retrospective US study by Rubio-Tapia et al. using stored serum reported a 4- to 4.5-fold increase in the rate of undiagnosed CD as compared to 50 years ago [9], and an increase in prevalence has been reported in other studies [10–13]. The cause of this increase is unknown and proposed modifying factors include breast-feeding [14], early exposure of infants to dietary gluten [15], and a change of bacterial gut flora [16–19], which could favor the evolution of CD in childhood. Recent reports also address the potential role of enteric infections in the pathogenesis of CD [13, 20–24], although this remains controversial.

E. Boettcher, M.D.
Clinical Fellow, Department of Medicine, Division of Gastroenterology, University of California, San Diego, La Jolla, CA, USA

S.E. Crowe, M.D. (✉)
Department of Medicine, University of California, San Diego, 9500 Gilman Drive, Mail Code 0063, La Jolla, CA 92093, USA
e-mail: secrowe@ucsd.edu

S.D. Rampertab and G.E. Mullin (eds.), *Celiac Disease*, Clinical Gastroenterology,
DOI 10.1007/978-1-4614-8560-5_17,

Table 17.1 Conditions or disorders associated with celiac disease

Family history
First- and second-degree relative(s) with celiac disease
Associated conditions
Autoimmune endocrine disorders
Type 1 diabetes mellitus
Autoimmune thyroid disease
Autoimmune adrenal disease
Autoimmune connective tissue disorders
Sjögren syndrome
Juvenile rheumatoid arthritis
Systemic lupus erythematosus
Autoimmune dermatological disorders
Psoriasis
Alopecia areata
Autoimmune hepatobiliary disorders
Primary sclerosing cholangitis
Primary biliary cirrhosis
Autoimmune hepatitis
Other digestive system disorders
Eosinophilic esophagitis
Microscopic colitis
Lymphocytic gastritis
Inflammatory bowel disease
Miscellaneous conditions
IgA deficiency
IgA nephropathy
Down syndrome
Turner syndrome

Misconception #2: Only Symptomatic Individuals Should Be Tested for Celiac Disease

There are several conditions associated with an elevated risk of CD supporting screening in asymptomatic individuals (Table 17.1). First- and second-degree family members of biopsy-proven CD patients are at increased risk of the disease with a prevalence estimated at 10 % [2, 25] and 2.6–5.5 % [2, 25], respectively. Type 1 diabetics have a clustered prevalence of CD estimated at 2–5 % in adults and 8 % in children [25–36], and patients with autoimmune thyroid disease have a pooled prevalence of 3 % [25]. These and other disorders that warrant screening include autoimmune adrenal disease [37–39] autoimmune connective tissue disorders such as Sjögren syndrome [40, 41], juvenile rheumatoid arthritis [42], and systemic lupus erythematosus [43]; autoimmune dermatological disorders including psoriasis [44] and alopecia areata [45]; autoimmune hepatobiliary disorders comprising autoimmune hepatitis, primary biliary cirrhosis, and primary sclerosing cholangitis [46]; IgA deficiency [47]; IgA nephropathy [48]; Down syndrome [49]; and Turner syndrome [50].

Misconception #3: Only Caucasians Are Susceptible to Celiac Disease

Genetic background plays a pivotal role in the predisposition to CD. There is an established association between celiac disease and specific human leukocyte antigen (HLA) class II genes, known as HLA-DQ2 and HLA-DQ8, located on chromosome 6p21. Most CD patients express genes encoding the major histocompatibility complex (MHC) class II protein HLA-DQ2; the remainder express HLA-DQ8.

HLA-DQ2 and -DQ8 haplotypes are common and are carried by approximately 30–40 % of Caucasian individuals implying that the presence of such alleles are necessary for disease development, but not sufficient on their own to cause celiac disease [51]. HLA-DQ2 and -DQ8 are not unique to Caucasians, however, and similar seroprevalence rates of CD in countries with such haplotypes are reported, including North Africa [52, 53], the Middle East [54, 55], and South Asia including India [56, 57] and Pakistan.

Little is known about the prevalence of CD among minorities in the USA as minority groups have, to date, been included in few prevalence studies. Additionally, these groups often comprise mixed racial and genetic backgrounds, which make it difficult to determine precise information about disease prevalence. In one of the first reported US studies of CD prevalence, Not et al. [58] included 230 African American patients among 2,000 healthy blood donors, one of whom (0.4 %) had a positive endomysial antibody. Fasano et al.'s [3] large multicenter trial of 13,145 patients comprised 395 African Americans and reported a prevalence among symptomatic African Americans of 1:48, similar to that of Caucasians. The overall prevalence of CD among all asymptomatic minorities (African American, Hispanic, and Asian) was 1:236. Rubio-Tapia et al.'s recent cross-sectional analysis [5] of 7,798 patients, in contrast, reported a much lower prevalence of 1:1,394 for African Americans and 1:2,519 for Hispanics.

Despite the few number of trials investigating the prevalence of CD among minorities, recent data suggest that physicians are less likely to consider the diagnosis among African American patients. Lebwohl et al.'s [59] multicenter study reported that among 13,091 individuals (9 % African American) undergoing upper endoscopy for the indication of diarrhea, anemia, iron deficiency, or weight loss, African Americans underwent duodenal biopsy in 28 % compared to 44 % of Caucasians ($p<0.0001$).

Misconception #4: Women Are More Often Affected by Celiac Disease

Multiple epidemiological studies in the USA and elsewhere have found that women are more likely to be diagnosed with CD [60, 61], and many studies of patients with CD have a female-to-male ratio of approximately 2:1 [62, 63]. Most seroprevalence studies of CD, however, have found a similar prevalence among men and women [3, 5, 9]. This cause for this discrepancy is unknown but may be in part due to increased rates of women accessing health care compared to men which is found in other conditions [64].

Misconception #5: You Cannot Have Celiac Disease if You Are Overweight

It is well established that many CD patients have a high or normal BMI at diagnosis [65–68]. The diagnosis of CD can be delayed by a low suspicion in patients with a normal or high body mass index (BMI) on initial presentation.

In Dickey et al.'s [66] single-center retrospective review of 371 patients with newly diagnosed CD on duodenal biopsy over a 10-year period, 143 (39 %) were overweight (BMI $\geq$ 25) including 48 (13 %) obese (BMI $\geq$ 30) patients. Similarly, Kabbani et al. [68] found that of 679 of patients with newly diagnosed CD, 217 (32 %) were overweight including 78 (11.5 %) with obesity.

Misconception #6: Celiac Disease Is Not a Serious Condition

A retrospective US study by Rubio-Tapia et al. indicates that the mortality of untreated CD is increased fourfold over control populations [9]. Similarly, a recent meta-analysis found an increased all-cause mortality odds ratio (OR) of 1.24 [69]. There was an excess risk of death from cardiovascular disease (OR 1.19, 95 % CI 1.01–4.01) and lymphoproliferative disease or malignancy (OR 2.53, 95 % CI 1.59–4.04). It has been proposed that mortality in CD is increased if gluten intake is high both before and after the diagnosis [70]. The greatest risk of malignancy is for non-Hodgkin's lymphoma including enteropathy-associated T-cell lymphoma (EATL) [71].

Misconception #7: Celiac Disease Signs and Symptoms Are Easy to Recognize

There are varying forms and many clinical presentations of CD, which can pose a serious challenge for clinicians. CD can present as "classical" disease in childhood, "nonclassical"/atypical disease with nonspecific gastrointestinal or extraintestinal manifestations, dermatitis herpetiformis, silent/asymptomatic disease, or latent/potential disease [72].

Classical celiac disease presents with symptoms of malabsorption and dramatic response to GFD. Nonclassical CD presents later with a potential range of symptoms,

Table 17.2 Symptoms or syndromes prompting consideration of celiac disease

Digestive system symptoms/syndromes
Gastrointestinal
Abdominal pain
Bloating
Weight loss
Diarrhea
Steatorrhea
Irritable bowel syndrome-like symptoms
Flatus
Altered bowel habits
Lactose intolerance
Heartburn
Dyspepsia
Recurrent aphthous ulcers
Atrophic glossitis
Hepatobiliary
Elevated aminotransferase levels
Extraintestinal symptoms/syndromes
Dermatitis herpetiformis
Iron deficiency
Folate deficiency
Infertility
Recurrent fetal loss
Low birth weight
Metabolic bone disease
Osteoporosis
Cerebellar ataxia
Unexplained or idiopathic peripheral neuropathy

including less severe gastrointestinal symptoms or extraintestinal manifestations. Asymptomatic or silent CD patients do not manifest any overt symptoms commonly associated with CD and are defined as having no symptoms that respond to gluten withdrawal. However, a recent study by Kurppa et al. [73] indicated that so-called asymptomatic relatives randomized to a GFD did experience improvements in health suggesting that they had subclinical disease. Potential or latent CD refers to patients with normal small intestinal biopsies who are at risk of developing CD as indicated by genetic susceptibility and positive CD serology. Both asymptomatic and potential patients are often diagnosed through testing of populations enrolled in screening programs or in case-finding strategies.

The classical presentation of celiac disease is relatively rare in current times. More commonly, CD presents later in life, with an average age of diagnosis in the fifth decade. Nonspecific presenting gastrointestinal symptoms include altered bowel habits with diarrhea, constipation, or a combination of both, abdominal pain, flatus, bloating, dyspepsia [74], and heartburn [75] (Table 17.2).

Some studies purport that a subset of patients diagnosed with irritable bowel syndrome (IBS) may in fact have celiac disease [76, 77], and decision analysis studies suggest that there is an acceptable cost of testing patients with diarrhea-predominant IBS [78, 79]. In support of this, a recent systematic review and meta-analysis of 14 studies found that the likelihood of biopsy-proven celiac disease in patients meeting criteria for IBS was increased more than fourfold compared with non-IBS controls [80]. Another study, however, reported a prevalence of CD in non-IBS-constipation predominant patients similar to controls [81]. Whether findings truly reflect an increased association between these two common clinical entities remains a matter of debate.

Other digestive system manifestations of CD that generally improve with GFD include a pattern of asymptomatic cryptogenic transaminitis with nonspecific histologic changes on liver biopsy [82] and disturbances of the oral cavity, such as recurrent aphthous ulcers [83] and atrophic glossitis [83, 84] (see Table 17.2). Digestive disorders that can coexist with CD and merit consideration, but in general, do not improve with GFD comprise eosinophilic esophagitis [85], microscopic colitis [86, 87], lymphocytic gastritis [88, 89], and inflammatory bowel disease [90, 91] (see Table 17.1).

While gastrointestinal symptoms are a dominant feature of CD, virtually any body system can be affected, with dermatologic, hematologic, reproductive, musculoskeletal, and neurologic systems most commonly involved (see Table 17.2). Many of the non-digestive conditions improve or resolve with a GFD underscoring the importance of early diagnosis and treatment.

The most common dermatologic manifestation of celiac disease is dermatitis herpetiformis (DH), a blistering, intensely pruritic papulovesicular rash typically distributed on extensor surfaces.

Although DH is highly associated with CD, the gastrointestinal symptoms in DH tend to be mild or can be completely absent. DH is the result of intestinal gluten sensitivity as opposed to a direct dermal response, and treatment with a GFD resolves both the intestinal and skin manifestations [92].

Anemia is the most common hematologic disorder in CD and may be the only presenting feature. Most often, the anemia is caused by iron deficiency, but it can also be due to folate or rarely vitamin B_{12} deficiency or a combination of several deficiencies. The iron deficiency in CD primarily results from impaired absorption of iron in the proximal small intestine. CD should be considered in the differential diagnosis of unexplained iron deficiency, especially if resistant to oral iron supplementation.

Reproductive disorders including delayed menarche, early menopause, secondary amenorrhea, infertility, recurrent miscarriages and intrauterine growth restriction, low birth weight, or preterm deliveries have all been reported [93, 94] in association with CD. Treating CD seems to improve fertility in women and men and pregnancy outcomes though systematic follow-up studies are lacking. Women and men with unexplained infertility and women with recurrent miscarriages should be considered for CD testing.

Celiac disease can result in vitamin D and calcium malabsorption and can impact the musculoskeletal system at any age [95]. Patients with unexplained metabolic bone disease or severe osteoporosis should be assessed for CD [96]. A GFD corrects bone loss in patients with mild disease and provides significant improvement in patients with severe malabsorption [95].

There are several links between neuropsychiatric and behavioral disorders and CD [97]. Classic associations that should prompt serologic assessment of CD include cerebellar ataxia [98, 99] and idiopathic peripheral neuropathy [100, 101]. These disorders have a variable response to a GFD.

Misconception #8: Celiac Disease Is Easy to Diagnose

Deciding when to test for CD is challenging. Furthermore the decision of when to refer a patient for further evaluation is equally difficult. These clinical challenges contribute to an average of 11 years of symptoms prior to diagnosis [102, 103] and often, a complete failure to test for the disease.

Based on the available data, it is recommended that patients with gastrointestinal or extraintestinal symptoms or syndromes suggestive of celiac disease (see Table 17.2) be tested. In addition, asymptomatic individuals with an associated condition as well as those with first- or second-degree family member(s) with biopsy-confirmed celiac disease should be screened for CD (see Table 17.1). The strategy varies depending on the clinical situation and is described below [80, 104, 105].

The initial screening for asymptomatic patients with associated conditions and testing for symptomatic older children and adults consuming gluten for greater than 1 year begins with the serological measurement of IgA anti-tissue transglutaminase (TTG) antibodies [25]. Serum TTG IgA has high sensitivity (89 %) and very high specificity (98 %) for CD in patients with abdominal symptoms [105]. A related antibody, anti-endomysial IgA antibody (EMA), which detects the same TTG protein as TTG antibodies by immunofluorescence assay, has a similar sensitivity (90 %) and specificity (99 %) [105]; however, this test is more expensive, complex, and operator-dependent [106]. In a meta-analysis of both symptomatic and asymptomatic patients, EMA IgA and TTG IgA had equally high sensitivities (93 % for both) and specificities (>99 % and >98 %, respectively), and again, due to cost and ease of administration, TTG IgA is recommended as the preferred test [107]. Although the absence of HLA DQ2 or DQ8 makes CD highly unlikely, adding genetic testing to either TTG IgA or EMA IgA antibody measurement in this clinical scenario does not change test performance [108], thus genetic testing is not recommended.

Antigliadin (AGA) IgG and IgA were previously used to screen for celiac disease but are no longer recommended in adults due to low sensitivities and specificities [109]. Recently available tests for IgG and IgA antibodies to deamidated gliadin peptide (DGP) were initially reported to match the performance of TTG and EMA antibody tests [110]. In a recent meta-analysis, however, DGP was found to be less sensitive and specific than TTG IgA [111].

While routine total IgA serum levels are not recommended in screening for CD, in the case of a low TTG IgA, total IgA levels should be obtained, and if IgA deficiency is confirmed, an IgG-based serological test such as TTG IgG is recommended [47, 112]. If TTG IgA is low and total IgA levels are normal, then CD is unlikely to be the cause of the symptoms. However, since the false negative rate of serological testing can be as high as one in ten cases, it is important to proceed to intestinal biopsy in patients with features that warrant further assessment such as unexplained diarrhea, steatorrhea, weight loss, and iron deficiency.

Genetic testing is recommended as the initial screening for an asymptomatic individual at increased risk of celiac disease due to family history [113]. If positive for either HLA DQ2 or HLA DQ8, the family member should have serum TTG IgA screening, which should begin after 2 years of age on a gluten-containing diet [113], although there is no scientific evidence to suggest the precise amount of gluten that needs to be ingested to elicit a measureable serological and/or intestinal mucosal response [113]. Since CD can develop at any age, identifying family members who are actually at risk for CD by using HLA DQ testing is recommended to prevent unnecessary TTG IgA testing in those with no risk [96]. The interval at which family members should be screened is not clear, but recent European Society of Pediatric Gastroenterology, Hepatology and Nutrition guidelines suggest every 2–3 years [113]. Given that the average age of diagnosis occurs in the fifth decade, screening of family members may be carried out through adult life.

If a patient has positive serologic testing or if results are negative but clinical suspicion is high, patients should be referred to a gastroenterologist for upper endoscopy with duodenal biopsies based on American Gastroenterological Association [25] and National Institutes of Health [114] guidelines.

Misconception #9: Everyone Knows How to Biopsy for Celiac Disease

A recent retrospective study using data from a national pathology service in 43 states found that among 132,352 subjects without known CD undergoing upper endoscopy with duodenal biopsy, only 35 % had the recommended minimum of four specimens submitted, despite the finding that adherence to this standard led to a doubling of the CD diagnosis rates [115]. This study also showed that the rate of diagnosis of CD increased as the number of biopsies increased up to as high as ≥8. Furthermore an analysis of the Clinical Outcomes Research Initiative (CORI) National Endoscopy Database found that, among individuals undergoing upper endoscopy for indications including symptoms of CD, the majority (89 %) did not undergo a duodenal biopsy during the procedure [116]. It is important to note, however, that the time span of this study predates the seroprevalence study revealing that CD is common [3].

Misconception #10: Celiac Disease Is Easy to Treat

The GFD is complex and difficult to adhere to, and patient motivation and education are paramount, particularly because there is no alternative treatment. Nonadherence is common and potential triggering factors include eating out of the home, peer pressure for children and teens [117], inadvertent consumption of gluten, the less acceptable taste and texture, and the increased cost and limited availability of gluten-free foods [118]. Furthermore, it is unclear how much gluten, if any, is safe for consumption. The lowest amount of daily gluten that causes damage to the intestinal mucosa over time is 10–50 mg per day (a 25-g slice of bread contains approximately 1.6 g of gluten) [119]. The Food and Drug Administration is in the process of defining safe gluten thresholds, and in their newest guidelines, they endorse a maximum gluten contamination of 20 parts per million in gluten-free products [120].

Once a GFD is initiated, symptoms may resolve in days to weeks and patients may incorrectly believe that the absence of symptoms when eating gluten-containing foods indicates that in can be consumed without harm. Accordingly, patients should be encouraged to strictly adhere to the diet to avoid potential complications.

Misconception #11: A Positive Response to Gluten-Free Diet Is Suggestive of CD

With the ever-increasing popularity and availability of gluten-free products, patients may present for diagnosis and treatment having already initiated a GFD. Further, an empiric trial of GFD without a biopsy-established diagnosis of CD is not recommended because a beneficial response may be seen in other disorders. Many dietary components in addition to gluten are eliminated in a GFD, which may also provide relief in such functional gastrointestinal disorders such as IBS, gastroesophageal reflux, functional dyspepsia, and a newly described condition, non-celiac gluten sensitivity (NCGS). In one study, the positive predictive value of a beneficial response after gluten withdrawal resulting from CD was only 36 % [121]. Differentiating between CD and other disorders that may respond to a GFD is important to help determine if a lifelong GFD is required and because of the implications for long-term management and risk assessment of relatives if celiac disease is present. There are also implications for family members to have a conclusive diagnosis of CD in the index case given their two- to threefold increased risk of CD.

Misconception #12: Getting Information About a Gluten-Free Diet Is Straightforward

Following the diagnosis of CD, patients should be referred to a dietitian, preferably one with clinical expertise in the GFD. Patients should also be directed to their local celiac organization chapter. Very few clinicians, including gastroenterologists, have

Table 17.3 Grains/seeds/flours/ingredients containing gluten (must be avoided)

Wheat
- Wheat starch, wheat bran, wheat germ, cracked wheat, hydrolyzed wheat protein
- Bulgur
- Couscous
- Durum
- Einkorn
- Emmer
- Spelt (Dinkel)
- Kamut
- Farina
- Farro
- Semolina

Barley
- Barley
- Barley malt

Rye

Triticale (cross between wheat and rye)

Processed foods that may contain wheat, barley, or rye
- Beer
- Bouillon cubes
- Brown rice syrup
- Candy
- Licorice
- Malt (malt syrup, malted milk, and malt vinegar)
- Soy sauce
- Modified food starch
- Brewer's yeast
- Cold cuts, hot dogs, salami, sausage
- Seasoned snack foods (tortilla chips, potato chips)
- Communion wafers
- French fries
- Gravy
- Imitation fish
- Matzo
- Rice mixes
- Sauces
- Self-basting turkey
- Soups
- Vegetables in sauce

a comprehensive understanding of food ingredients (Tables 17.3 and 17.4) or time to effectively counsel patients. Important topics to address include identifying hidden sources of gluten, maintaining adequate nutrition, focusing on what can be eaten as opposed to what cannot (Table 17.5), as well as counseling on the increased cost of prepared gluten-free foods and the importance of lifelong adherence. Depending on the geographical location, however, expert dietitians may not be accessible, and patients may seek outside sources of information such as the Internet which can provide outdated or erroneous data, including but not limited to the following myths. Expert advice is needed to direct patients to reputable and helpful sources of dietary information (books, online resources) and gluten-free foods (stores and online ordering).

Table 17.4 Gluten-free grains/seeds/flours (safe to eat)

Grains
Pure oats
Amaranth
Corn
Rice, rice flour, rice bran
Sorghum
Teff
Millet
Quinoa
Plant foods/starches
Arrowroot
Buckwheat (kasha)
Flax
Indian ricegrass (Montina)
Legume flours (bean, garbanzo bean, lentil, pea)
Mesquite flour
Potato flour, potato starch
Nut flours (almond, hazelnut, pecan)
Soybean flour
Sweet potato flour
Tapioca (cassava, manioc)
Wild rice
Yucca
Sago

Table 17.5 General nutritional advice for patients with celiac disease

- Maintain a gluten-free diet for life
- Choose naturally gluten-free foods (meat, poultry, fish, seafood, egg, vegetable, potato, rice)
- Minimize packaged or processed gluten-free foods
- Plan meals and snacks ahead
- Avoid lactose-containing dairy products temporarily after starting a gluten-free diet
- Continue to eat naturally low-lactose dairy products such as lactose-free yogurt and aged cheeses if lactose intolerance persists
- Choose foods rich in bioavailable iron such as red meat, dark poultry, and fishes

Myths of Management: You Cannot Use Gluten-Containing Beauty Products if You Have Celiac Disease

The only way to trigger an immune response in CD, including the skin manifestations, is by ingesting gluten, so as long as shampoos, creams, lotions, and other body products stay out of the mouth, they will not cause problems. Since lipsticks are ingested, albeit in small amounts, patients can be instructed to choose a gluten-free product.

Myths of Management: The Consumption of Oats Can Trigger Celiac Disease

At one time, the consensus was that oats were immunogenic to those with CD, but a large number of studies in adults and children have demonstrated that oats can be safely consumed [122–126]. However, only pure oats are safe to eat and until recently, most food manufacturers milled oats in the same facility as gluten-containing grains, leading to gluten contamination of commercial oat products [127]. Fortunately, pure oat-containing food products are becoming increasingly available, both at specialty food stores and larger grocery chains.

Myths of Management: A Separate Set of Utensils, Dishes, Appliances, and Other Kitchen Goods Are Necessary

In reality, as long as cooking utensils are thoroughly washed before using, it is acceptable to share cooking implements, with the exception of upright toasters and other items that are difficult to clean.

Myths of Management: Gluten-Free Cleaning Products Are Recommended

Again, the only way to trigger an immune response in CD is by ingesting glute, so gluten-containing cleaning products are fine as long as they do not come in contact with the mouth.

Myths of Management: Pets Should Eat Gluten-Free Food

In the same vein, as long as pet food is not consumed by patients with CD, they are safe to feed.

Conclusion

CD is one of the most common immune-mediated disorders in genetically prone individuals, affecting 1:100 to 1:300 individuals. It has gone largely undiagnosed in the USA and should be considered in patients with a number of gastrointestinal and non-gastrointestinal symptoms, as well as in high-risk groups including those with a family history of CD or with an associated condition or disorder. Given the varying forms and many clinical presentations of CD, deciding when to test for CD is challenging, and deciding when to refer a patient to a gastroenterologist is equally difficult. Biopsy remains the gold standard in diagnosis, but serological tests are important in determining who should undergo endoscopy and biopsy. Genetic testing is used to rule out the condition. Once the diagnosis is confirmed, counseling on lifelong adherence to a GFD from an expert dietitian is crucial as ongoing gluten consumption may predispose patients to complications or associated disorders.

Conflict of Interest Dr. S.E.Crowe is a Principal Investigator in the "Clinical Evaluation of Three Celiac Disease-Specific Patient Reported Outcome Instruments in Established and Newly Diagnosed Celiac Disease Patients" study sponsored by Alvine Pharmaceuticals, Inc. She is also the author of Celiac Disease for Dummies and receives royalties from John Wiley & Sons Publishers.

References

1. Mustalahti K, Catassi C, Reunanen A, Fabiani E, Heier M, McMillan S, et al. The prevalence of celiac disease in Europe: results of a centralized, international mass screening project. Ann Med. 2010;42(8):587–95.
2. Dube C, Rostom A, Sy R, Cranney A, Saloojee N, Garritty C, et al. The prevalence of celiac disease in average-risk and at-risk Western European populations: a systematic review. Gastroenterology. 2005;128(4 Suppl 1):S57–67.
3. Fasano A, Berti I, Gerarduzzi T, Not T, Colletti RB, Drago S, et al. Prevalence of celiac disease in at-risk and not-at-risk groups in the United States: a large multicenter study. Arch Intern Med. 2003;163(3):286–92.
4. Godfrey JD, Brantner TL, Brinjikji W, Christensen KN, Brogan DL, Van Dyke CT, et al. Morbidity and mortality among older individuals with undiagnosed celiac disease. Gastroenterology. 2010;139(3):763–9.
5. Rubio-Tapia A, Ludvigsson JF, Brantner TL, Murray JA, Everhart JE. The prevalence of celiac disease in the United States. Am J Gastroenterol. 2012;107(10):1538–44.
6. Virta LJ, Kaukinen K, Collin P. Incidence and prevalence of diagnosed coeliac disease in Finland: results of effective case finding in adults. Scand J Gastroenterol. 2009;44(8): 933–8.
7. Biagi F, Klersy C, Balduzzi D, Corazza GR. Are we not over-estimating the prevalence of coeliac disease in the general population? Ann Med. 2010;42(8):557–61.
8. Katz KD, Rashtak S, Lahr BD, Melton 3rd LJ, Krause PK, Maggi K, et al. Screening for celiac disease in a North American population: sequential serology and gastrointestinal symptoms. Am J Gastroenterol. 2011;106(7):1333–9.
9. Rubio-Tapia A, Kyle RA, Kaplan EL, Johnson DR, Page W, Erdtmann F, et al. Increased prevalence and mortality in undiagnosed celiac disease. Gastroenterology. 2009;137(1): 88–93.
10. Lohi S, Mustalahti K, Kaukinen K, Laurila K, Collin P, Rissanen H, et al. Increasing prevalence of coeliac disease over time. Aliment Pharmacol Ther. 2007;26(9):1217–25.
11. Vilppula A, Kaukinen K, Luostarinen L, Krekela I, Patrikainen H, Valve R, et al. Increasing prevalence and high incidence of celiac disease in elderly people: a population-based study. BMC Gastroenterol. 2009;9:49.
12. Dydensborg S, Toftedal P, Biaggi M, Lillevang ST, Hansen DG, Husby S. Increasing prevalence of coeliac disease in Denmark: a linkage study combining national registries. Acta Paediatr. 2012;101(2):179–84.

13. Riddle MS, Murray JA, Porter CK. The incidence and risk of celiac disease in a healthy US adult population. Am J Gastroenterol. 2012;107(8):1248–55.
14. Szajewska H, Chmielewska A, Piescik-Lech M, Ivarsson A, Kolacek S, Koletzko S, et al. Systematic review: early infant feeding and the prevention of coeliac disease. Aliment Pharmacol Ther. 2012;36(7):607–18.
15. Norris JM, Barriga K, Hoffenberg EJ, Taki I, Miao D, Haas JE, et al. Risk of celiac disease autoimmunity and timing of gluten introduction in the diet of infants at increased risk of disease. JAMA. 2005;293(19):2343–51.
16. Collado MC, Calabuig M, Sanz Y. Differences between the fecal microbiota of coeliac infants and healthy controls. Curr Issues Intest Microbiol. 2007;8(1):9–14.
17. Collado MC, Donat E, Ribes-Koninckx C, Calabuig M, Sanz Y. Imbalances in faecal and duodenal Bifidobacterium species composition in active and non-active coeliac disease. BMC Microbiol. 2008;8:232.
18. Collado MC, Donat E, Ribes-Koninckx C, Calabuig M, Sanz Y. Specific duodenal and faecal bacterial groups associated with paediatric coeliac disease. J Clin Pathol. 2009;62(3):264–9.
19. Sellitto M, Bai G, Serena G, Fricke WF, Sturgeon C, Gajer P, et al. Proof of concept of microbiome-metabolome analysis and delayed gluten exposure on celiac disease autoimmunity in genetically at-risk infants. PLoS One. 2012;7(3):e33387.
20. Landzberg BR, Connor BA. Persistent diarrhea in the returning traveler: think beyond persistent infection. Scand J Gastroenterol. 2005;40(1):112–4.
21. Verdu EF, Mauro M, Bourgeois J, Armstrong D. Clinical onset of celiac disease after an episode of Campylobacter jejuni enteritis. Can J Gastroenterol. 2007;21(7):453–5.
22. Smits SL, van Leeuwen M, van der Eijk AA, Fraaij PL, Escher JC, Simon JH, et al. Human astrovirus infection in a patient with new-onset celiac disease. J Clin Microbiol. 2010;48(9): 3416–8.
23. Pal N, Sharma R, Sharma B, Suman R. A case of Cryptosporidium infection in a child of celiac disease. J Postgrad Med. 2012;58(2):160.
24. Edling L, Rathsman S, Eriksson S, Bohr J. Celiac disease and giardiasis: a case report. Eur J Gastroenterol Hepatol. 2012;24(8):984–7.
25. Rostom A, Murray JA, Kagnoff MF. American Gastroenterological Association (AGA) Institute technical review on the diagnosis and management of celiac disease. Gastroenterology. 2006;131(6):1981–2002.
26. Li Voon Chong JS, Leong KS, Wallymahmed M, Sturgess R, MacFarlane IA. Is coeliac disease more prevalent in young adults with coexisting Type 1 diabetes mellitus and autoimmune thyroid disease compared with those with Type 1 diabetes mellitus alone? Diabet Med. 2002;19(4):334–7.
27. Lorini R, Scotta MS, Cortona L, Avanzini MA, Vitali L, De Giacomo C, et al. Celiac disease and type 1 (insulin-dependent) diabetes mellitus in childhood: follow-up study. J Diabetes Complications. 1996;10(3):154–9.
28. Lampasona V, Bonfanti R, Bazzigaluppi E, Venerando A, Chiumello G, Bosi E, et al. Antibodies to tissue transglutaminase C in type 1 diabetes. Diabetologia. 1999;42(10): 1195–8.
29. Sjoberg K, Eriksson KF, Bredberg A, Wassmuth R, Eriksson S. Screening for coeliac disease in adult insulin-dependent diabetes mellitus. J Intern Med. 1998;243(2):133–40.
30. Talal AH, Murray JA, Goeken JA, Sivitz WI. Celiac disease in an adult population with insulin-dependent diabetes mellitus: use of endomysial antibody testing. Am J Gastroenterol. 1997;92(8):1280–4.
31. Saukkonen T, Savilahti E, Reijonen H, Ilonen J, Tuomilehto-Wolf E, Akerblom HK. Coeliac disease: frequent occurrence after clinical onset of insulin-dependent diabetes mellitus. Childhood Diabetes in Finland Study Group. Diabet Med. 1996;13(5):464–70.
32. Spiekerkoetter U, Seissler J, Wendel U. General screening for celiac disease is advisable in children with type 1 diabetes. Horm Metab Res. 2002;34(4):192–5.
33. Kordonouri O, Dieterich W, Schuppan D, Webert G, Muller C, Sarioglu N, et al. Autoantibodies to tissue transglutaminase are sensitive serological parameters for detecting

silent coeliac disease in patients with Type 1 diabetes mellitus. Diabet Med. 2000;17(6): 441–4.
34. Page SR, Lloyd CA, Hill PG, Peacock I, Holmes GK. The prevalence of coeliac disease in adult diabetes mellitus. QJM. 1994;87(10):631–7.
35. De Vitis I, Ghirlanda G, Gasbarrini G. Prevalence of coeliac disease in type 1 diabetes: a multicentre study. Acta Paediatr Suppl. 1996;412:56–7.
36. Not T, Tommasini A, Tonini G, Buratti E, Pocecco M, Tortul C, et al. Undiagnosed coeliac disease and risk of autoimmune disorders in subjects with Type 1 diabetes mellitus. Diabetologia. 2001;44(2):151–5.
37. Myhre AG, Aarsetoy H, Undlien DE, Hovdenak N, Aksnes L, Husebye ES. High frequency of coeliac disease among patients with autoimmune adrenocortical failure. Scand J Gastroenterol. 2003;38(5):511–5.
38. O'Leary C, Walsh CH, Wieneke P, O'Regan P, Buckley B, O'Halloran DJ, et al. Coeliac disease and autoimmune Addison's disease: a clinical pitfall. QJM. 2002;95(2):79–82.
39. Biagi F, Campanella J, Soriani A, Vailati A, Corazza GR. Prevalence of coeliac disease in Italian patients affected by Addison's disease. Scand J Gastroenterol. 2006;41(3):302–5.
40. Iltanen S, Collin P, Korpela M, Holm K, Partanen J, Polvi A, et al. Celiac disease and markers of celiac disease latency in patients with primary Sjogren's syndrome. Am J Gastroenterol. 1999;94(4):1042–6.
41. Szodoray P, Barta Z, Lakos G, Szakall S, Zeher M. Coeliac disease in Sjogren's syndrome–a study of 111 Hungarian patients. Rheumatol Int. 2004;24(5):278–82.
42. Neuhausen SL, Steele L, Ryan S, Mousavi M, Pinto M, Osann KE, et al. Co-occurrence of celiac disease and other autoimmune diseases in celiacs and their first-degree relatives. J Autoimmun. 2008;31(2):160–5.
43. Ludvigsson JF, Rubio-Tapia A, Chowdhary V, Murray JA, Simard JF. Increased risk of systemic lupus erythematosus in 29,000 patients with biopsy-verified celiac disease. J Rheumatol. 2012;39(10):1964–70.
44. Ludvigsson JF, Lindelof B, Zingone F, Ciacci C. Psoriasis in a nationwide cohort study of patients with celiac disease. J Invest Dermatol. 2011;131(10):2010–6.
45. Collin P, Reunala T. Recognition and management of the cutaneous manifestations of celiac disease: a guide for dermatologists. Am J Clin Dermatol. 2003;4(1):13–20.
46. Rubio-Tapia A, Murray JA. The liver in celiac disease. Hepatology. 2007;46(5):1650–8.
47. Chow MA, Lebwohl B, Reilly NR, Green PH. Immunoglobulin A deficiency in celiac disease. J Clin Gastroenterol. 2012;46(10):850–4.
48. Collin P, Syrjanen J, Partanen J, Pasternack A, Kaukinen K, Mustonen J. Celiac disease and HLA DQ in patients with IgA nephropathy. Am J Gastroenterol. 2002;97(10):2572–6.
49. Nisihara RM, Kotze LM, Utiyama SR, Oliveira NP, Fiedler PT, Messias-Reason IT. Celiac disease in children and adolescents with Down syndrome. J Pediatr. 2005;81(5):373–6.
50. Bonamico M, Pasquino AM, Mariani P, Danesi HM, Culasso F, Mazzanti L, et al. Prevalence and clinical picture of celiac disease in Turner syndrome. J Clin Endocrinol Metab. 2002;87(12):5495–8.
51. Karell K, Louka AS, Moodie SJ, Ascher H, Clot F, Greco L, et al. HLA types in celiac disease patients not carrying the DQA1*05-DQB1*02 (DQ2) heterodimer: results from the European Genetics Cluster on Celiac Disease. Hum Immunol. 2003;64(4):469–77.
52. Alarida K, Harown J, Ahmaida A, Marinelli L, Venturini C, Kodermaz G, et al. Coeliac disease in Libyan children: a screening study based on the rapid determination of anti-transglutaminase antibodies. Dig Liver Dis. 2011;43(9):688–91.
53. Catassi C, Ratsch IM, Gandolfi L, Pratesi R, Fabiani E, El Asmar R, et al. Why is coeliac disease endemic in the people of the Sahara? Lancet. 1999;354(9179):647–8.
54. Dalgic B, Sari S, Basturk B, Ensari A, Egritas O, Bukulmez A, et al. Prevalence of celiac disease in healthy Turkish school children. Am J Gastroenterol. 2011;106(8):1512–7.
55. Shahbazkhani B, Malekzadeh R, Sotoudeh M, Moghadam KF, Farhadi M, Ansari R, et al. High prevalence of coeliac disease in apparently healthy Iranian blood donors. Eur J Gastroenterol Hepatol. 2003;15(5):475–8.

56. Kochhar R, Sachdev S, Kochhar R, Aggarwal A, Sharma V, Prasad KK, et al. Prevalence of coeliac disease in healthy blood donors: a study from north India. Dig Liver Dis. 2012;44(6):530–2.
57. Makharia GK, Verma AK, Amarchand R, Bhatnagar S, Das P, Goswami A, et al. Prevalence of celiac disease in the northern part of India: a community based study. J Gastroenterol Hepatol. 2011;26(5):894–900.
58. Not T, Horvath K, Hill ID, Partanen J, Hammed A, Magazzu G, et al. Celiac disease risk in the USA: high prevalence of antiendomysium antibodies in healthy blood donors. Scand J Gastroenterol. 1998;33(5):494–8.
59. Lebwohl B, Tennyson CA, Holub JL, Lieberman DA, Neugut AI, Green PH. Sex and racial disparities in duodenal biopsy to evaluate for celiac disease. Gastrointest Endosc. 2012;76(4):779–85.
60. Ludvigsson JF, Montgomery SM, Ekbom A, Brandt L, Granath F. Small-intestinal histopathology and mortality risk in celiac disease. JAMA. 2009;302(11):1171–8.
61. Murray JA, Van Dyke C, Plevak MF, Dierkhising RA, Zinsmeister AR, Melton 3rd LJ. Trends in the identification and clinical features of celiac disease in a North American community, 1950-2001. Clin Gastroenterol Hepatol. 2003;1(1):19–27.
62. Lebwohl B, Stavsky E, Neugut AI, Green PH. Risk of colorectal adenomas in patients with coeliac disease. Aliment Pharmacol Ther. 2010;32(8):1037–43.
63. Leffler DA, Edwards-George J, Dennis M, Schuppan D, Cook F, Franko DL, et al. Factors that influence adherence to a gluten-free diet in adults with celiac disease. Dig Dis Sci. 2008;53(6):1573–81.
64. Mustard CA, Kaufert P, Kozyrskyj A, Mayer T. Sex differences in the use of health care services. N Engl J Med. 1998;338(23):1678–83.
65. Olen O, Montgomery SM, Marcus C, Ekbom A, Ludvigsson JF. Coeliac disease and body mass index: a study of two Swedish general population-based registers. Scand J Gastroenterol. 2009;44(10):1198–206.
66. Dickey W, Kearney N. Overweight in celiac disease: prevalence, clinical characteristics, and effect of a gluten-free diet. Am J Gastroenterol. 2006;101(10):2356–9.
67. Cheng J, Brar PS, Lee AR, Green PH. Body mass index in celiac disease: beneficial effect of a gluten-free diet. J Clin Gastroenterol. 2010;44(4):267–71.
68. Kabbani TA, Goldberg A, Kelly CP, Pallav K, Tariq S, Peer A, et al. Body mass index and the risk of obesity in coeliac disease treated with the gluten-free diet. Aliment Pharmacol Ther. 2012;35(6):723–9.
69. Tio M, Cox MR, Eslick GD. Meta-analysis: coeliac disease and the risk of all-cause mortality, any malignancy and lymphoid malignancy. Aliment Pharmacol Ther. 2012;35(5): 540–51.
70. Biagi F, Corazza GR. Mortality in celiac disease. Nat Rev Gastroenterol Hepatol. 2010;7(3):158–62.
71. Grainge MJ, West J, Solaymani-Dodaran M, Card TR, Logan RF. The long-term risk of malignancy following a diagnosis of coeliac disease or dermatitis herpetiformis: a cohort study. Aliment Pharmacol Ther. 2012;35(6):730–9.
72. Ludvigsson JF, Leffler DA, Bai JC, Biagi F, Fasano A, Green PH, et al. The Oslo definitions for coeliac disease and related terms. Gut. 2013;62(1):43–52.
73. Kurppa K, Collin P, Lindfors K, Laurila K, Saavalainen P, Huhtala H, et al. Should screen-detected and asymptomatic celiac disease patients be treated? A prospective and randomized trial. Gastroenterology. 2011;140(5):S-112.
74. Santolaria Piedrafita S, Fernandez Banares F. Gluten-sensitive enteropathy and functional dyspepsia. Gastroenterol Hepatol. 2012;35(2):78–88.
75. Nachman F, Vazquez H, Gonzalez A, Andrenacci P, Compagni L, Reyes H, et al. Gastroesophageal reflux symptoms in patients with celiac disease and the effects of a gluten-free diet. Clin Gastroenterol Hepatol. 2011;9(3):214–9.
76. Wahnschaffe U, Ullrich R, Riecken EO, Schulzke JD. Celiac disease-like abnormalities in a subgroup of patients with irritable bowel syndrome. Gastroenterology. 2001;121(6): 1329–38.

77. Sanders DS, Carter MJ, Hurlstone DP, Pearce A, Ward AM, McAlindon ME, et al. Association of adult coeliac disease with irritable bowel syndrome: a case-control study in patients fulfilling ROME II criteria referred to secondary care. Lancet. 2001;358(9292):1504–8.
78. Spiegel BM, DeRosa VP, Gralnek IM, Wang V, Dulai GS. Testing for celiac sprue in irritable bowel syndrome with predominant diarrhea: a cost-effectiveness analysis. Gastroenterology. 2004;126(7):1721–32.
79. Mein SM, Ladabaum U. Serological testing for coeliac disease in patients with symptoms of irritable bowel syndrome: a cost-effectiveness analysis. Aliment Pharmacol Ther. 2004;19(11):1199–210.
80. Ford AC, Chey WD, Talley NJ, Malhotra A, Spiegel BM, Moayyedi P. Yield of diagnostic tests for celiac disease in individuals with symptoms suggestive of irritable bowel syndrome: systematic review and meta-analysis. Arch Intern Med. 2009;169(7):651–8.
81. Cash BD, Rubenstein JH, Young PE, Gentry A, Nojkov B, Lee D, et al. The prevalence of celiac disease among patients with nonconstipated irritable bowel syndrome is similar to controls. Gastroenterology. 2011;141(4):1187–93.
82. Prasad KK, Debi U, Sinha SK, Nain CK, Singh K. Hepatobiliary disorders in celiac disease: an update. Int J Hepatol. 2011;2011:438184.
83. Cheng J, Malahias T, Brar P, Minaya MT, Green PH. The association between celiac disease, dental enamel defects, and aphthous ulcers in a United States cohort. J Clin Gastroenterol. 2010;44(3):191–4.
84. Lucchese A, Guida A, Serpico R. Glossodynia and coeliac disease. Immunopharmacol Immunotoxicol. 2012;34(2):247–9.
85. Thompson JS, Lebwohl B, Reilly NR, Talley NJ, Bhagat G, Green PH. Increased incidence of eosinophilic esophagitis in children and adults with celiac disease. J Clin Gastroenterol. 2012;46(1):e6–e11.
86. Green PH, Yang J, Cheng J, Lee AR, Harper JW, Bhagat G. An association between microscopic colitis and celiac disease. Clin Gastroenterol Hepatol. 2009;7(11):1210–6.
87. Stewart M, Andrews CN, Urbanski S, Beck PL, Storr M. The association of coeliac disease and microscopic colitis: a large population-based study. Aliment Pharmacol Ther. 2011;33(12):1340–9.
88. Feeley KM, Heneghan MA, Stevens FM, McCarthy CF. Lymphocytic gastritis and coeliac disease: evidence of a positive association. J Clin Pathol. 1998;51(3):207–10.
89. Bhatti TR, Jatla M, Verma R, Bierly P, Russo PA, Ruchelli ED. Lymphocytic gastritis in pediatric celiac disease. Pediatr Dev Pathol. 2011;14(4):280–3.
90. Yang A, Chen Y, Scherl E, Neugut AI, Bhagat G, Green PH. Inflammatory bowel disease in patients with celiac disease. Inflamm Bowel Dis. 2005;11(6):528–32.
91. Cottone M, Marrone C, Casa A, Oliva L, Orlando A, Calabrese E, et al. Familial occurrence of inflammatory bowel disease in celiac disease. Inflamm Bowel Dis. 2003;9(5):321–3.
92. Nakajima K. Recent advances in dermatitis herpetiformis. Clin Dev Immunol. 2012;2012:914162.
93. Ozgor B, Selimoglu MA. Coeliac disease and reproductive disorders. Scand J Gastroenterol. 2010;45(4):395–402.
94. Soni S, Badawy SZ. Celiac disease and its effect on human reproduction: a review. J Reprod Med. 2010;55(1–2):3–8.
95. Bernstein CN, Leslie WD, Leboff MS. AGA technical review on osteoporosis in gastrointestinal diseases. Gastroenterology. 2003;124(3):795–841.
96. Crowe SE. In the clinic. Celiac disease. Ann Intern Med 2011;154(9):ITC5-1–15; quiz ITC5-16.
97. Bushara KO. Neurologic presentation of celiac disease. Gastroenterology. 2005;128(4 Suppl 1):S92–7.
98. Pellecchia MT, Scala R, Perretti A, De Michele G, Santoro L, Filla A, et al. Cerebellar ataxia associated with subclinical celiac disease responding to gluten-free diet. Neurology. 1999;53(7):1606–8.

99. Hadjivassiliou M, Davies-Jones GA, Sanders DS, Grunewald RA. Dietary treatment of gluten ataxia. J Neurol Neurosurg Psychiatry. 2003;74(9):1221–4.
100. Cicarelli G, Della Rocca G, Amboni M, Ciacci C, Mazzacca G, Filla A, et al. Clinical and neurological abnormalities in adult celiac disease. Neurol Sci. 2003;24(5):311–7.
101. Chin RL, Sander HW, Brannagan TH, Green PH, Hays AP, Alaedini A, et al. Celiac neuropathy. Neurology. 2003;60(10):1581–5.
102. Cranney A, Zarkadas M, Graham ID, Butzner JD, Rashid M, Warren R, et al. The Canadian celiac health survey. Dig Dis Sci. 2007;52(4):1087–95.
103. Green PHR, Stavropoulos SN, Panagi SG, Goldstein SL, Mcmahon DJ, Absan H, et al. Characteristics of adult celiac disease in the USA: results of a national survey. Am J Gastroenterol. 2001;96(1):126–31.
104. Turco R, Boccia G, Miele E, Giannetti E, Buonavolonta R, Quitadamo P, et al. The association of coeliac disease in childhood with functional gastrointestinal disorders: a prospective study in patients fulfilling Rome III criteria. Aliment Pharmacol Ther. 2011;34(7):783–9.
105. van der Windt DA, Jellema P, Mulder CJ, Kneepkens CM, van der Horst HE. Diagnostic testing for celiac disease among patients with abdominal symptoms: a systematic review. JAMA. 2010;303(17):1738–46.
106. Tesei N, Sugai E, Vazquez H, Smecuol E, Niveloni S, Mazure R, et al. Antibodies to human recombinant tissue transglutaminase may detect coeliac disease patients undiagnosed by endomysial antibodies. Aliment Pharmacol Ther. 2003;17(11):1415–23.
107. Lewis NR, Scott BB. Systematic review: the use of serology to exclude or diagnose coeliac disease (a comparison of the endomysial and tissue transglutaminase antibody tests). Aliment Pharmacol Ther. 2006;24(1):47–54.
108. Hadithi M, von Blomberg BM, Crusius JB, Bloemena E, Kostense PJ, Meijer JW, et al. Accuracy of serologic tests and HLA-DQ typing for diagnosing celiac disease. Ann Intern Med. 2007;147(5):294–302.
109. Rostom A, Dube C, Cranney A, Saloojee N, Sy R, Garritty C, et al. The diagnostic accuracy of serologic tests for celiac disease: a systematic review. Gastroenterology. 2005;128(4 Suppl 1):S38–46.
110. Kaukinen K, Collin P, Laurila K, Kaartinen T, Partanen J, Maki M. Resurrection of gliadin antibodies in coeliac disease. Deamidated gliadin peptide antibody test provides additional diagnostic benefit. Scand J Gastroenterol. 2007;42(12):1428–33.
111. Lewis NR, Scott BB. Meta-analysis: deamidated gliadin peptide antibody and tissue transglutaminase antibody compared as screening tests for coeliac disease. Aliment Pharmacol Ther. 2010;31(1):73–81.
112. Mozo L, Gomez J, Escanlar E, Bousono C, Gutierrez C. Diagnostic value of anti-deamidated gliadin peptide IgG antibodies for celiac disease in children and IgA-deficient patients. J Pediatr Gastroenterol Nutr. 2012;55(1):50–5.
113. Husby S, Koletzko S, Korponay-Szabo IR, Mearin ML, Phillips A, Shamir R, et al. European Society for Pediatric Gastroenterology, Hepatology, and Nutrition guidelines for the diagnosis of coeliac disease. J Pediatr Gastroenterol Nutr. 2012;54(1):136–60.
114. NIH Consensus Development Conference on Celiac Disease. NIH Consens State Sci Statements 2004;21(1):1–23.
115. Lebwohl B, Kapel RC, Neugut AI, Green PH, Genta RM. Adherence to biopsy guidelines increases celiac disease diagnosis. Gastrointest Endosc. 2011;74(1):103–9.
116. Harewood GC, Holub JL, Lieberman DA. Variation in small bowel biopsy performance among diverse endoscopy settings: results from a national endoscopic database. Am J Gastroenterol. 2004;99(9):1790–4.
117. Kurppa K, Lauronen O, Collin P, Ukkola A, Laurila K, Huhtala H, et al. Factors associated with dietary adherence in celiac disease: a nationwide study. Digestion. 2012;86(4):309–14.
118. Hall NJ, Rubin G, Charnock A. Systematic review: adherence to a gluten-free diet in adult patients with coeliac disease. Aliment Pharmacol Ther. 2009;30(4):315–30.

119. Catassi C, Fabiani E, Iacono G, D'Agate C, Francavilla R, Biagi F, et al. A prospective, double-blind, placebo-controlled trial to establish a safe gluten threshold for patients with celiac disease. Am J Clin Nutr. 2007;85(1):160–6.
120. Sharma GM. Immunoreactivity and detection of wheat proteins by commercial ELISA kits. J AOAC Int. 2012;95(2):364–71.
121. Campanella J, Biagi F, Bianchi PI, Zanellati G, Marchese A, Corazza GR. Clinical response to gluten withdrawal is not an indicator of coeliac disease. Scand J Gastroenterol. 2008;43(11):1311–4.
122. Janatuinen EK, Pikkarainen PH, Kemppainen TA, Kosma VM, Jarvinen RM, Uusitupa MI, et al. A comparison of diets with and without oats in adults with celiac disease. N Engl J Med. 1995;333(16):1033–7.
123. Janatuinen EK, Kemppainen TA, Pikkarainen PH, Holm KH, Kosma VM, Uusitupa MI, et al. Lack of cellular and humoral immunological responses to oats in adults with coeliac disease. Gut. 2000;46(3):327–31.
124. Janatuinen EK, Kemppainen TA, Julkunen RJ, Kosma VM, Maki M, Heikkinen M, et al. No harm from five year ingestion of oats in coeliac disease. Gut. 2002;50(3):332–5.
125. Hogberg L, Laurin P, Falth-Magnusson K, Grant C, Grodzinsky E, Jansson G, et al. Oats to children with newly diagnosed coeliac disease: a randomised double blind study. Gut. 2004;53(5):649–54.
126. Holm K, Maki M, Vuolteenaho N, Mustalahti K, Ashorn M, Ruuska T, et al. Oats in the treatment of childhood coeliac disease: a 2-year controlled trial and a long-term clinical follow-up study. Aliment Pharmacol Ther. 2006;23(10):1463–72.
127. Thompson T. Gluten contamination of commercial oat products in the United States. N Engl J Med. 2004;351(19):2021–2.

Chapter 18
Summary of Recommendations from the American College of Gastroenterology Celiac Disease Guidelines

Gerard E. Mullin and S. Devi Rampertab

1. Patients with symptoms, signs, or laboratory evidence suggestive of malabsorption, such as chronic diarrhea with weight loss, steatorrhea, postprandial abdominal pain, and bloating, should be tested for CD. (Strong recommendation, high level of evidence)
2. Patients with symptoms, signs, or laboratory evidence for which CD is a treatable cause should be considered for testing for CD. (Strong recommendation, moderate level of evidence)
3. Patients with a first-degree family member who has a confirmed diagnosis of CD should be tested if they show possible signs or symptoms or laboratory evidence of CD.
4. Consider testing of asymptomatic relatives with a first-degree family member who has a confirmed diagnosis of CD. (Conditional recommendation, high level of evidence)
5. CD should be sought among the explanations for elevated serum aminotransferase levels when no other etiology is found. (Strong recommendation, high level of evidence)
6. Patients with type I DM should be tested for CD if there are any digestive symptoms, or signs, or laboratory evidence suggestive of CD. (Strong recommendation, high level of evidence)

G.E. Mullin, M.D. (✉)
Division of Gastroenterology, Johns Hopkins University School of Medicine,
600 N Wolfe St. CARN 464 B, Baltimore, MD 21287, USA
e-mail: gmullin1@jhmi.edu

S.D. Rampertab, M.D., F.A.C.G. (✉)
Department of Medicine, Rutgers-Robert Wood Johnson Medical School,
One Robert Wood Johnson Place MEB 478, New Brunswick, NJ 08903, USA
e-mail: rampersd@rutgers.edu

S.D. Rampertab and G.E. Mullin (eds.), *Celiac Disease*, Clinical Gastroenterology,
DOI 10.1007/978-1-4614-8560-5_18, © Springer Science+Business Media New York 2014

7. IgA anti-TTG antibody is the preferred single test for detection of CD in individuals over the age of 2 years. (Strong recommendation, high level of evidence)
8. When there exists a high probability of CD wherein the possibility of IgA deficiency is considered, total IgA should be measured. An alternative approach is to include both IgA- and IgG-based testing, such as IgG DGPs, in these high-probability patients. (Strong recommendation, moderate level of evidence)
9. In patients in whom low IgA or selective IgA deficiency is identified, IgG-based testing (IgG DGPs and IgG TTG) should be performed. (Strong recommendation, moderate level of evidence)
10. If the suspicion of CD is high, intestinal biopsy should be pursued even if serologies are negative. (Strong recommendation, moderate level of evidence)
11. All diagnostic serologic testing should be done with patients on a gluten-containing diet. (Strong recommendation, high level of evidence)
12. Antibodies directed against native gliadin are not recommended for the primary detection of CD. (Strong recommendation, high level of evidence)
13. Combining several tests for CD in lieu of TTG IgA alone may marginally increase the sensitivity for CD but reduces specificity and therefore are not recommended in low-risk populations. (Conditional recommendation, moderate level of evidence)
14. When screening children younger than 2 years of age for CD, the IgA TTG test should be combined with DGPs (IgA and IgG). (Strong recommendation, moderate level of evidence)
15. The confirmation of a diagnosis of CD should be based on a combination of findings from the medical history, physical examination, serology, and upper endoscopy with histological analysis of multiple biopsies of the duodenum. (Strong recommendation, high level of evidence)
16. Upper endoscopy with small-bowel biopsy is a critical component of the diagnostic evaluation for persons with suspected CD and is recommended to confirm the diagnosis. (Strong recommendation, high level of evidence)
17. Multiple biopsies of the duodenum (one or two biopsies of the bulb and at least four biopsies of the distal duodenum) are recommended to confirm the diagnosis of CD. (Strong recommendation, high level of evidence)
18. Lymphocytic infiltration of the intestinal epithelium in the absence of villous atrophy is not specific for CD and other causes should also be considered. (Strong recommendation, high level of evidence)
19. HLA-DQ2/DQ8 testing should not be used routinely in the initial diagnosis of CD. (Strong recommendation, moderate level of evidence)
20. HLA-DQ2/DQ8 genotyping testing should be used to effectively rule out the disease in selected clinical situations. (Strong recommendation, moderate level of evidence) Examples of such clinical situations include but are not limited to:

    (a) Equivocal small-bowel histological finding (Marsh I–II) in seronegative patients
    (b) Evaluation of patients on a GFD in whom no testing for CD was done before GFD

(c) Patients with discrepant celiac-specific serology and histology
(d) Patients with suspicion of refractory CD where the original diagnosis of celiac remains in question
(e) Patients with Down's syndrome.

21. Capsule endoscopy should not be used for initial diagnosis except for patients with positive celiac-specific serology who are unwilling or unable to undergo upper endoscopy with biopsy. (Strong recommendation, moderate level of evidence)
22. Capsule endoscopy should be considered for the evaluation of small-bowel mucosa in patients with complicated CD. (Strong recommendation, moderate level of evidence)
23. Intestinal permeability tests, D-xylose, and small-bowel follow-through are neither specific nor sensitive and are not recommended for CD diagnosis. (Strong recommendation, moderate level of evidence)
24. Stool studies or salivary tests are neither validated nor recommended for use in the diagnosis of CD. (Strong recommendation, weak level of evidence)
25. Symptoms or symptom response to a GFD alone should not be used to diagnose CD, as these do not differentiate CD from non-celiac gluten sensitivity. (Strong recommendation, moderate level of evidence)
26. A diagnosis of non-celiac gluten sensitivity should be considered only after CD has been excluded with appropriate testing. (Strong recommendation, moderate level of evidence)
27. While standard diagnostic tests (specific serology and intestinal biopsy) have a high PPV for CD, they should not be relied upon to exclude CD in patients already adhering to a GFD. (Strong recommendation, high level of evidence)
28. HLA-DQ2/DQ8 genotyping should be used to try to exclude CD prior to embarking on a formal gluten challenge. (Strong recommendation, high level of evidence)
29. CD should be differentiated from non-celiac gluten sensitivity in order to identify the risk for nutritional deficiency states, complications of CD, risk for CD and associated disorders in family members, and to influence the degree and duration of adherence to the GFD. (Conditional recommendation, moderate level of evidence)
30. Formal gluten challenge should be considered, where necessary, to diagnose or exclude CD in patients already adhering to a GFD. (Strong recommendation, high level of evidence)
31. Despite the disadvantages of neither confirming nor excluding a diagnosis of CD, some patients will opt to continue on a strict GFD without undergoing formal gluten challenge; such patients should be managed in a similar fashion to those with known CD. (Conditional recommendation, low level of evidence)
32. People with CD should adhere to a GFD for life. A GFD entails strict avoidance of all products containing the proteins from wheat, barley, and rye. (Strong recommendation, high level of evidence)

33. While pure oats appear to be safely tolerated by the majority of people with CD, oats should be introduced into the diet with caution and patients should be monitored closely for evidence of adverse reaction. (Strong recommendation, moderate level of evidence)
34. People with CD should be referred to a registered dietitian who is knowledgeable about CD in order to receive a thorough nutritional assessment and education on the GFD. (Strong recommendation, moderate level of evidence)
35. People with newly diagnosed CD should undergo testing and treatment for micronutrient deficiencies. Deficiencies to be considered for testing should include, but not be limited to, iron, folic acid, vitamin D, and vitamin B12. (Conditional recommendation, low level of evidence)
36. People with CD should be monitored regularly for residual or new symptoms, adherence to GFD, and assessment for complications. In children, special attention to assure normal growth and development is recommended. (Strong recommendation, moderate level of evidence)
37. Periodic medical follow-up should be performed by a health-care practitioner with knowledge of CD. Consultation with a dietitian should be offered if gluten contamination is suspected. (Strong recommendation, moderate level of evidence)
38. Monitoring of adherence to GFD should be based on a combination of history and serology (IgA TTG or IgA (or IgG) DGP antibodies). (Strong recommendation, moderate level of evidence)
39. Upper endoscopy with intestinal biopsies is recommended for monitoring in cases with lack of clinical response or relapse of symptoms despite a GFD. (Strong recommendation, moderate level of evidence)
40. Monitoring of people with CD should include verification of normalization of laboratory abnormalities detected during initial laboratory investigation. (Strong recommendation, moderate level of evidence)
41. Patients with NRCD should be evaluated carefully to identify and treat the specific etiology in each patient. (Strong recommendation, high level of evidence)
42. Early steps in the evaluation should include measurement of celiac serologies and a thorough review of the patient's diet by a dietitian who is experienced in CD management. (Strong recommendation, high level of evidence)
43. Differentiation should be made between type I and type II refractory CD as this is important for management and prognosis. (Strong recommendation, moderate level of evidence)
44. Treatment with medication, as an adjunct to the GFD, should be considered in refractory CD. (Conditional recommendation, moderate level of evidence)
45. Patients with RCD should be monitored closely and receive aggressive nutritional support, including parenteral nutrition whenever indicated. (Strong recommendation, high level of evidence)

Appendix A
Resources for Celiac Disease Practitioners and Patients

Patient Advocacy Organizations and Support Groups

Academy of Nutrition and Dietetics—http://www.eatright.org
American College of Gastroenterology (ACG)—http://www.acg.gi.org
American Celiac Disease Alliance—http://www.americanceliac.org
American Celiac Society—http://www.americanceliacsociety.org/
American Gastroenterological Association—http://www.gastro.org
Celiac Disease Awareness Campaign—http://www.celiac.nih.gov/
Celiac Central, National Foundation for Celiac Awareness—http://www.celiaccentral.org
Celiac Disease Foundation—http://www.celiac.org
Celiac Disease Association/USA—http://www.csaceliacs.info/
Celiac Sprue Association—http://www.csaceliacs.org
Gluten-Free Certification Organizations—http://www.gfco.org
Gluten Intolerance Group of North America—http://www.gluten.net/
North American Society for Pediatric Gastroenterology, Hepatology and Nutrition—http://www.naspghan.org
R.O.C.K. (Raising Our Celiac Kids)—http://www.celiackids.com

Online Resources

Primary Care CME

The National Foundation for Celiac Awareness (NFCA) offers a free online continuing education program for primary care providers. The course teaches how to detect, diagnose, and manage celiac disease (http://www.CeliacCMECentral.com).

S.D. Rampertab and G.E. Mullin (eds.), *Celiac Disease*, Clinical Gastroenterology,
DOI 10.1007/978-1-4614-8560-5, © Springer Science+Business Media New York 2014

GREAT Pharmacists

NFCA offers a free online continuing education course for pharmacy professionals on the topic of celiac disease. This continuing education activity provides pharmacists with a reliable understanding of celiac disease and their role in dealing with patients with gluten-related disorders (http://www.proce.com/activities/activity_detail?id=7).

Celiac Disease Symptoms Checklist

After submitting this simple online checklist, you will be able to download a printer-friendly form for your doctor that includes information on celiac disease testing (http://www.CeliacCentral.org/checklist).

NFCA Monthly e-Newsletter

NFCA's monthly e-newsletter covers a variety of topics, including health and wellness articles, food and lifestyle tips, gluten-free product reviews, recipes, and new updates (http://www.CeliacCentral.org/newsletter).

NFCA Free Webinars

NFCA hosts monthly webinars that provide gluten-free individuals and dietitians with valuable information and resources to help manage celiac disease and the gluten-free diet, as well as improve general health and wellness. Webinars are a free service to the community (http://www.CeliacCentral.org/webinars).

Non-Celiac Gluten Sensitivity

Find answers to frequently asked questions about non-celiac gluten sensitivity, with input from expert researchers (http://www.CeliacCentral.org/ncgs).

Gluten Free in College

College students face a unique set of challenges when living gluten free on campus. This special web section includes blogs, articles, and a digital magazine authored by students with gluten-related disorders (http://www.CeliacCentral.org/college).

Gluten-Free Labeling Updates

This section of NFCA's Web site includes the latest updates on gluten-free labeling regulations. Read FAQs and browse blog posts on this important topic in the gluten-free community (http://www.CeliacCentral.org/FDA).

Gluten in Medications

Current US regulations do NOT require manufacturers to label the inactive ingredients in drugs. Learn all about the inactive ingredients in medications and NFCA's FDA-funded research (http://www.CeliacCentral.org/medications).

GREAT Kitchens (Gluten-Free Resource Education and Awareness Training)

NFCA offers comprehensive, online gluten-free training for foodservice professionals through the GREAT Kitchens program. Courses are available for restaurants, hospitality, caterers, schools, universities and colleges, and camps (http://www.CeliacCentral.org/GREAT).

Gluten-Free Recipes

NFCA posts a new gluten-free recipe each Monday. Also find recipe boxes featuring meal ideas that use popular gluten-free products (http://www.CeliacCentral.org/recipes).

Gluten-Free Resource Directory

This Directory includes a database of gluten-free products and resources, categorized by type for convenient browsing (http://www.glutenfreeresourcedirectory.com).

Gluten-Free Drugs

This list is maintained by Steven Plogsted, PharmD, a pharmacist at Nationwide Children's Hospital in Columbus, OH (http://www.GlutenFreeDrugs.com).

Gluten-Free Dietitian

Tricia Thompson, MS, RD, is a food manufacturing and gluten-free labeling expert. Her blog shares insights on issues affecting the celiac disease population (http://www.glutenfreedietitian.com).

Triumph Dining

Triumph Dining publishes a variety of resources, including a grocery guide and dining guide. The company also makes gluten-free dining cards to assist in communication with waitstaff and chefs (http://www.triumphdining.com).

Find Me Gluten Free

Find Me Gluten Free is a mobile app that helps users find local restaurants that serve gluten-free food (http://www.FindMeGlutenFree.com).

North American Society for the Study of Celiac Disease (NASSCD)

North American Society for the Study of Celiac Disease's (NASSCD's) overall mission is to advance the fields of celiac disease and gluten-related disorders by fostering research and by promoting excellence in clinical care, including diagnosis and treatment of patients with these conditions (http://www.nasscd.org).

National Institute of Diabetes and Digestive and Kidney Diseases (NIDDK)

The NIDDK conducts and supports medical research and research training and disseminates science-based information on digestive diseases, including celiac disease (http://www.niddk.nih.gov).

Celiac Disease Centers

Celiac Center at Beth Israel Deaconess Medical Center—http://www.CeliacNow.org

Celiac Center at Paoli Hospital—http://www.mainlinehealth.org/paoliceliac

Celiac Disease Center at Columbia University—http://www.celiacdiseasecenter.org/CF-HOME.htm

Center for Celiac Disease at The Children's Hospital of Philadelphia—http://www.chop.edu/service/center-for-celiac-disease/home.html

Center for Celiac Research and Treatment at Mass General Hospital for Children—http://www.celiaccenter.org

Jefferson Celiac Center—http://www.jeffersonhospital.org/departments-and-services/celiac-center.aspx

Mayo Clinic Celiac Center—http://www.mayoclinic.org/celiac-disease/

Stanford Celiac Disease Clinic—http://www.stanfordhospital.org/digestivehealth/celiacdisease/

University of Chicago Celiac Disease Center—http://www.cureceliacdisease.org/

Appendix B
Taxonomic Relationships of the Major Cereal Grains

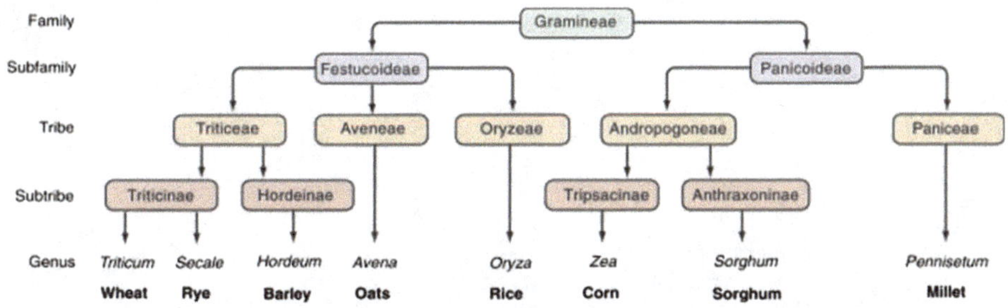

The prolamins of wheat are referred to as *gliadins*. Prolamins from other cereals also are considered to be gluten and are named according to their source (*secalins* from rye, *hordeins* from barley, *avenins* from oats, and *zeins* from corn). The taxonomic relationships of the major cereal grain families provide a framework on which their toxicities in celiac disease can be predicted. Wheat, rye, and barley belong to the tribe known as Triticeae, and oats belong to a neighboring tribe known as Aveneae. Avenin is genetically less similar to gliadin than gliadin is to secalin and hordein. Despite their genetic differences, however, prolamins from oats, barley, wheat, and rye still have immunologic cross-reactivity because of their common ancestry. Grains that do not activate disease (rice, corn, sorghum, and millet) are separated still further from wheat, rye, and barley in terms of their derivation from the primitive grasses. Reprinted with permission from Farrell RJ, Kelly CP. Celiac disease and refractory celiac disease. In: Feldman M, Friedman LS, Brandt LJ, editors. Sleisenger and Fordtrans Gastrointestinal and Liver Disease—Pathophysiology Diagnosis Management. 9th ed. Philadelphia: Elsevier: 2010; with permission from Elsevier.

S.D. Rampertab and G.E. Mullin (eds.), *Celiac Disease*, Clinical Gastroenterology,
DOI 10.1007/978-1-4614-8560-5, © Springer Science+Business Media New York 2014

Appendix C
Some Potential Sources of Hidden Gluten[1]

Beers, ales, other fermented beverages (distilled beverages are acceptable)
Bouillon and soups
Candy
Communion wafers
Drink mixes
Gravy and sauces
Herbal tea
Imitation meat and seafood
Lipstick and lip balms
Medications (pills and capsules)
Nutritional supplements
Play-Doh
Salad dressings and marinades
Self-basting turkeys
Soy sauce
Toothpaste

[1] Reprinted with permission from Farrell RJ, Kelly CP. Celiac disease and refractory celiac disease. In: Feldman M, Friedman LS, Brandt LJ, editors. Sleisenger and Fordtrans Gastrointestinal and Liver Disease—Pathophysiology Diagnosis Management. 9th ed. Philadelphia: Elsevier: 2010; with permission from Elsevier.

S.D. Rampertab and G.E. Mullin (eds.), *Celiac Disease*, Clinical Gastroenterology, DOI 10.1007/978-1-4614-8560-5, © Springer Science+Business Media New York 2014

Appendix D
Key Elements in the Management of Celiac Disease[2]

*C*onsultation with a skilled dietitian
*E*ducation about the disease
*L*ifelong adherence to a gluten-free diet
*I*dentification and treatment of nutritional deficiencies
*A*ccess to an advocacy group
*C*ontinuous long-term follow-up by a multidisciplinary team

[2]Reprinted from the National Institutes of Health Consensus Development Conference Statement on Celiac Disease, June 28–30, 2004. Gastroenterology 2005;128:S1–S9.

S.D. Rampertab and G.E. Mullin (eds.), *Celiac Disease*, Clinical Gastroenterology,
DOI 10.1007/978-1-4614-8560-5, © Springer Science+Business Media New York 2014

Appendix E
Celiac Iceberg[3]

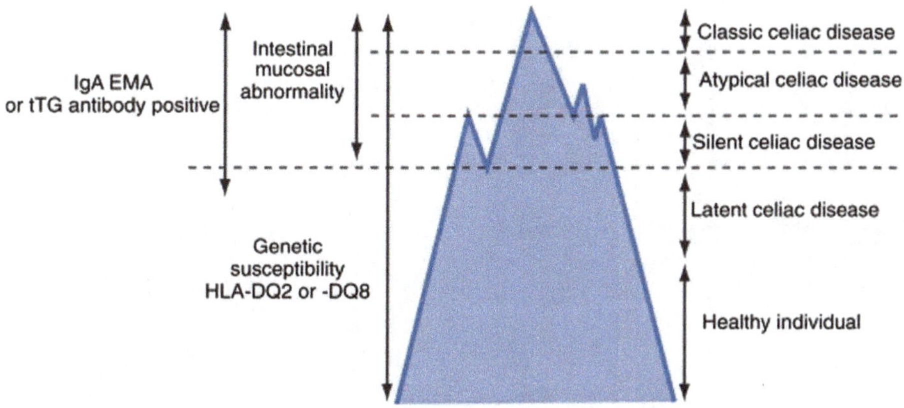

[3] Reprinted with permission from Farrell RJ, Kelly CP. Celiac disease and refractory celiac disease. In: Feldman M, Friedman LS, Brandt LJ, editors. Sleisenger and Fordtrans Gastrointestinal and Liver Disease—Pathophysiology Diagnosis Management. 9th ed. Philadelphia: Elsevier;2010; Chapter 104, p 1801. Figure 104–3, with permission from Elsevier.

S.D. Rampertab and G.E. Mullin (eds.), *Celiac Disease*, Clinical Gastroenterology,
DOI 10.1007/978-1-4614-8560-5, © Springer Science+Business Media New York 2014

Appendix F
An Approach to Gluten Challenge for the Diagnosis or Exclusion of Celiac Disease[4]

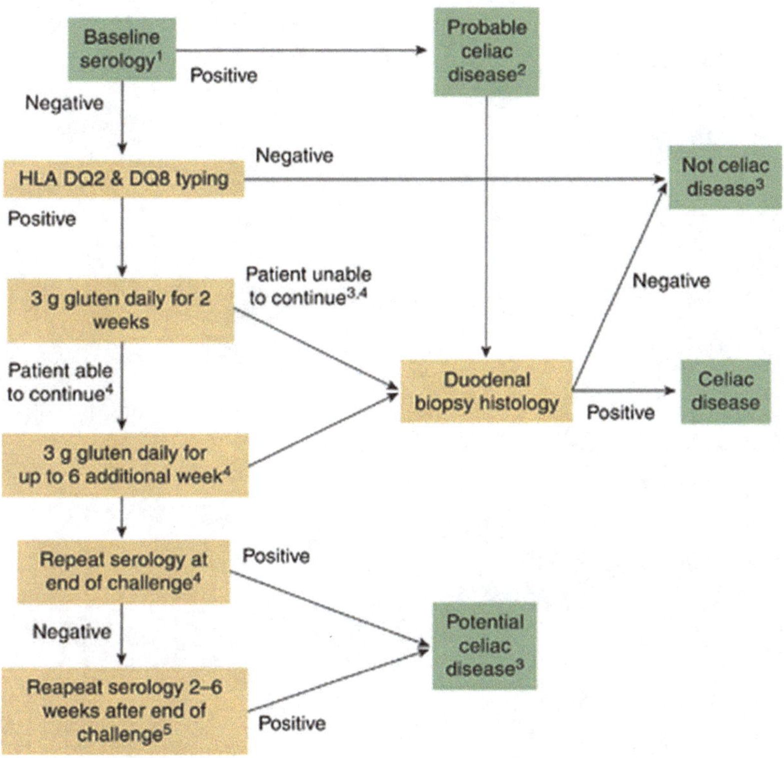

[4]Reprinted by permission from Macmillan Publishers Ltd: Rubio-Tapia A, Hill ID, Kelly CP, Calderwood AH, Murray JA. ACG Clinical Guidelines: Diagnosis and Management of Celiac Disease. Am J Gastroenterol. 2013 May;108(5):656–76, copyright 2013.

S.D. Rampertab and G.E. Mullin (eds.), *Celiac Disease*, Clinical Gastroenterology, DOI 10.1007/978-1-4614-8560-5, © Springer Science+Business Media New York 2014

Appendix G
An Approach to the Monitoring of Celiac Disease[5]

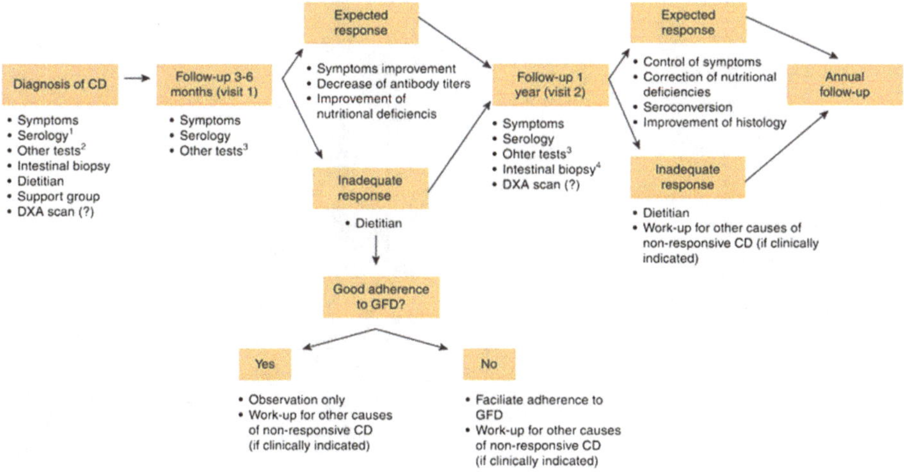

[5] Reprinted by permission from Macmillan Publishers Ltd: Rubio-Tapia A, Hill ID, Kelly CP, Calderwood AH, Murray JA. ACG Clinical Guidelines: Diagnosis and Management of Celiac Disease. Am J Gastroenterol. 2013 May;108(5):656-76, copyright 2013.

S.D. Rampertab and G.E. Mullin (eds.), *Celiac Disease*, Clinical Gastroenterology, DOI 10.1007/978-1-4614-8560-5, © Springer Science+Business Media New York 2014

Appendix H
An Approach to the Diagnosis of Celiac Disease[6]

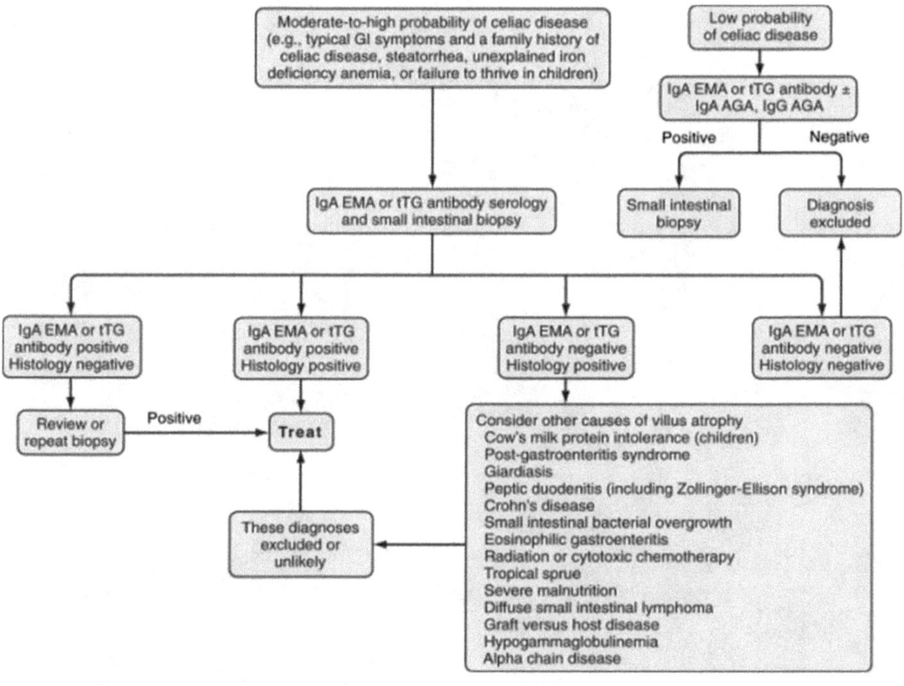

[6]Reprinted by permission from Macmillan Publishers Ltd: Rubio-Tapia A, Hill ID, Kelly CP, Calderwood AH, Murray JA. ACG Clinical Guidelines: Diagnosis and Management of Celiac Disease. Am J Gastroenterol. 2013 May;108(5):656-76, copyright 2013.

S.D. Rampertab and G.E. Mullin (eds.), *Celiac Disease*, Clinical Gastroenterology, DOI 10.1007/978-1-4614-8560-5, © Springer Science+Business Media New York 2014

Appendix I
An Approach to the Patient with Non-Responsive Celiac Disease[7]

[7] Reprinted with permission from Farrell RJ, Kelly CP. Celiac disease and refractory celiac disease. In: Feldman M, Friedman LS, Brandt LJ, editors. Sleisenger and Fordtrans Gastrointestinal and Liver Disease - Pathophysiology Diagnosis Management. 9th ed. Philadelphia: Elsevier; 2010; with permission from Elsevier.

S.D. Rampertab and G.E. Mullin (eds.), *Celiac Disease*, Clinical Gastroenterology, DOI 10.1007/978-1-4614-8560-5, © Springer Science+Business Media New York 2014

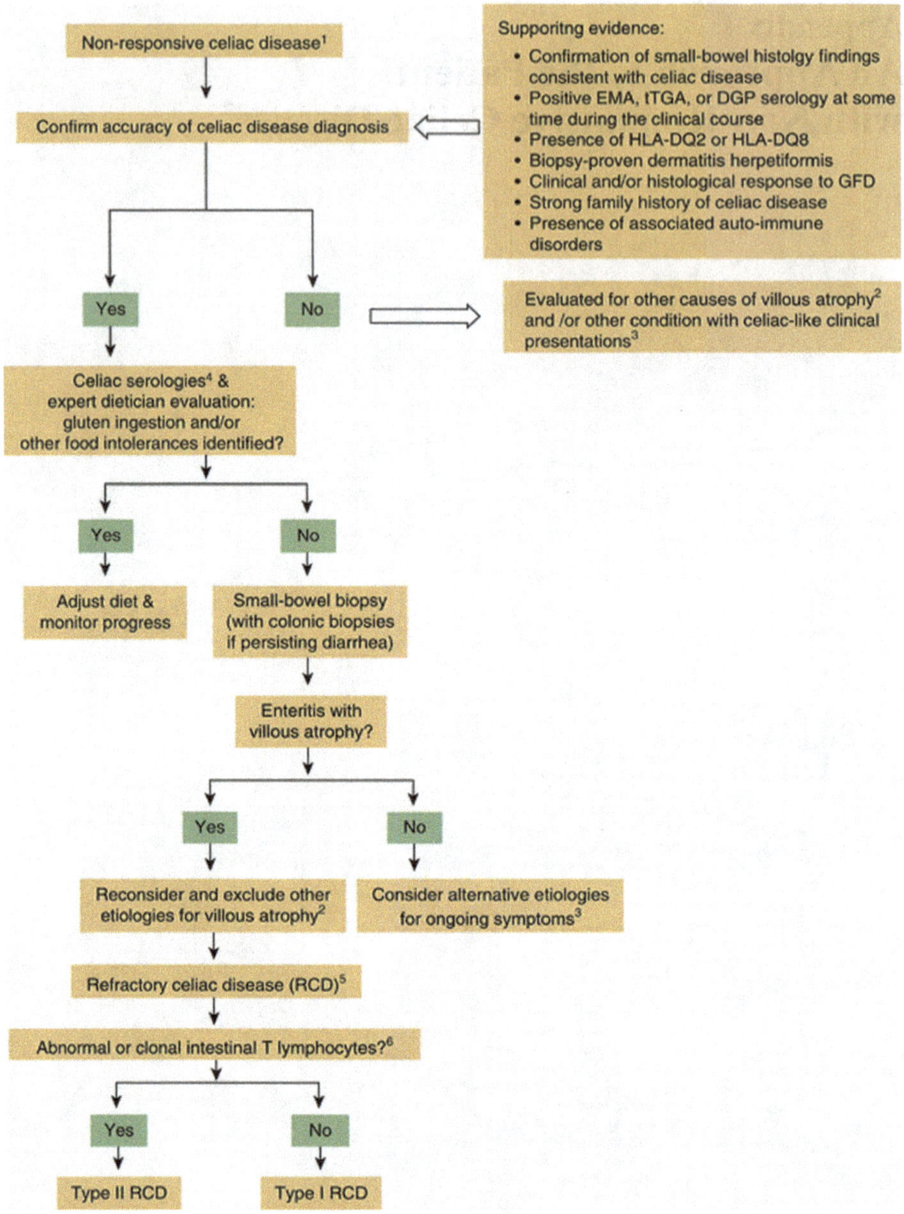
Non-responsive celiac disease[1]
Confirm accuracy of celiac disease diagnosis
Supporitng evidence:
• Confirmation of small-bowel histolgy findings consistent with celiac disease
• Positive EMA, tTGA, or DGP serology at some time during the clinical course
• Presence of HLA-DQ2 or HLA-DQ8
• Biopsy-proven dermatitis herpetiformis
• Clinical and/or histological response to GFD
• Strong family history of celiac disease
• Presence of associated auto-immune disorders
Yes
No
Evaluated for other causes of villous atrophy[2] and /or other condition with celiac-like clinical presentations[3]
Celiac serologies[4] & expert dietician evaluation: gluten ingestion and/or other food intolerances identified?
Yes
No
Adjust diet & monitor progress
Small-bowel biopsy (with colonic biopsies if persisting diarrhea)
Enteritis with villous atrophy?
Yes
No
Reconsider and exclude other etiologies for villous atrophy[2]
Consider alternative etiologies for ongoing symptoms[3]
Refractory celiac disease (RCD)[5]
Abnormal or clonal intestinal T lymphocytes?[6]
Yes
No
Type II RCD
Type I RCD

Appendix J
Dietary Reference Intakes (DRIs): Recommended Dietary Allowances and Adequate Intakes, Vitamins and Elements

S.D. Rampertab and G.E. Mullin (eds.), *Celiac Disease*, Clinical Gastroenterology, DOI 10.1007/978-1-4614-8560-5, © Springer Science+Business Media New York 2014

Food and Nutrition Board, Institute of Medicine, National Academies

Life stage group	Vitamin A (μg/ day)[a]	Vitamin C (mg/ day)	Vitamin D (μg/ day)[b,c]	Vitamin E (mg/day)[d]	Vitamin K (μg/ day)	Thiamin (mg/day)	Riboflavin (mg/day)	Niacin (mg/ day)[e]	Vitamin B_6 (mg/ day)	Folate (μg/ day)[f]	Vitamin B_{12} (μg/ day)	Pantothenic Acid (mg/ day)	Biotin (μg/ day)	Choline (mg/ day)[g]
Infants														
0–6 months	400*	40*	10	4*	2.0*	0.2*	0.3*	2*	0.1*	65*	0.4*	1.7*	5*	125*
6–12 months	500*	50*	10	5*	2.5*	0.3*	0.4*	4*	0.3*	80*	0.5*	1.8*	6*	150*
Children														
1–3 years	**300**	**15**	**15**	**6**	30*	**0.5**	**0.5**	**6**	**0.5**	**150**	**0.9**	2*	8*	200*
4–8 years	**400**	**25**	**15**	**7**	55*	0.6	0.6	**8**	**0.6**	**200**	**1.2**	3*	12*	250*
Males														
9–13 years	**600**	**45**	**15**	**11**	60*	**0.9**	**0.9**	**12**	**1.0**	**300**	**1.8**	4*	20*	375*
14–18 years	**900**	**75**	**15**	**15**	75*	**1.2**	**1.3**	**16**	**1.3**	**400**	**2.4**	5*	25*	550*
19–30 years	**900**	**90**	**15**	**15**	120*	**1.2**	**1.3**	**16**	**1.3**	**400**	**2.4**	5*	30*	550*
31–50 years	**900**	**90**	**15**	**15**	120*	**1.2**	**1.3**	**16**	**1.3**	**400**	**2.4**	5*	30*	550*
51–70 years	**900**	**90**	**15**	**15**	120*	**1.2**	**1.3**	**16**	**1.7**	**400**	**2.4**[h]	5*	30*	550*
>70 years	**900**	**90**	**20**	**15**	120*	**1.2**	**1.3**	**16**	**1.7**	**400**	**2.4**[h]	5*	30*	550*
Females														
9–13 years	**600**	**45**	**15**	**11**	60*	**0.9**	**0.9**	**12**	**1.0**	**300**	**1.8**	4*	20*	375*
14–18 years	**700**	**65**	**15**	**15**	75*	**1.0**	**1.0**	**14**	**1.2**	**400**[i]	**2.4**	5*	25*	400*
19–30 years	**700**	**75**	**15**	**15**	90*	**1.1**	**1.1**	**14**	**1.3**	**400**[i]	**2.4**	5*	30*	425*
31–50 years	**700**	**75**	**15**	**15**	90*	**1.1**	**1.1**	**14**	**1.3**	**400**[i]	**2.4**	5*	30*	425*
51–70 years	**700**	**75**	**15**	**15**	90*	**1.1**	**1.1**	**14**	**1.5**	**400**	**2.4**[h]	5*	30*	425*
>70 years	**700**	**75**	**20**	**15**	90*	**1.1**	**1.1**	**14**	**1.5**	**400**	**2.4**[h]	5*	30*	425*
Pregnancy														
14–18 years	**750**	**80**	**15**	**15**	75*	**1.4**	**1.4**	**18**	**1.9**	**600**[j]	**2.6**	6*	30*	450*
19–30 years	**770**	**85**	**15**	**15**	90*	**1.4**	**1.4**	**18**	**1.9**	**600**[j]	**2.6**	6*	30*	450*
31–50 years	**770**	**85**	**15**	**15**	90*	**1.4**	**1.4**	**18**	**1.9**	**600**[j]	**2.6**	6*	30*	450*

Lactation														
14–18 years	**1,200**	**115**	**15**	**19**	75*	**1.4**	**1.6**	**17**	**2.0**	**500**	**2.8**	7*	35*	550*
19–30 years	**1,300**	**120**	**15**	**19**	90*	**1.4**	**1.6**	**17**	**2.0**	**500**	**2.8**	7*	35*	550*
31–50 years	**1,300**	**120**	**15**	**19**	90*	**1.4**	**1.6**	**17**	**2.0**	**500**	**2.8**	7*	35*	550*

Note: This table (taken from the DRI reports, see http://www.nap.edu) presents Recommended Dietary Allowances (RDAs) in bold type and Adequate Intakes (AIs) in ordinary type followed by an asterisk (*). An RDA is the average daily dietary intake level sufficient to meet the nutrient requirements of nearly all (97–98 %) healthy individuals in a group. It is calculated from an Estimated Average Requirement (EAR). If sufficient scientific evidence is not available to establish an EAR, and thus calculate an RDA, an AI is usually developed. For healthy breastfed infants, an AI is the mean intake. The AI for other life stage and gender groups is believed to cover the needs of all healthy individuals in the groups, but lack of data or uncertainty in the data prevent being able to specify with confidence the percentage of individuals covered by this intake.

[a] As retinol activity equivalents (RAEs). 1 RAE = 1 μg retinol, 12 μg β-carotene, 24 μg α-carotene, or 24 μg β-cryptoxanthin. The RAE for dietary provitamin A carotenoids is twofold greater than retinol equivalents (RE), whereas the RAE for preformed vitamin A is the same as RE

[b] As cholecalciferol. 1 μg cholecalciferol = 40 IU vitamin D

[c] Under the assumption of minimal sunlight

[d] As α-tocopherol. α-Tocopherol includes *RRR*-α-tocopherol, the only form of α-tocopherol that occurs naturally in foods, and the 2*R*-stereoisomeric forms of α-tocopherol (*RRR*-, *RSR*-, *RRS*-, and *RSS*-α-tocopherol) that occur in fortified foods and supplements. It does not include the 2*S*-stereoisomeric forms of α-tocopherol (*SRR*-, *SSR*-, *SRS*-, and *SSS*-α-tocopherol), also found in fortified foods and supplements

[e] As niacin equivalents (NE). 1 mg of niacin = 60 mg of tryptophan; 0–6 months = preformed niacin (not NE)

[f] As dietary folate equivalents (DFE). 1 DFE = 1 μg food folate = 0.6 μg of folic acid from fortified food or as a supplement consumed with food = 0.5 μg of a supplement taken on an empty stomach

[g] Although AIs have been set for choline, there are few data to assess whether a dietary supply of choline is needed at all stages of the life cycle, and it may be that the choline requirement can be met by endogenous synthesis at some of these stages

[h] Because 10–30 % of older people may malabsorb food-bound B_{12}, it is advisable for those older than 50 years to meet their RDA mainly by consuming foods fortified with B_{12} or a supplement containing B_{12}

[i] In view of evidence linking folate intake with neural tube defects in the fetus, it is recommended that all women capable of becoming pregnant consume 400 μg from supplements or fortified foods in addition to intake of food folate from a varied diet

[j] It is assumed that women will continue consuming 400 μg from supplements or fortified food until their pregnancy is confirmed and they enter prenatal care, which ordinarily occurs after the end of the periconceptional period—the critical time for formation of the neural tube

Sources: *Dietary Reference Intakes for Calcium, Phosphorous, Magnesium, Vitamin D, and Fluoride* (1997); *Dietary Reference Intakes for Thiamin, Riboflavin, Niacin, Vitamin* B_6, *Folate, Vitamin* B_{12}, *Pantothenic Acid, Biotin, and Choline* (1998); *Dietary Reference Intakes for Vitamin C, Vitamin E, Selenium, and Carotenoids* (2000); *Dietary Reference Intakes for Vitamin A, Vitamin K, Arsenic, Boron, Chromium, Copper, Iodine, Iron, Manganese, Molybdenum, Nickel, Silicon, Vanadium, and Zinc* (2001); *Dietary Reference Intakes for Water, Potassium, Sodium, Chloride, and* Sulfate (2005); and *Dietary Reference Intakes for Calcium and Vitamin D* (2011). These reports may be accessed via http://www.nap.edu

Dietary Reference Intakes (DRIs): Recommended Dietary Allowances and Adequate Intakes, Elements

Food and Nutrition Board, Institute of Medicine, National Academies

Life Stage Group	Calcium (mg/day)	Chromium (μg/day)	Copper (μg/day)	Fluoride (mg/day)	Iodine (Hg/day)	Iron (mg/day)	Magnesium (mg/day)	Manganese (mg/day)	Molybdenum (Hg/day)	Phosphorus (mg/day)	Selenium (μg/day)	Zinc (mg/day)	Potassium (g/day)	Sodium (g/day)	Chloride (g/day)
Infants															
0–6 months	200*	0.2*	200*	0.01*	110*	0.27*	30*	0.003*	2*	100*	15*	2*	0.4*	0.12*	0.18*
6–12 months	260*	5.5*	220*	0.5*	130*	11	75*	0.6*	3*	275*	20*	3	0.7*	0.37*	0.57*
Children															
1–3 years	700	11*	340	0.7*	90	7	80	1.2*	17	460	20	3	3.0*	1.0*	1.5*
4–8 years	1,000	15*	440	1*	90	10	130	1.5*	22	500	30	5	3.8*	1.2*	1.9*
Males															
9–13 years	1,300	25*	700	2*	120	8	240	1.9*	34	1,250	40	8	4.5*	1.5*	2.3*
14–18 years	1,300	35*	890	3*	150	11	410	2.2*	43	1,250	55	11	4.7*	1.5*	2.3*
19–30 years	1,000	35*	900	4*	150	8	400	2.3*	45	700	55	11	4.7*	1.5*	2.3*
31–50 years	1,000	35*	900	4*	150	8	420	2.3*	45	700	55	11	4.7*	1.5*	2.3*
51–70 years	1,000	30*	900	4*	150	8	420	2.3*	45	700	55	11	4.7*	1.3*	2.0*
>70 years	1,200	30*	900	4*	150	8	420	2.3*	45	700	55	11	4.7*	1.2*	1.8*
Females															
9–13 years	1,300	21*	700	2*	120	8	240	1.6*	34	1,250	40	8	4.5*	1.5*	2.3*
14–18 years	1,300	24*	890	3*	150	15	360	1.6*	43	1,250	55	9	4.7*	1.5*	2.3*
19–30 years	1,000	25*	900	3*	150	18	310	1.8*	45	700	55	8	4.7*	1.5*	2.3*
31–50 years	1,000	25*	900	3*	150	18	320	1.8*	45	700	55	8	4.7*	1.5*	2.3*
51–70 years	1,200	20*	900	3*	150	8	320	1.8*	45	700	55	8	4.7*	1.3*	2.0*
>70years	1,200	20*	900	3*	150	8	320	1.8*	45	700	55	8	4.7*	1.2*	1.8*
Pregnancy															
14–18 years	1,300	29*	1,000	3*	220	27	400	2.0*	50	1,250	60	12	4.7*	1.5*	2.3*
19–30 years	1,000	30*	1,000	3*	220	27	350	2.0*	50	700	60	11	4.7*	1.5*	2.3*
31–50 years	1,000	30*	1,000	3*	220	27	360	2.0*	50	700	60	11	4.7*	1.5*	2.3*

Lactation															
14–18 years	**1,300**	44*	**1,300**	3*	**290**	**10**	**360**	2.6*	**50**	**1,250**	**70**	**13**	5.1*	1.5*	2.3*
19–30 years	**1,000**	45*	**1,300**	3*	**290**	**9**	**310**	2.6*	**50**	**700**	**70**	**12**	5.1*	1.5*	2.3*
31–50 years	**1,000**	45*	**1,300**	3*	**290**	**9**	**320**	2.6*	**50**	**700**	**70**	**12**	5.1*	1.5*	2.3*

Note: This table (taken from the DRI reports, see http://www.nap.edu) presents Recommended Dietary Allowances (RDAs) in **bold type** and Adequate Intakes (AIs) in ordinary type followed by an asterisk (*). An RDA is the average daily dietary intake level sufficient to meet the nutrient requirements of nearly all (97–98 %) healthy individuals in a group. It is calculated from an Estimated Average Requirement (EAR). If sufficient scientific evidence is not available to establish an EAR, and thus calculate an RDA, an AI is usually developed. For healthy breastfed infants, an AI is the mean intake. The AI for other life stage and gender groups is believed to cover the needs of all healthy individuals in the groups, but lack of data or uncertainty in the data prevent being able to specify with confidence the percentage of individuals covered by this intake

Sources: *Dietary Reference Intakes for Calcium, Phosphorous, Magnesium, Vitamin D, and Fluoride* (1997); *Dietary Reference Intakes for Thiamin, Riboflavin, Niacin, Vitamin* B_6, *Folate, Vitamin* B_{12}, *Pantothenic Acid, Biotin, and Choline* (1998); *Dietary Reference Intakes for Vitamin C, Vitamin E, Selenium, and Carotenoids* (2000); and *Dietary Reference Intakes for Vitamin A, Vitamin K, Arsenic, Boron, Chromium, Copper, Iodine, Iron, Manganese, Molybdenum, Nickel, Silicon, Vanadium, and Zinc* (2001); *Dietary Reference Intakes for Water, Potassium, Sodium, Chloride, and* Sulfate (2005); and *Dietary Reference Intakes for Calcium and Vitamin D* (2011). These reports maybe accessed via http://www.nap.edu.

Appendix K
Dietary Reference Intakes (DRIs): Tolerable Upper Intake Levels, Vitamins and Elements

S.D. Rampertab and G.E. Mullin (eds.), *Celiac Disease*, Clinical Gastroenterology, DOI 10.1007/978-1-4614-8560-5, © Springer Science+Business Media New York 2014

Food and Nutrition Board, Institute of Medicine, National Academies

Life Stage Group	Vitamin A (μg/day)[a]	Vitamin C (mg/day)	Vitamin D (μg/day)	Vitamin E (mg/day)[b,c]	Vitamin K	Thiamin	Riboflavin	Niacin (mg/day)[c]	Vitamin B_6 (mg/day)	Folate (μg/day)[c]	Vitamin B_{12}	Pantothenic Acid	Biotin	Choline (g/day)	Carotenoids[d]
Infants															
0–6 months	600	ND[e]	25	ND	ND	ND	ND	ND	ND	ND	ND	ND	ND	ND	ND
6–12 months	600	ND	38	ND	ND	ND	ND	ND	ND	ND	ND	ND	ND	ND	ND
Children															
1–3 years	600	400	63	200	ND	ND	ND	10	30	300	ND	ND	ND	1.0	ND
4–8 years	900	650	75	300	ND	ND	ND	15	40	400	ND	ND	ND	1.0	ND
Males															
9–13 years	1,700	1,200	100	600	ND	ND	ND	20	60	600	ND	ND	ND	2.0	ND
14–18 years	2,800	1,800	100	800	ND	ND	ND	30	80	800	ND	ND	ND	3.0	ND
19–30 years	3,000	2,000	100	1,000	ND	ND	ND	35	100	1,000	ND	ND	ND	3.5	ND
31–50 years	3,000	2,000	100	1,000	ND	ND	ND	35	100	1,000	ND	ND	ND	3.5	ND
51–70 years	3,000	2,000	100	1,000	ND	ND	ND	35	100	1,000	ND	ND	ND	3.5	ND
>70 years	3,000	2,000	100	1,000	ND	ND	ND	35	100	1,000	ND	ND	ND	3.5	ND
Females															
9–13 years	1,700	1,200	100	600	ND	ND	ND	20	60	600	ND	ND	ND	2.0	ND
14–18 years	2,800	1,800	100	800	ND	ND	ND	30	80	800	ND	ND	ND	3.0	ND
19–30 years	3,000	2,000	100	1,000	ND	ND	ND	35	100	1,000	ND	ND	ND	3.5	ND
31–50 years	3,000	2,000	100	1,000	ND	ND	ND	35	100	1,000	ND	ND	ND	3.5	ND
51–70 years	3,000	2,000	100	1,000	ND	ND	ND	35	100	1,000	ND	ND	ND	3.5	ND
>70 years	3,000	2,000	100	1,000	ND	ND	ND	35	100	1,000	ND	ND	ND	3.5	ND
Pregnancy															
14–18 years	2,800	1,800	100	800	ND	ND	ND	30	80	800	ND	ND	ND	3.0	ND
19–30 years	3,000	2,000	100	1,000	ND	ND	ND	35	100	1,000	ND	ND	ND	3.5	ND
31–50 years	3,000	2,000	100	1,000	ND	ND	ND	35	100	1,000	ND	ND	ND	3.5	ND

Lactation															
14–18 years	2,800	1,800	100	800	ND	ND	ND	30	80	800	ND	ND	ND	3.0	ND
19–30 years	3,000	2,000	100	1,000	ND	ND	ND	35	100	1,000	ND	ND	ND	3.5	ND
31–50 years	3,000	2,000	100	1,000	ND	ND	ND	35	100	1,000	ND	ND	ND	3.5	ND

Note: A Tolerable Upper Intake Level (UL) is the highest level of daily nutrient intake that is likely to pose no risk of adverse health effects to almost all individuals in the general population. Unless otherwise specified, the UL represents total intake from food, water, and supplements. Due to a lack of suitable data, ULs could not be established for vitamin K, thiamin, riboflavin, vitamin B_{12}, pantothenic acid, biotin, and carotenoids. In the absence of a UL, extra caution may be warranted in consuming levels above recommended intakes. Members of the general population should be advised not to routinely exceed the UL. The UL is not meant to apply to individuals who are treated with the nutrient under medical supervision or to individuals with predisposing conditions that modify their sensitivity to the nutrient

[a]As preformed vitamin A only

[b]As α-tocopherol; applies to any form of supplemental α-tocopherol

[c]The ULs for vitamin E, niacin, and folate apply to synthetic forms obtained from supplements, fortified foods, or a combination of the two

[d]β-Carotene supplements are advised only to serve as a provitamin A source for individuals at risk of vitamin A deficiency

[e]ND=Not determinable due to lack of data of adverse effects in this age group and concern with regard to lack of ability to handle excess amounts. Source of intake should be from food only to prevent high levels of intake

Sources: *Dietary Reference Intakes for Calcium, Phosphorous, Magnesium, Vitamin D, and Fluoride* (1997); *Dietary Reference Intakes for Thiamin, Riboflavin, Niacin, Vitamin B_6, Folate, Vitamin B_{12}, Pantothenic Acid, Biotin, and Choline* (1998); *Dietary Reference Intakes for Vitamin C, Vitamin E, Selenium, and Carotenoids* (2000); *Dietary Reference Intakes for Vitamin A, Vitamin K, Arsenic, Boron, Chromium, Copper, Iodine, Iron, Manganese, Molybdenum, Nickel, Silicon, Vanadium, and Zinc* (2001); *and Dietary Reference Intakes for Calcium and Vitamin D* (2011). These reports may be accessed via http://www.nap.edu.

Dietary Reference Intakes (DRIs): Tolerable Upper Intake Levels, Elements

Food and Nutrition Board, Institute of Medicine, National Academies

Life Stage Group	Arsenic[a]	Boron (mg/day)	Calcium (mg/day)	Chromium	Copper (μg/day)	Fluoride (mg/day)	Iodine (μg/day)	Iron (mg/day)	Magnesium (mg/day)[b]	Manganese (mg/day)	Molybdenum (μg/day)	Nickel (mg/day)	Phosphorus (g/day)	Selenium (μg/day)	Silicon[c]	Vanadium (mg/day)[d]	Zinc (mg/day)	Sodium (g/day)	Chloride (g/day)
Infants																			
0–6 months	ND[e]	ND	1,000	ND	ND	0.7	ND	40	ND	ND	ND	ND	ND	45	ND	ND	4	ND	ND
6–12 months	ND	ND	1,500	ND	ND	0.9	ND	40	ND	ND	ND	ND	ND	60	ND	ND	5	ND	ND
Children																			
1–3 years	ND	3	2,500	ND	1,000	1.3	200	40	65	2	300	0.2	3	90	ND	ND	7	1.5	2.3
4–8 years	ND	6	2,500	ND	3,000	2.2	300	40	110	3	600	0.3	3	150	ND	ND	12	1.9	2.9
Males																			
9–13 years	ND	11	3,000	ND	5,000	10	600	40	350	6	1,100	0.6	4	280	ND	ND	23	2.2	3.4
14–18 years	ND	17	3,000	ND	8,000	10	900	45	350	9	1,700	1.0	4	400	ND	ND	34	2.3	3.6
19–30 years	ND	20	2,500	ND	10,000	10	1,100	45	350	11	2,000	1.0	4	400	ND	1.8	40	2.3	3.6
31–50 years	ND	20	2,500	ND	10,000	10	1,100	45	350	11	2,000	1.0	4	400	ND	1.8	40	2.3	3.6
51–70 years	ND	20	2,000	ND	10,000	10	1,100	45	350	11	2,000	1.0	4	400	ND	1.8	40	2.3	3.6
> 70 years	ND	20	2,000	ND	10,000	10	1,100	45	350	11	2,000	1.0	3	400	ND	1.8	40	2.3	3.6
Females																			
9–13 years	ND	11	3,000	ND	5,000	10	600	40	350	6	1,100	0.6	4	280	ND	ND	23	2.2	3.4
14–18 years	ND	17	3,000	ND	8,000	10	900	45	350	9	1,700	1.0	4	400	ND	ND	34	2.3	3.6
19–30 years	ND	20	2,500	ND	10,000	10	1,100	45	350	11	2,000	1.0	4	400	ND	1.8	40	2.3	3.6
31–50 years	ND	20	2,500	ND	10,000	10	1,100	45	350	11	2,000	1.0	4	400	ND	1.8	40	2.3	3.6
51–70 years	ND	20	2,000	ND	10,000	10	1,100	45	350	11	2,000	1.0	4	400	ND	1.8	40	2.3	3.6
>70 years	ND	20	2,000	ND	10,000	10	1,100	45	350	11	2,000	1.0	3	400	ND	1.8	40	2.3	3.6
Pregnancy																			
14–18 years	ND	17	3,000	ND	8,000	10	900	45	350	9	1,700	1.0	3.5	400	ND	ND	34	2.3	3.6
19–30 years	ND	20	2,500	ND	10,000	10	1,100	45	350	11	2,000	1.0	3.5	400	ND	ND	40	2.3	3.6
61–50 years	ND	20	2,500	ND	10,000	10	1,100	45	350	11	2,000	1.0	3.5	400	ND	ND	40	2.3	3.6

Lactation																		
14–18 years[ND]	17	3,000	ND	8,000	10	900	45	350	9	1,700	1.0	4	400	ND	ND	34	2.3	3.6
19–30 years[ND]	20	2,500	ND	10,000	10	1,100	45	350	11	2,000	1.0	4	400	ND	ND	40	2.3	3.6
31–50 years[ND]	20	2,500	ND	10,000	10	1,100	45	350	11	2,000	1.0	4	400	ND	ND	40	2.3	3.6

Note: A Tolerable Upper Intake Level (UL) is the highest level of daily nutrient intake that is likely to pose no risk of adverse health effects to almost all individuals in the general population. Unless otherwise specified, the UL represents total intake from food, water, and supplements. Due to a lack of suitable data, ULs could not be established for vitamin K, thiamin, riboflavin, vitamin B_{12}, pantothenic acid, biotin, and carotenoids. In the absence of a UL, extra caution may be warranted in consuming levels above recommended intakes. Members of the general population should be advised not to routinely exceed the UL. The UL is not meant to apply to individuals who are treated with the nutrient under medical supervision or to individuals with predisposing conditions that modify their sensitivity to the nutrient

[a]Although the UL was not determined for arsenic, there is no justification for adding arsenic to food or supplements

[b]The ULs for magnesium represent intake from a pharmacological agent only and do not include intake from food and water

[c]Although silicon has not been shown to cause adverse effects in humans, there is no justification for adding silicon to supplements

[d]Although vanadium in food has not been shown to cause adverse effects in humans, there is no justification for adding vanadium to food and vanadium supplements should be used with caution. The UL is based on adverse effects in laboratory animals and this data could be used to set a UL for adults but not children and adolescents

[e]ND=Not determinable due to lack of data of adverse effects in this age group and concern with regard to lack of ability to handle excess amounts. Source of intake should be from food only to prevent high levels of intake

Sources: *Dietary Reference Intakes for Calcium, Phosphorous, Magnesium, Vitamin D, and Fluoride* (1997); *Dietary Reference Intakes for Thiamin, Riboflavin, Niacin, Vitamin B6, Folate, Vitamin B12, Pantothenic Acid, Biotin, and Choline* (1998); *Dietary Reference Intakes for Vitamin C, Vitamin E, Selenium, and Carotenoids* (2000); *Dietary Reference Intakes for Vitamin A, Vitamin K, Arsenic, Boron, Chromium, Copper, Iodine, Iron, Manganese, Molybdenum, Nickel, Silicon, Vanadium, and Zinc* (2001); *Dietary Reference Intakes for Water, Potassium, Sodium, Chloride, and Sulfate* (2005); and *Dietary Reference Intakes for Calcium and Vitamin D* (2011). These reports may be accessed via http://www.nap.edu

Index

S.D. Rampertab and G.E. Mullin (eds.), *Celiac Disease*, Clinical Gastroenterology,
DOI 10.1007/978-1-4614-8560-5, © Springer Science+Business Media New York 2014